Critical Sports Studies

A Document Reader

Critical Sports Studies

A Document Reader

Edited by Nicholas Villanueva, Jr.

First Edition

cognella
SAN DIEGO

Bassim Hamadeh, CEO and Publisher
Alisa Munoz, Project Editor
Celeste Paed, Associate Production Editor
Jess Estrella, Senior Graphic Designer
Greg Isales, Licensing Associate
Natalie Piccotti, Director of Marketing
Kassie Graves, Vice President of Editorial
Jamie Giganti, Director of Academic Publishing

Printed in the United States of America.

cognella® | ACADEMIC PUBLISHING
3970 Sorrento Valley Blvd., Ste. 500, San Diego, CA 92121

CONTENTS

ACKNOWLEDGMENTS

The editor would like to thank photographer Ryan Villanueva for his contributions.

INTRODUCTION

BY NICHOLAS VILLANUEVA, JR.

THE SOCIAL WORLD OF SPORT AND WHY WE STUDY IT

Sports are a global phenomenon. The sports industry is a billion-dollar industry that brings people together, divides the populace of a nation-state, and can lead to off-the-field conflict that has at times resulted in death. Moreover, some want to trivialize sport as merely the games we play. If you are reading this book, you most likely have an interest in sport and are taking a college course in critical sports studies, kinesiology, the sociology of sport, or an academic field related to the history and culture of sport. This chapter sets up a framework for understanding what critical sports studies are. This academic discipline examines social interaction and cultural understanding of the world of sport and looks at social problems that exist in sport and society. When reading the following chapters, be aware that the additional articles accessed through QR codes are not expected to be optional reading; they reinforce the essays with the stories of athletes.

Many students of sport have an interest because of current or previous sporting participation. If their experience was positive, then they might believe that this is true for all who participate. This is part of a theory that sociologist Jay Coakley developed: "The **Great Sports Myth**—the widespread assumption that sport is, inherently, a force of good—even though it can both empower and humiliate, build bonds and destroy them, blur boundaries and marginalize."[1]

The following chapters contain a collection of essays that examine social problems in sport. When examining social problems that exist in sport, there are essential critical thinking skills necessary to be successful in scrutinizing what we believe is genuine about sport. First, **biases**: be able to recognize a personal bias and suspend that judgment to examine the rationality of a concept, proposition, or debate. Second, **perspectives**: take the time to consider various perspectives related to the concept, proposition, or debate. Third, **outcomes**: think through the concept, proposition, or debate, and identify the consequences of a belief or action. Fourth, **evidence**: when examining the concepts, propositions, or debates presented in this text, use reliable evidence and sources to explain your view of the topics presented, and avoid relying on feelings or emotions. Fifth, **self-reflection**: take what you have learned from the readings and reassess your original assumptions about the concept, proposition, or debate presented in each chapter. Critical thinking is not as easy as it sounds when presented with a topic that might trigger a strong emotional response. However, your ability to think critically will help you understand sport and society in new and much more sophisticated ways.

Chapter one is an introduction to the critical study of sport. This chapter explains the significance of the study of sport in society as an academic discipline. Chapter two discusses amateurism in sport and takes a close look at the National Collegiate Athletic Association (NCAA). Chapter three explores politics and sports. When did sports become a political tool and who has control of sports? Chapter four looks into the role media plays in sports and how it influences and, at times, controls

1 Brian J. Barth, "Stadiums and Other Sacred Cows: Why Questioning the Value of Sports Is Seen as Blasphemy," *Nautilus*, August 18, 2016.

our understanding of what we witnessed. Chapter five presents readers with documents about race and racism in sports. From the first black men and women in sports to current advocates such as Colin Kaepernick, this chapter reveals a division that remains in sports today. Chapter six examines the role sporting institutions and fans play in cultural appropriation of Native American images in sports. Chapter seven explores gender participation in sports and the role Title IX played in the participation of women and girls in sports. Chapter eight provides documents for a discussion about the inclusion of LGBTQ athletes in sports. Chapter nine examines the dangers of disordered eating and body image in sports. Chapter ten looks into violence and aggression in sports. This chapter explains how an appreciation for violence by athletes and spectators reinforces toxic masculinity that exists in the social world of sports. Chapter eleven identifies the dangers of team bonding through hazing, and the personal and financial losses as a result of these events. Chapter twelve continues to unpack the "Great Sports Myth" through the coach and athlete relationship. The documents presented in this chapter examine why physical and sexual violence by authority figures in sports is largely unreported. Finally, chapter thirteen provides possible steps to make sports a more inclusive space.

The goal of this text is to provide documents for discussion that supplement class lectures and/or other reading documents provided by your instructor. Critical sports studies can be intellectually challenging and surprisingly fun at the same time, as long as students allow themselves to critically think about the topics presented.

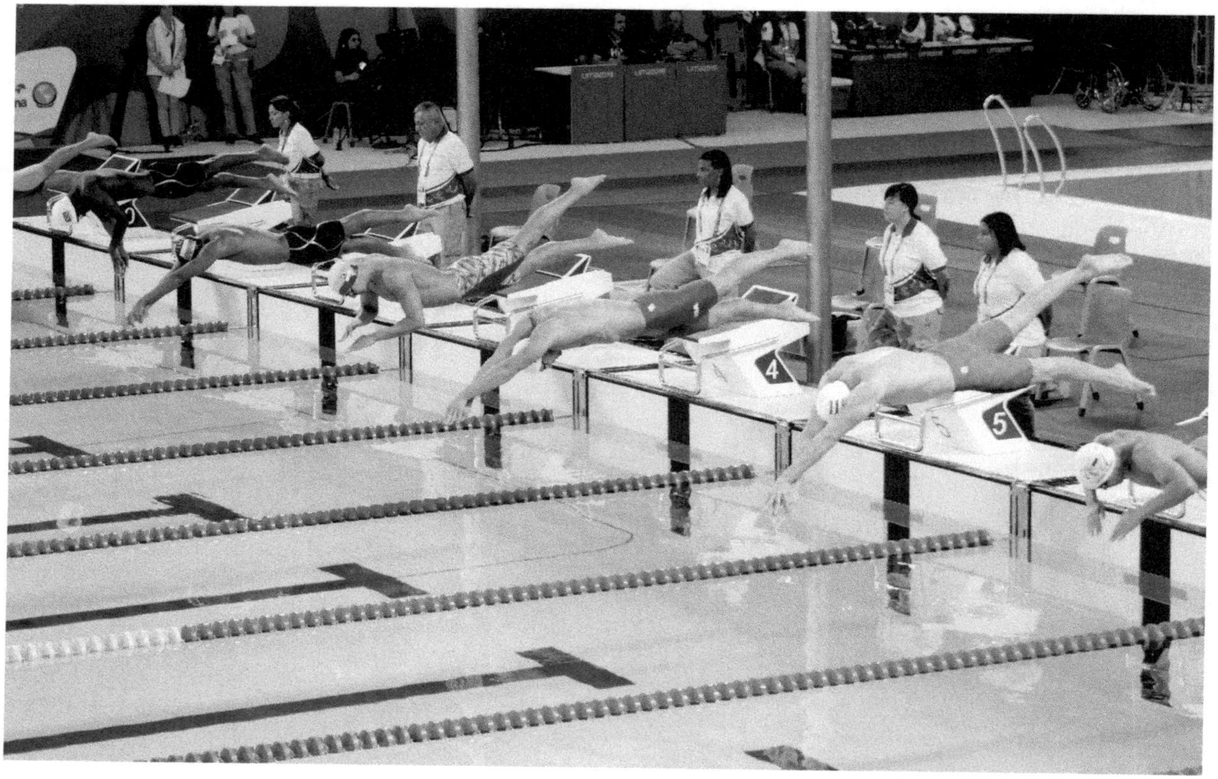
4
5

CHAPTER 1

WHAT IS CRITICAL SPORT STUDIES?

On Friday, April 26, 2019, while on a research trip in Little Rock, Arkansas, I purchased a ticket to a minor league baseball game—The Arkansas Travelers. As I approached the stadium, I saw a giant Mexican sombrero suspended in the air near the entryway into the park. Inside I found advertisements for tequila shots near the south entry and churros sold at the peanuts and popcorn stand. I learned that this was a new plan by Major League Baseball to attract the growing Latinx population in the United States to minor league baseball games. Minor league ballparks around the country reserve an average of ten games each season where the host organization creates a Latinx atmosphere. On these nights, the Travelers become "el Diamantes de Arkansas."

Between the second and third innings, I walked around the entire stadium and observed the fans and ballpark staff. To my surprise, the majority of the people in attendance were white men, women, and children. Some of the attendees wore red and green ponchos and sombreros. The only Latinx people I met were working the concessions. Upon further inspection, I found the Traveler's other mascot, an opossum wearing a Mexican poncho. Earlier that evening, my critical eye for sport and society brought my attention to a group of men and women, dressed in their Travelers' jerseys, who had all purchased shots of tequila. As the group simultaneously licked their salt, slammed their shots, and bit into their limes, one woman coughed from the unpleasant experience, one man spat most of the alcohol out of his mouth, and the remaining four companions laughed uncontrollably. The group's playful event, witnessed by many people in the concession area, drowned out the sound of the United States national anthem. At a time in sports history when Americans were highly critical of athletes making a somber statement by taking a knee during the playing of this song, I found it hypocritical that dozens of people in the area saw this behavior as acceptable. Later, before the start of the fifth inning, the announcer asked everyone to turn their attention to a man standing at home plate. The man, dressed in uniform, was recognized that night for his military service in Afghanistan as a supply clerk for the U.S. Army. Finally, during the seventh-inning stretch, that moment during mid-inning when fans are asked to sing "Take Me Out to the Ballgame," we were all instructed to stand for the playing of "God Bless America." Without being told, most of the people who were standing held their hand over their hearts. I attended this game to see home runs, stolen bases, and ninety-mile-per-hour fastball pitches. What I found was that baseball is no longer only about baseball.

The purpose of critical sports studies is to study human behavior in the social world of sports and ask essential questions about how and why games can have ever-changing meanings.

Students should ask these questions while reading the documents in these chapters. Sports are social constructions, and the meaning of sports change over time and are understood in different ways depending on the region or the country. The documents in chapter one will prepare you for the subsequent chapters. Think critically, and do not hesitate to ask questions that might contradict what you thought you knew about sports.

1

SPORT, CULTURE, AND SOCIETY

AN INTRODUCTION

Grant Jarvie

It is impossible to fully understand contemporary society and culture without acknowledging the place of sport. We inhabit a world in which sport is an international phenomenon, it is important for politicians and world leaders to be associated with sports personalities; it contributes to the economy, some of the most visible international spectacles are associated with sporting events; it is part of the social and cultural fabric of different localities, regions and nations, its transformative potential is evident in some of the poorest areas of the world; it is important to the television and film industry, the tourist industry; and it is regularly associated with social problems and issues such as crime, health, violence, social division, labor migration, economic and social regeneration and poverty.

We also live in a world in which some of the richest and poorest people identify with forms of sport in some way. This can be said without denying the fact that an immense gap exists between rich and poor parts of the world or accepting uncritically the myth of global sport. In some ways global sport has never been more successful. The Sydney 2000 Olympic Games involved 10,300 athletes from 200 countries, attracted more than US $600 million in sponsorship and was viewed on TV by more than 3.7 billion people. Sport's social and commercial power makes it a potentially potent force in the modern world, for good and for bad. It can be a tool of dictatorship, a symbol of democratic change, it has helped to start wars and promote international reconciliation. Almost every government around the world commits public resources to sporting infrastructure because of sport's perceived benefits to improving health, education, creating jobs and preventing crime. Sport matters to people. The competing notions of identity, internationalization, national tradition and global solidarity that are contested within sport all matter far beyond the reach of sport. At the same time, some have suggested that there is a legitimate crisis of confidence in global sport and those dealing with the pressures of its transformation cannot handle the reform that is required within twenty-first-century sport.

Modern sport has been described as (i) a ritual sacrifice of human energy; (ii) providing a common cultural currency between peoples; (iii) a means of compensating for deficiencies in life; (iv) a mechanism for the affirmation of identity and difference; (v) business rather than sport;

(vi) a social product; (vii) a contested arena shaped by struggles both on and off the field of play and (viii) being a euphemism for Western or capitalist sport.

Sport Theory and the Problem of Values

While it is important to explain and understand sport in society, the more important intellectual and practical questions emanate from questions relating to social change. Raising awareness about social issues within sport and answering social problems that arise out of and between different sporting worlds may occur at different levels or entry points.

How does theory help us to understand sport? Theory and empirical research provide ways of explaining and understanding sport. The constant interplay between theory and evidence helps to examine taken-for-granted sporting assumptions. Sporting myths need to be constantly challenged and re-evaluated. How these particular tools, theory and evidence, are used and for what purpose should not be the exclusive prerogative of researchers and students themselves but used in specific social contexts and on behalf of the individual's or group's values and interests. It is important that the accuracy, rigor and relevance of theory and evidence provide a basis for not only critically examining popular and unpopular sports issues but also providing students with solutions and explanation to particular sporting problems.

In approaching the study of sport for the first time it is useful to begin thinking about some of the many popular theoretical approaches to the study of sport, culture and society. Despite the burgeoning interest in sport, culture and society, one of the peculiarities of most general books in this area is that many, not all, are still discussed largely in isolation from a broader context and to a lesser extent the society of which they are part. Many popular sporting texts are not written from the standpoint of the critical thinker, sociologist, historian, geographer, anthropologist, feminist, economist or political scientist, all of whom have used concepts and theories as a basis for explaining and understanding sport as part of social life.

It is no coincidence that the thinker who evokes the promise of sociology to think about sport will draw upon political science, economics, social policy, history and other bodies of knowledge in practicing and developing a critical and practical understanding of sporting problems, practices and issues. At the same time, those studies of sport which have helped to provide insights into different ways of understanding the world of sport or some part of it have all made domain assumptions, adopted starting points, prioritized certain questions and marginalized others. In this sense a number of competing problematics have emerged. Some of the most common have been Marxism, feminism, post-modernism, cultural studies, figurational or process sociology, social anthropology, interpretative sociology, positivism, humanism, structuralism and post-colonialism.

It would be a mistake to suggest that the above problematics are simply ideology. There is no agreed understanding of many of the concepts and ideas introduced here. Notions of justice, rights, equality, authority and poverty are all essentially contested concepts. The contests over different solutions, policies and approaches to sport that occur between different sports administrators, participants, researchers or teachers may also occur between any two people who subscribe to different political ideologies. The claim that any position can be dismissed on the grounds of ideology does in fact remove the possibility of having any healthy debate over any particular sports issue.

All of the aforementioned themes have contributed to the scope and understanding of sport. One of the fundamental roles of the student of sport is to question critically and understand the very nature of why sport is the way it is and what it could or should be. The promise of fully understanding and grasping the complexity of sport, culture and society necessitates a broader understanding of sport and theory which in itself helps to inform not only the sociological imagination, but also the policy advisor, political activist, public speaker or student of sport who wants to think and reflect socially about sport, culture and society.

The Value of Theory to the Analysis of Sport, Culture and Society

Sport, culture and society, like other bodies of knowledge, has its own perspectives, ways of seeing things and of analyzing human actions, as well as its own set of principles for interpretation. It is first and foremost a distinct body of knowledge, but it also has fluid boundaries in that it draws upon other bodies of knowledge, for example in the search for solving classical sociological problems. Fundamentally, both practical and scholastic social questions are not about interpreting the world of sport, but about how to change it. As a tentative summation of what is entailed in thinking sociologically about sport it is important to develop the habit of viewing human actions as elements of wider figurations. Sport does not exist in a value-free, neutral social, cultural or political context but is influenced by all of these contexts. The value of sociology to the study of sport, culture and society is primarily that it provides a multitude of different ways of thinking about the human world. The way one chooses to think about sport will ultimately depend upon the values and political standpoint from which one views the human world. Thinking sociologically about sport is more than just adopting a common-sense approach to sport, in that the art of thinking sociologically may help the student of sport to be more sensitive to the human conditions that constitute the different worlds of sport. Thinking sociologically about sport may help us to understand that an individual's personal experience of sport is ultimately connected to broader public issues.

In the same way that the relationship between sport and capitalism was a common theme within much of the critical Marxist or socialist literature on sport produced towards the end of the twentieth century, the notion of global sport and the accompanying language of globalization have increasingly and uncritically dominated social, cultural and political debates about the nature of sport in the early part of the twenty-first century. It is as if at some point a resolution between the inherent tensions brought about by globalization and capitalism has been achieved and that sport and its relationship to capitalism has lost its meaningfulness as a way of thinking about sport in the world today. If we reduce the various theoretical forms of appeal to sport—globalization, capitalism, the third way, or post-colonialism—as a basis for simple abstraction about the social world, then we need to jettison such an approach. If we view theory as useful shorthand for a set of collectively practiced prompts to reflection—in other words, if we raise sport through all its activities and forms as a basis for reflexivity about the very nature of sport and the world itself, then we are subjecting sport and the world we live in to a qualitative assessment. Theory can help to lay the foundations for this assessment that in turn may extend to the notion of a critique of sport that is often ignored by mainstream, orthodox and traditional sports practitioners. This is but one of the core healthy progressive functions of theory—the function of criticism.

One of the fundamental functions of theory and sociology is that it contributes to a form of critique of existing forms of culture and society. Putting aside the issues of a sociology dominated by Western thinking, which is itself problematic, there is much credibility in the enduring claim that the practice of sociology demands invoking what C. Wright Mills (1970) referred to as the sociological imagination. This is a threefold exercise that involves an historical, anthropological and a critical sensitivity. The first effort of the sociological imagination involves recovering our own immediate past and understanding the basis of how historical transformation has influenced the social and cultural dimensions of life. The second effort entails the cultivation of an anthropological insight. This is particularly helpful in that it lends itself to an appreciation of the diversity of different modes of human existence and cultures throughout the world and not just those associated with the materiality of life in the West or advancing modern capitalist societies. Through a better understanding of the variety of human cultures and societies it is asserted that we can learn or facilitate a better understanding of ourselves. The third aspect of the imagination is but a combination of the first two in that the exercise of the sociological imagination avoids a critical analysis based upon the here and now and involves the potential of grasping an understanding of social relations between societies throughout the world.

Since at least the 1960s the scope and significance of the study of sport, culture and society has expanded rapidly. The breadth of perspectives that have been brought to bear upon sport has led some to be critical of the multi-paradigmatic rivalry which has been viewed as a source of potential weakness, while others have welcomed the breadth of perspectives as a basis for strengthening sociology's position as an integrative force for research into all social and developmental aspects of sport. While the importance of particular approaches and ways of knowing about sport will ultimately become less eclectic as one develops, in the first instance it is important for students of sport, culture and society to be familiar with some of the main epistemological developments which have shaped the area of study.

Sport in Social Thought

One of the tasks and promises of sociological theory has always been to help us draw bigger diagnostic pictures of sport, culture and society. With these pictures students and researchers can begin to understand and comprehend the socially and politically situated nature of their work and being. The jostling of divergent theoretical approaches will be viewed here as an expression of vitality. The coverage of various theoretical developments should not simply limit itself to sociology since other trends and influences such as post-colonialism and postmodernism are as much a product of social history and social geography as they are of sociology. Nor is what follows meant to be a simple chronology of the main developments in sociology reflected through sport.

Functionalism

Functionalist perspectives tend to be based upon the notion that social events can best be explained in terms of the function they perform. Society is viewed as a complex system whose various parts work in relationship to each other. Functionalist theories in both sociology and anthropology help to explain social institutions primarily in terms of functions and, consequently, if sport were viewed within this problematic one of the core questions would be what is the function of sport as a social institution today? Some of the central areas of debate have concerned the treatment of social order, power, social conflict and social change with the assertion being that functionalism overemphasizes the socialized conception of sport in society at the expense of the human subject or individual agency. The idea of studying social life in terms of its social functions was adopted in the early twentieth century by social anthropology. Society was seen as being made up of different interdependent parts that operated together to meet different social needs.

Symbolic Interactionism

Symbolic interactionism places a strong emphasis on the role of symbols and language as core elements of all human interaction. The definitions that people use are constructed from the symbols that are available to them throughout their culture and society. Symbols convey information and are used by people to convey meaning to the situations in which they find themselves. These symbols are learned and communicated through interaction with others.

The theory highlights the way in which human beings distinctly manipulate symbols. It is through symbols that they alone are capable of producing culture and transmitting history. A further theme relates to the notion of process and emergence in the sense that the social world is viewed as a dynamic and dialectical web in which attention is paid not to rigid structures, but to a fluid process of interaction between self and society. Any understanding of, for example, an athlete's career and the extent to which sport contributes to personal identity or feelings of loss or achievement might be open to a symbolic interactionist approach. A further theme is emphasis on the fact that the social world is interactive and from this point of view there is no such thing as a solitary individual, only an understanding of the self in relation to other humans. Finally, certain strands have stressed that any interaction is very much a dynamic process that is not necessarily harmonious. It involves the expression of meanings in a multi-layered exchange between social actors that is reciprocal and not simply linear or one-way. Symbolic interactionists may study the life experiences of footballers or baseball players or swimmers or dancers or sports administrators as distinct groups, but they would also detect common processes at work in all these groups, perhaps in terms of how status is negotiated or loss of status is dealt with.

Interpretative Sociology

Interpretative sociology has tended to incorporate symbolic interactionism as a basis for looking at core issues, such as meaning, action, status, *Verstehen*, rationality and cultural relativism. While symbolic interactionism mounted an increasingly successful challenge to the excessive claims made by functionalism, it too was challenged in the 1960s by what was claimed to be a more radical perspective on interaction, namely phenomenology and ethnomethodology. Interpretative sociology has been associated with Weber, Simmel, Garfinkel, Schultz and the early work of Anthony Giddens. Phenomenological approaches have focused attention upon the taken-for-granted content of everyday consciousness. When reified these allegedly form the external constraining realities of society. Ethnomethodology attempts to take this one step further by examining the processes through which people sustain a taken-for-granted sense of reality in their everyday lives. It is not difficult to see the potential connections here with more contemporary perspectives such as post-modernism.

Process Sociology

Figurational, sometimes referred to as process or developmental, sociology has grown out of the work of Norbert Elias. Its impact upon the sociology of sport has been sustained in a number of projects in the latter half of the twentieth century and the early part of the twenty-first century. A central facet of figurational sociology has been the notion of figuration that Elias (1978) referred to as a structure of mutually orientated and interdependent people. Figurations of interdependent people make up many webs of interdependence, which are characterized in part by different balances of power of many sorts, such as families, states, towns or simply groups. Elias used the word figuration as a processual or dynamic term in contrast with more static expressions, such as social system or social structure. Elias preferred to talk of process sociology rather than figurational sociology and this primacy of process, according to Goudsblom (1977:105), has four principled points of departure, namely that sociology is about people in the plural and that people's lives develop within and between the social figurations they form together; these figurations are continually in flux; the long-term developments taking place in human beings have and continue to be unplanned and the development of human knowledge is one important aspect of overall development. The primacy of process then has given rise to the notion of process sociology although the term figurational sociology is what is often referred to within the sport, culture and society literature.

Figurational accounts of sport have been supportive of the links between history and sociology, namely that a developmental approach to sport has made and continues to make an important contribution to historical sociology. The coverage of sport which has been informed by figurational sociology has included studies of the development of rugby in Britain, fox-hunting, global sport, boxing, Highland Games, football hooliganism and violence in sport in general.

Political Economy

Classical Marxist and liberal theories of political economy have tended to provide a basis for a socio-economic analysis of sport. In short what is the politics that arises out of an analysis of sporting economics? Liberal political economy as opposed to Marxist political economy also developed around several themes more closely associated with the discipline of economics or more precisely the inter-relationship between economic theory and political action. It encompassed several broad themes, such as an economic theory of historical progress; a theory of accumulation and economic growth through the division of labor; a redefinition of wealth as comprised of commerce and not just treasure; a theory of individual behavior which reconciled the pursuit of self-interest with the collective good and a labor theory of value which argued for labor as a measure and sometimes a source of value.

Culture and Power

It is to its credit that much of the research into sport, culture and society since at least the 1980s has acknowledged the importance of a cultural politics that moves far beyond analysis of the nation-state. The Gramscian notion of hegemony has been a clarion call for a significant amount of research into sport. In its traditional sense hegemony has literally been taken to mean the ideological/cultural domination of one class by another achieved by engineering consensus through controlling the content of cultural forms and major institutions. In *Sport, Power and Culture*, John Hargreaves (1986) rejected a 'common-sense' approach to British sport on the grounds that it helped to sustain and reproduce rather than challenge particular notions of sport. It was argued throughout that it is precisely because sport played different roles in relation to different cultures that it was able to reproduce existing power relations. Culture, in the sense that we can identify working-class culture, men's and women's culture, black culture, bourgeois culture and youth culture, must be sensitive to the fact that the function and significance of sport within different cultures may vary. The point emphasized by Hargreaves (1986:9) was that the significance of sports varied within and between cultures, and that a comprehensive account of sport, power and culture had to make reference to other forms of culture such as popular culture and consumer culture, more specifically, the relationship between the populist attraction of sport and capitalism. Analysis of sport, power and culture consequently had to acknowledge the transformative potential of sport.

Over the past three decades one of the undoubted strengths of feminist work in the area of sport, power and culture has been the presence of significant differences and, consequently, rich substantive empirical work that has told us so many different stories about women's experiences of sport. These have acknowledged the fact that power is everywhere and that power is not simply an institution or a structure, but rather it is exercised through innumerable points, rather than a single political centre. Foucault (1988) was concerned with an analysis of power within detailed studies of social practices. This approach to power dealt directly with the antagonistic struggles of social movements, arguing that one of the most important aspects of these struggles in contemporary society was the way in which they challenged subjectification. These might include struggles against the power of men over women in sport or the coach over the child or parents over children or of the power of sporting administrative bodies over national sports plans or the way people experience sport.

The advantage of this approach to the study of sport, culture and society is that it allows the student to move beyond the conventional analysis of politics at the level of the state or the ways in which, for example, governments use sport as an instrument of nation-building or as a facet of health policy. This does not mean that the study of the way in which the state uses sport is irrelevant, but that the cultural politics in civil societies, between civil society and the state and within the practices and institutions considered to be of the state must also be taken into account when analyzing the politics of sport. Cultural politics is understood to be potentially everywhere and therefore it has a broad social context.

Cultural and Social Anthropology

A resurgence of anthropological studies of sport has emerged from different parts of the world during the late twentieth century. The essential core of culture consists of traditional ideas and especially their attached values. The frequent use of cross-cultural comparative field studies provides for a substantive and empirical attention to how sport, games and play have evolved as part of the process of cultural change in different cultures. The study of objective cultural artifacts that contribute to a particular culture, tradition or set of customs is referred to as cultural materialism or etymology. A value of any etymological study of sport is the potential richness that can be found in the collection and analysis of those cultural artifacts such as songs, rituals, medals, flags, team colors and equipment associated with any grounded study of the sport. Any analysis of the cultural materials that make up sporting settings can contribute to an understanding of the social and cultural fabric of sport in both a contemporary and a historical sense.

Recent anthropological approaches to the study of sport have made a valuable contribution to the ethnography of sport, culture and society and yet such an approach has not been without criticism. In a critique of the anthropological studies of football, King (2002) argued that the failure to situate the ethnography within any critical anthropological or sociological framework led to a descent into forms of uncritical journalism. Anthropological approaches to sport have had the tendency to be all consuming and fail to differentiate and theorize adequately the notion of sport, power and culture. An all-consuming evolutionary approach to culture tends to marginalize issues of power and social differentiation between and within groups or sub-cultures. If everything within a particular way of life is seen as culture it is difficult to distinguish between different aspects of culture or the relationship between sub-cultures. The notions of power or social inequality or social differentiation or social inclusion and exclusion need not be silent within all-embracing anthropological notions of culture. King (2002:14) observes that thinking critically about sport necessitates researchers continually to question why they think the way they do and never taking for granted that the way they think is the correct way. This provides a starting point for any self-conscious reflection.

Feminism

Feminism, according to Ahmed (2000), is not simply one set of struggles in that it has mobilized different women in different places at different times, all of whom are seeking social transformation but who are not necessarily seeking the same thing nor even responding to the same situation. Feminism and theories of feminism therefore speak to different women for different reasons and for different political aims. It is not a single theory or a united political movement, nor is it a static body of knowledge. Certain key notions might include sexuality, patriarchy, gender logic, gender roles, space, femininity, engendered power relations, notions of the body, social difference and oppression. Just as it is misrepresentative to talk of feminist theory and not theories, it is also misguided to state that feminism is a just a matter of women's equality. Yet in the sporting imagination this definition of feminism is persistent within the popular imagination. It is a testament to the ongoing reflexivity inherent in feminism that there is at least recognition of the fact that women may oppress others. Consequently women can be both oppressed and oppressor.

Racism and Ethnicity

Racism is any political or social belief that justifies treating people differently according to their racial origins. Ethnicity refers to a sometimes complex combination of racial, cultural and historical characteristics by which societies are occasionally divided into separate and often hostile political families. Ethnicity often raises the question of national identity, which is why ethnic politics are often at their most virulent when they are attached to the politics of territory, space and place. Popular arguments about sport, racism and ethnicity have contributed to a number of racist beliefs about different people's sporting abilities. Sport has often been implicated in campaigns against racism and sporting organizations in many countries are subject to Race Relations Acts aimed at combating racism. Historically sport played a central role in bringing about change in South Africa during the period of apartheid rule. The African National Congress slogan, 'you cannot have normal sport in an abnormal society', specifically referred to the way in which the politics of apartheid or separateness mitigated against the possibility of multi-racial or anti-racial sport in South Africa. The 1968 Black Power demonstration by black American athletes at the 1968 Mexico Olympic Games was in part a protest against the treatment of black American people, but also an attempt to raise consciousness about the politics of participation in sport by talented black athletes, who were deemed to be first class citizens while running for their country on the athletic track, and second class citizens when they walked out of the athletic stadium. The politics of ethnic identity are evident in the emergence of the Maccabbi Games which is often referred to as the Jewish Olympic Games.

Both racism and ethnicity are closely associated with imperialism and post-colonialism. During the 1990s what were termed the new politics of race and racism displayed a deep ambivalence towards what was termed Eurocentric discourses and the politics of otherness. This approach challenged whiteness as the universal norm and what was at stake was the attempt to create a different vocabulary for representing racism, race and border relations—that is, the relationships that often cross national boundaries.

Globalization

Globalization theories in relation to sport have tended to focus upon the spread of sport across the globe in economic, cultural and political terms. A particular strand of this process has been to argue that the nation-state and the national are no longer as important as the global or the European or indeed broader configurations such as the Celtic. There are two competing concepts of globalization. One encompasses a community of human citizens for which a group of environmentalists might work, who talk in terms of thinking global and acting local. The other is of an unregulated free market where capital is king or queen and the poor are left to struggle with the consequences of deregulation, privatization, and the international plundering by international corporations. Proponents of globalization typically argue that we live in an age in which a new kind of international world has emerged, one that is characteristic of global competition for markets, consumers and culture. A facet of the free-market driven form of globalization has been that markets have decided whether we will have pensions in our old age; whether people suffering from ill-health in Africa will be treated and what forms of games and sports will be supported or even whether certain regions will have football clubs or not.

Critics of globalization insist that the process and development of global sport has neither been created completely nor produced a world that may be defined by rampant free markets or passive nation-states. While globalization may exist as a process it has not been achieved as an end point. The movement for global change is often referred to as an anti-globalization or anti-capitalist movement. There are two competing concepts of anti-globalization, one termed radical and one moderate. The radical wing views globalization as a process largely designed to ensure that wealthy elites become wealthier at the expense of poorer countries. The moderate wing, although more difficult to define, tends to share the view that globalization has the potential to be good or bad. It has the potential to provide for a sharing of cultures paid for out of the economic growth provided by free trade. However because the institutions and rules that govern the world are currently controlled by wealthy elites, inequality, instability and injustice are inevitable. In a sporting context a corollary of this might be to argue that traditional cultural rights and sporting traditions need to be at least equally recognized as socially and culturally, if not economically, as important as market-supported forms of commercialized sport.

Post-modernism

The belief that society is no longer governed by history or progress is one of the central tenets of post-modernism. Post-modern epistemology is highly pluralistic and diverse with no grand narrative directing its development. Although the history of the concept of post-modernism might be traced back to the 1960s, the post-modernist and subsequent post-structural influence on sport, culture and society emerged in the late 1980s and 1990s. It has hardly touched the Islamic countries, Asia or Latin America. The post-modern perspective is characterized by the rejection of grand theory and an emphasis on human difference. This potentially distances post-modernism from structuralism with its base in grand theory and a potential emphasis on the capitalist mode of production. Post-modern work on the body demonstrates that commodities do not necessarily have to be consumed, you merely have to gaze at them and be seduced into desiring them. Hence the post-modern body becomes a signifier of desire and you get bodies for aerobics, bodies for fashion, bodies for vacations, bodies for everything in the sense that the body can be seen to be an all-consuming metaphysical object of signs and desires. It signifies an unreal world of commodity signs rather than the real world of capital, production, consumption and exploitation.

The centrality of the symbolic value of post-modernism or post-structuralism is evident in Wynsberghe and Ritchie's (1998) analysis of the five-ring logo associated with the Olympic Games. Rather than being appropriated with the pseudo-sacred symbols and ideals associated with the modern Olympics signification, they argue that the logo has become a hyper commercial signifier used to signify virtually any product around which advertisers want to construct a story. They also argue that it signifies something for diverse groups of different people. In the same way Slowikowski's (1993) studies of sporting mascots, in particular those referred to as Native American mascots, are discussed or framed as a nostalgic, hyper, real, post-modern American culture that is absolutely fake.

Post-modernist writers tend to distance themselves from grand narratives or universal law-like statements. This emphasis on the need to study sport, culture and society from a number of viewpoints of diverse individuals and groups has been reflected in studies of gender differences as well as in studies of spaces of exclusion from and in sport occupied by minority groups defined by class, marital status, sexuality, race, age and disability. A major criticism directed at the post-modern approach to sport, culture and society is its unlimited approach to relativism. Because it privileges the views of all individuals, it appears that there is no limit to the range of possible interpretations to any given situation. In other words, there is no real world because everything is a signifier. This in particular has attracted concern from socially committed sports researchers and activists who decry postmodernism's inability to add anything to the real problem of sport's contribution to alleviating poverty and disadvantage.

Post-democracy

The idea of post-democracy describes situations in which boredom, frustration and disillusion with late twentieth-century forms of democracy exist. Such situations reflect the fact that in some places powerful minority interests have become far more influential than the wishes of ordinary people. Furthermore we live in a world in which many people have to be persuaded to exercise their vote because of a lack of trust and suspicion of political elites or oligarchies manipulating the system. Post-democracy is in part characterized by shifting patterns of irreverence and deference in which politicians anxiously seek to discover what their customers want in order to stay in business. It is part of the family of post-worlds in which it is increasingly difficult to distinguish appearance from reality because appearance is the only reality and the alleged end of ideology politics means that there are big ideas to hold on to. The disengagement of ordinary people from politics, which is developing across the world, is a further characteristic of a shift to a post-democratic period. The global or international firm has become the key institution in the post-democratic world. Social class is no longer a driving force behind democracy while the gap between rich and poor remains. The geography of anti-globalization protests signals that a new world political landscape and international social forums have replaced national civil societies as the political ground for questioning neoliberal globalization.

Historical Sociology

Historical sociological studies of sport have in some cases attempted to fill the middle ground between overtly theoretical sociological accounts of sport and dense micro-empirical historical accounts of sport. At least three types of concern constitute the focus of historical sociological studies of sport, namely a specific concern with explaining how sport has been affected by transition of one form of society to another; a further concern with tracing patterns of freedom and constraint in the life-histories of sports personnel and the relationship between these and broader public issues, and, finally, an insistence that historical studies of sport which are insensitive to sociological concerns are just as inadequate as those sociological studies of sport that do not pay due attention to historical or developmental concerns.

Conclusion: In Search of Common Ground and Social Change

It might be useful to elaborate upon the term *problematic* at this point. Each of the approaches outlined above and all other forms of analysis are *problematic*, not in the sense that they are wrong or unethical, but that at various levels of sophistication they have provided the basis for the organization of a field of knowledge or research about sport. In this sense a problematic is a definite structuring of knowledge about sport which organizes a particular research enquiry into making certain kinds of questions about sport possible or permissible, and making other questions suppressed or marginalized. In other words, the problematic in which one chooses to operate as a student or researcher will in part determine the sorts of questions that are asked about sport. At the same time it will also highlight what questions are not being asked and why.

Each of the major approaches mentioned, and many others, can claim to illuminate some part of the complexity that is sport, culture and society. Writing better histories and more inclusive progressive theory means the pursuit of complexity rather than totality. Whatever position or story that the student of sport, culture and society wants to tell about the changing nature of sport in different cultures or societies, they can always be more complex and always partial. The student of sport needs to provide more reality-congruent bodies of knowledge by continually evaluating the continual interplay between theory, evidence and the broader context.

In reality just as sociology needs history (and geography) so does theory need evidence. Purely theoretical accounts of sport, culture and society are just as unsatisfactory as those empirical accounts of sport that exude findings without any theoretical grounding or explanation. The constant interaction between theory and evidence remains one of the best defenses against the imposition of grand theory or dogma or empiricism without explanation. The student of sport, culture and society should never be value-free or far less value-neutral. It is impossible to develop theoretical or problematic frameworks by which one can understand sport, culture and society in contemporary life by adopting a value-free position.

In a sensitive and socially committed conclusion to *Sport, Leisure and Culture in Twentieth Century Britain*, Hill (2002:183–185) comments that there is an immense chasm between the grand all-consuming narrative informing sport and studies of sport that offer a smaller focus that might be traditionally empirical in their orientation. The search for whatever the truth might be perhaps lies somewhere in between these two polarities, but there is no escaping the idea that sport, culture and society is an important popular ideological battleground over values and therefore can never be neutral. Ultimately, the student of sport, culture and society needs to decide upon an entry point into the battleground over the particular issue, debate or social phenomena being studied. In all of this, critical social and historical analysts should acknowledge the socially situated nature of their work. The process of producing social change necessitates the need for multi-layered committed perspectives that move beyond just an explanation of what is going on in sport, culture and society.

Discussion Questions

1. Choose 2 of the problematics outlined above and write 2–3 possible research questions that would arise from each approach.
2. Why is the study of sport important?
3. Why is theory important to the study of sport, culture and society?

References

Ahmed, A. (2000). *Post-modernism and Islam.* London: Routledge.
Elias, N. (1978). *What is Sociology?* London: Hutchinson.
Foucault, M. (1988). *The History of Sexuality, Volume 1: An Introduction.* New York: Vintage.
Goudsblom, J. (1977). *Sociology in the Balance.* Blackwell: Oxford.
Gruneau, R. (1999). *Class, Sports and Social Development.* Illinois: Human Kinetics.
Hargreaves, John (1986). *Sport, Power and Culture.* Cambridge: Polity Press.
Hill, J. (2002). *Sport, Leisure and Culture in Twentieth Century Britain.* Basingstoke: Palgrave.
King, A. (2002). *The End of the Terraces.* London: Leicester University Press.
Mills, C. W. (1970). *The Sociological Imagination.* Middlesex: Penguin Books.
Slowikowski, S. (1993). 'Cultural Performance and Sport Mascots'. *Journal of Sport and Social Issues,* 17(1): 23–33.
Wynsberghe, R. and Ritchie, I. (1998). '(Ir)relevant Ring: The Symbolic Consumption of the Olympic Logo in Postmodern Media Culture'. In Rail, G. (ed.) *Sport and Postmodern Times.* New York: State University of New York Press, 367–384.

SPORT AS A REFLECTION OF SOCIETY

Angela Lumpkin

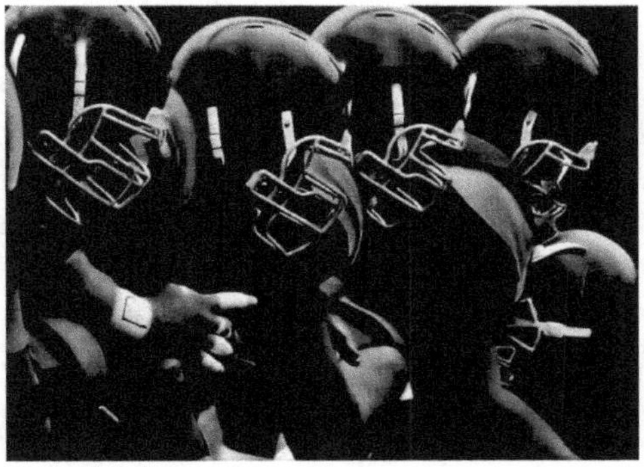

The pervasiveness of sports in the United States today is undeniable. Athletics have become so interwoven into the fabric of families, friendships, and business connections in this country, it can be argued that sport plays a role in shaping the minds and lives of individuals of all ages.

Social and cultural bonding through athletics, which extends beyond the playing field to activities such as parents playing sports with their children or families and friends tailgating before their favorite team's game, helps shape the values of those involved. Conversely, it could be argued that sports journalism describes athletics in ways that reflect people's cultural, economic, and moral values.

So, in a social climate characterized by corporate executives fabricating financial records, employees cheating employers, and thousands falsifying their reported taxes, it should come as no surprise that many athletes, coaches, sport administrators, and owners choose to cheat in sports—whether in class, during games, while recruiting, or in gaining economic and competitive advantages. Today, looking out for one's own self-interest often seems to trump everything else inside, and outside of, sports. Many coaches, athletes, sport administrators, and owners even claim that "if you are not cheating, then you are not trying hard enough to win."

Yet, sports also have been praised for teaching values. Parents, coaches, school and college administrators, and many fans claim that young people can learn respect, responsibility, self-discipline, sportsmanship, and teamwork through participation in sports. However, it is when winning becomes the primary or only goal for coaches, athletes, and parents that the potential for developing character disappears and is replaced by a "win-at-all-cost" mentality. Taught at a young age to grab the competitive edge, young athletes can learn how to cheat and gain unfair advantages that will allegedly improve the chances of winning. Many athletes have even

Angela Lumpkin, "Sport as a Reflection of Society," *Phi Kappa Phi Forum*, vol. 88, no. 4, pp. 34-35.

> Many coaches, athletes, sport administrators, and owners even claim that 'if you are not cheating, then you are not trying hard enough to win.'

acknowledged that their coaches taught them how to cheat or engage in other unethical behaviors in pursuit of glory.

Intercollegiate athletics today, and especially football and men's basketball, threaten to make a travesty of the claim that sports are educational at their core. For example, when colleges preferentially admit students based on athletic prowess, spend millions of dollars on state-of-the-art athletic facilities in an athletic "arms race," and pay coaches more than college presidents, they are using athletics and the sports media to promote their institutions while trying to keep up with or surpass other, equally-motivated schools. Many institutions charge fees to all students, take resources away from academic purposes or become, in essence, commercialized businesses to fund their expensive intercollegiate athletics programs. Playing a zero-sum game, these institutions continue to spend more and circumvent rules in order to elevate their institution's status through athletics.

In the headlong pursuit of championships and national recognition, many directors of athletics prostrate themselves to corporate sponsors who demand rule changes and scheduling accommodations that reduce athletes' abilities to be serious students. Athletes, with dreams of million-dollar contracts despite the infinitesimal odds against this goal, are encouraged by coaches to lie about the number of hours they spend engaged in their sports. Parents invest thousands of dollars in the elusive pursuit of elusive grants-in-aid for their children, even though the trade-offs physically, psychologically, and pharmacologically are often harmful. Spectators demand more victories, as if blinded to the cheating that occurs in recruiting top athletes and keeping them academically eligible.

Athletes, coaches, and boosters know that cheating has helped CEOs, lawyers, accountants, and other wealthy individuals get ahead in life by prioritizing themselves, regardless of how much harm they may cause to others. Athletes and coaches frequently see the successful perpetrators of white-collar crime profit handsomely; so, they may argue, this justifies their cheating, too.

Why shouldn't they? Told they are exceptional from an early age, many upper-echelon athletes see themselves as the next superstars in their chosen sports, but only if they can stay in the game until they sign lucrative contracts. Athletes thrive on the cheers of fans and encouragement of coaches to help them on their journeys, even as the echo of "everybody cheats" rings in their ears and unethical behaviors to get ahead become their models.

Many athletes, coaches, directors of athletics, and educational administrators believe that only chumps play by the rules. These self-promoting individuals believe the way to get ahead is to do whatever it takes to win. These individuals are reflecting—and enjoying the rewards of—sports as seen through the prism of today's attitudes, beliefs, and values of society.

FURTHER READING

Stadiums and Other Sacred Cows

Brian J. Barth

If you have a digital edition of this book, please click on the link below to access the article:

http://nautil.us/issue/39/sport/stadiums-and-other-sacred-cows

If you have a print edition of this book, please use your cell phone to scan the QR code below to access the article:

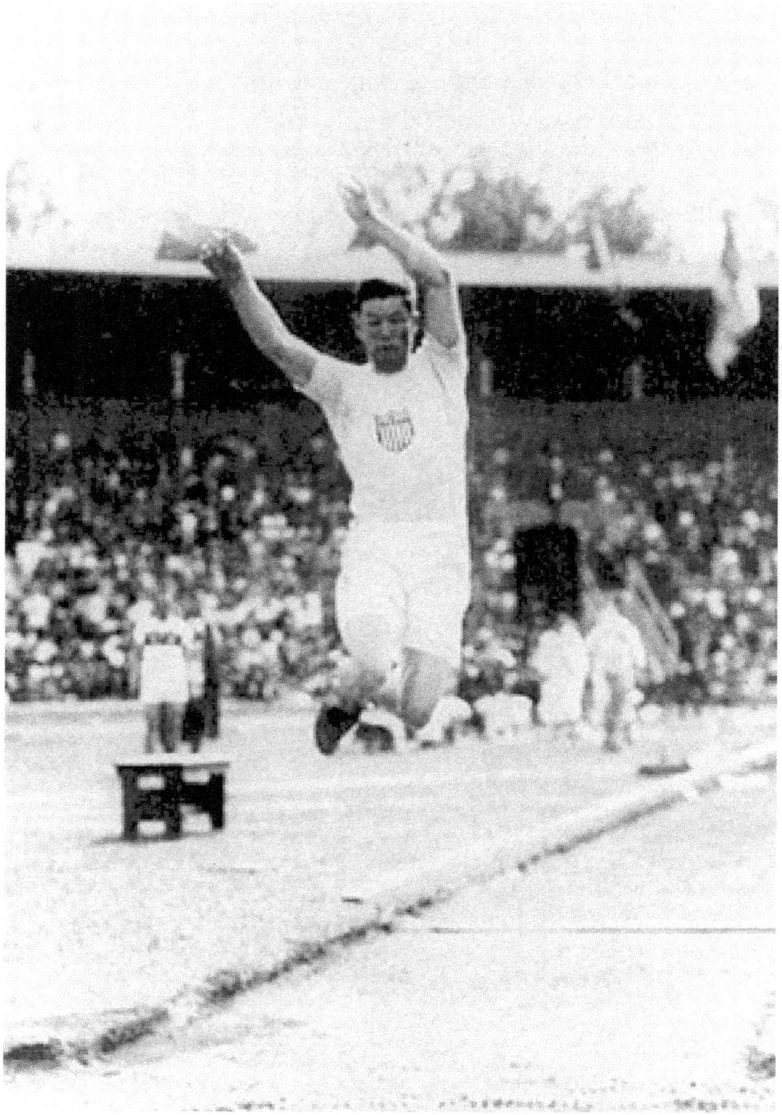

CHAPTER 2
AMATEUR ATHLETES

A**mateurism** in sport is a topic of contestation today. The National Collegiate Athletics Association administrates intercollegiate athletics within the principles of amateurism. If the NCAA earns billions of dollars from the efforts of amateur athletes, should college athletes earn some type of compensation? If so, what would that look like? These are questions that have recently become topics of conversation on sports radio and in critical sports studies classes. They intensify during college football's postseason bowl games and the NCAA men's and women's basketball tournaments. Amateurism and pay for these athletes are not new topics of conversation. Social media recently played a part in the increased awareness of this debate as well as provided a place for athletes to voice frustrations. However, we can see these topics discussed over a century ago when we examine Native American athlete James Francis Thorpe (Jim Thorpe, seen here in Chapter Two) and his accomplishments at the 1912 Summer Olympic Games in Stockholm, Sweden. Thorpe won two gold medals and set a record in the decathlon. After returning to the United States, he signed a well-paid contract to play professional baseball. An incredible athlete, Thorpe was a two-time all-American in football when he played for the Carlisle Indian Industrial School. With success came notoriety, and newspaper journalists reported that Thorpe earned a paycheck playing baseball in 1909 and 1910. This should have concluded his amateur status and made him ineligible to compete in the 1912 Olympic Games. Thorpe was stripped of his medals, and officials removed his decathlon record from the books. Historian Lars Anderson argues that this "caused his fall from grace as one of the nation's top athletes in history."[1] Chapter 2 examines amateurism and the NCAA.

Figure Credit

Fig. 2.1: Source: https://commons.wikimedia.org/wiki/File:Jim_Thorpe1912_Olympics.jpg.

1 Lars Anderson, *Carlisle vs. Army: Jim Thorpe, Dwight Eisenhower, Pop Warner, and the Forgotten Story of Football's Greatest Battle* (New York: Random House, 2007), 316.

3

AMATEURISM AND THE NCAA CARTEL

Robert Scott Lemons

Key Terms

- Amateur student athlete
- Collegiate athletics
- Cartel economics
- Monopsony/Monopoly
- Athletic scholarship

Economics of the Cartel

The National Collegiate Athletic Association (NCAA) is the organizing body of a cartel comprising over 1,100 colleges and universities (NCAA, 2014a). Over the past 25 years, university presidents have largely taken over the administration of the NCAA (Igel & Boland, 2011).

To understand the economics of college sports requires an analysis of the market power of the NCAA and its member schools. In essence, market power is the capacity to increase the market price over the marginal costs. In other words, firms with significant market power become "price makers," because they set the price. In contrast, firms in a competitive market act as "price takers," because they must take the price arrived at by the competitive market. In general, market power leads to socially undesirable results as price increases and quantity decreases. In economic terms, this would be called inefficiency or deadweight loss, resultant from excessive market power.

The NCAA member schools enjoy market power by controlling a large portion of the market. College sports, excluding junior colleges, are controlled by three distinct organizations: (1) the NCAA, (2) the National Association of Intercollegiate Athletics (NAIA), and (3) the United States Collegiate Athletic Association (USCAA). The NCAA claims 460,000 college athletes (NCAA, 2014a). The NAIA has 65,000 collegiate athletes ("About the NAIA," 2016). The USCAA probably has around 14,000 athletes. Thus, the NCAA controls 85 percent of the shares, with the

NAIA and the USCAA controlling 12 percent and 3 percent, respectively. Because the NCAA doesn't control the entire market, it cannot be described as a monopoly, but since they control 85 percent of the market, the NCAA schools can be described as having monopoly power. As the NCAA sells the product of college sports entertainment to various buyers, especially television networks, it acts as a monopolist, from the Greek "single seller." In his memoir entitled *Unsportsmanlike Conduct,* Walter Byers, the famed, first, full-time executive director of the NCAA, proclaimed, "Amateurism is not a moral issue; it is an economic camouflage for monopoly practice" (Huma & Staurowsky, 2012, p. 8).

The NCAA also behaves as a monopsonist (Greek for "one" and "purchasing food"). In contrast to a monopoly, where there is only one seller, monopsony describes a situation where there is a single buyer of a particular good or service in a given market. As the NCAA member schools acquire college athletes through the recruitment and scholarship process, they are effectively a single buyer of athletes. Any attempt to monopolize or monopsonize is illegal in the United States, according to section 2 of the Sherman Antitrust Act of 1890.

How do the NCAA member schools gain monopoly and monopsony power? The NCAA serves as a catalyst to foster collusion. Put another way, the NCAA operates as a collusive monopsony when "purchasing" athletes and a collusive monopoly when selling college sports. From an economic perspective, the NCAA promotes explicit collusion, because its members openly cooperate to make mutually beneficial pricing and production decisions. In many ways, the NCAA functions like OPEC (Organization of Petroleum Exporting Countries), as both collude, price-fix, and manipulate production (Nocera, 2011).

Judge Richard A. Posner, of the US Court of Appeals for the Seventh Circuit in Chicago and a leading antitrust scholar, agrees that the NCAA behaves monopsonistically. He says, "Although cartels, including monopsonistic ones, are generally deemed to be illegal per se under American antitrust law, the NCAA's monopsonistic behavior has thus far not been successfully challenged" (Posner, 2011, p. 1). Posner posits that colleges and the NCAA have avoided legal sanctions for their monopsonistic behavior for two reasons: 1) collegiate athletes are students, and their educational mission would be corrupted by compensation; 2) colleges and the NCAA are nonprofit institutions. Ironically, if colleges paid athletes, the schools would be engaged in a business unrelated to their academic mission and no longer immune from taxation.

Typically, cartels make agreements concerning prices, outputs, market areas, the use/construction of productive capacity, and advertising expenditures (Koch, 1973). The enterprise of college sports differs significantly from other cartel-driven industries; therefore, the cartel of NCAA member colleges functions differently from typical cartels. The NCAA functions as the head of a cartel in the following ways: (1) it fixes the compensation of college athletes; (2) it controls the supply of athletes; (3) it distributes profits in a fashion that satisfies its members; (4) it protects cartel rents; and (5) it enforces rules on athletes and member colleges (Miller, 2013).

The NCAA Fixes the Compensation of College Athletes

The NCAA requires that collegiate athletes must compete without salary to maintain their amateur status. Any compromise to this amateur status disqualifies the athlete from all future collegiate competition. According to the NCAA, "No student shall represent a college or university in any intercollegiate game or contest ... who has at any time received, either directly or indirectly, money, or any other consideration" (NCAA, 2013a, p. 1).

Amateurism mandates that athletic scholarships represent the sole remuneration to college athletes (Zola, 2013). Colleges cannot award to a college athlete financial aid that exceeds the "cost of attendance" (the amount calculated by a campus financial aid office, using federal regulations that include transportation and other expenses in addition to tuition and fees, room and board, and books) or the full "grant-in-aid" limit (defined by the NCAA as tuition and fees, room and board, and required textbooks), whichever is lower (Murray & Burton, 2003). These athletes are strictly prohibited from receiving compensation for non-athletic services that might be understood to reflect on their athletic ability. In essence, this represents a twofold restriction on player remuneration: (1) it caps the total amount of compensation; and (2) it restricts the form of remuneration, because scholarships can only purchase academic units.

College athletes differ from other scholarship students, who can use their talents to earn extra money while in school. For example, music students can play concerts and get paid, and science students can work in laboratories for a salary (Wharton, 2013). No similar options are made available to college athletes.

The NCAA effectively creates a price ceiling (compensation ceiling) for student-athletes by the limitations of their scholarships and by limitations on other compensation that student-athletes could receive. Price ceilings typically result in economic inefficiency, including deadweight loss. In figure 3.1, notice the disparity between the college (consumer) surplus and college athlete (producer) surplus, suggesting a significant advantage for the colleges from the price ceiling.

Beyond setting a price ceiling on scholarship compensation, the NCAA further fixes the compensation of college athletes by fixing their commercial rights at zero (O'Bannon, 2009). The NCAA accomplishes this by completely controlling the exposure of athletes in perpetuity. In essence, the NCAA controls if and when these college athletes will be exposed and retains all profits related to this exposure.

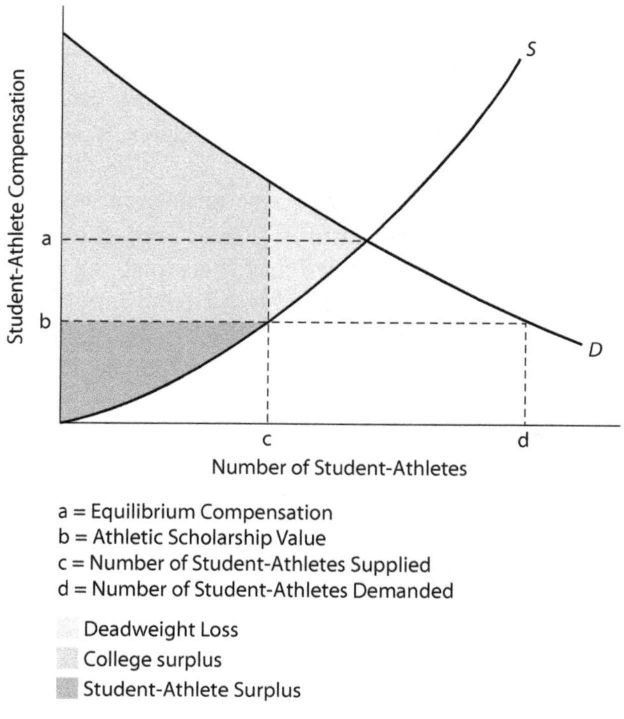

FIGURE 3.1 Comparison of College (Consumer) Surplus and College Athlete (Producer) Surplus

The NCAA Controls the Supply of College Athletes

Figure 3.1 also demonstrates that a price ceiling lowers the quantity of inputs, meaning fewer college students have the opportunity to participate in college sports. Thus, the price ceiling limits opportunities for potential college athletes, with too many talented/qualified athletes chasing too few athletic scholarships. If the NCAA allowed a progressively larger supply of athletes and events, the price of the events would decline. Therefore, the NCAA must control the quantity of athletes and competitions.

The NCAA limits the number of college athletes by limiting the number of scholarships per sport per college. In Division I basketball, each school is allowed just 13 scholarships. Football Bowl Subdivision (FBS) schools can award 85 football players with athletic scholarships.

The supply of college athletes is also controlled by the five-year eligibility rule, NCAA Bylaw 14.2.1 (NCAA, 2014b, p. 3). This rule mandates that college athletes only have five years of athletic eligibility to complete their four-year college athletic career. Simply put, they have just five years to play four seasons.

The NCAA Distributes Profits in a Fashion that Satisfies its Members

As with any cartel, the NCAA members expect that the NCAA revenue will be distributed to the membership, with the most successful members receiving the most revenue. In the 2012–13 school year, the NCAA revenue totaled $484,046,000 (NCAA, 2013c). In reality, the bulk of this revenue comes from the men's basketball tournament. March Madness captures almost 140 million viewers, and, according to NCAA president Mark Emmert, "Ninety percent of the revenue that flows into the NCAA comes from the media rights and ticket sales for the NCAA men's basketball tournament" (Bergman, 2011, p. 1). After the NCAA covers its overhead, all the remaining revenue is distributed to the member schools. The NCAA claims that 96 percent of all revenue collected returns to member colleges. As figure 3.2 demonstrates, the NCAA's largest distribution (39 percent of total revenue distributed) goes into the "basketball fund" (NCAA, 2014a). This fund "provides moneys to be distributed to Division I Men's Basketball Championships over a six-year rolling period. Independent institutions receive a full unit share based on their tournament participation over the same rolling six-year period ... In 2012–2013, each basketball unit will be approximately $245,500" (NCAA, 2014a, p. 1). What does that mean? As an example, consider the tournament revenue generated by the University of Connecticut Huskies, who played in five tournament games in 2011 and seven tournament games over the previous five years. This gave Connecticut 12 "game units." In 2011, each game unit was worth $239,664 (Smith, 2012). Therefore, from 2006 to 2011, the university generated $2,875,968 ($239,664 × 12) for its Big East Conference (Smith, 2012).

From the above, a couple of points become clear. First, it pays to be successful in college basketball, especially if the team qualifies for the NCAA tournament. Second, the revenue-distribution process seems complicated. Third, the member schools must be satisfied with the terms of the distribution process, as no schools have threatened to leave the NCAA cartel and no universities have filed public grievances against the NCAA's distribution process.

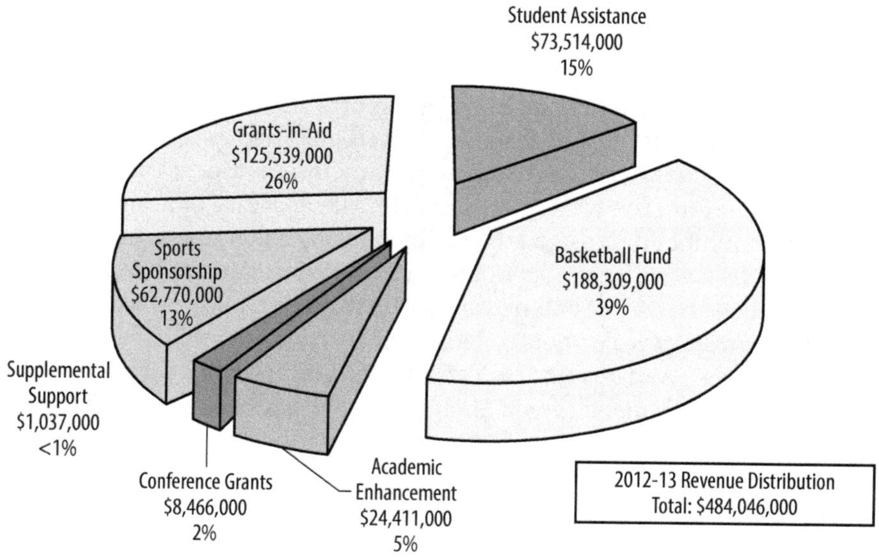

FIGURE 3.2 NCAA Revenue Distribution, 2012–13. Source: NCAA, 2013b

The NCAA Protects Cartel Rents

The actions taken by the NCAA to protect cartel rents represent another indicator that it functions as the head of a cartel. The NCAA has swallowed up any potential rivals. Consider how Walter Byers exploited the National Invitational Tournament (NIT) cheating scandal of 1951, elevating the NCAA basketball tournament into its premier position (Barra, 2012). Further consider how the NCAA eliminated the Association of Intercollegiate Athletics for Women (AIAW) in 1982 (Kahn, 2006). The NAIA may be the NCAA's next victim. Ever since the NCAA formed Division II and Division III levels of play in the mid-1970s, the NAIA's membership has steadily declined, with exiting members joining the NCAA ("The NAIA to NCAA," 2013, p. 2).

The NCAA Enforces Rules on Athletes and Member Colleges

Nobel laureate George Stigler described two challenges that successful cartels must overcome: (1) the cartel must be able to reach a consensus on its terms, and (2) the cartel must be able to police its collusive agents and punish those who have strayed from the agreed terms (Stigler, 1964). In the above section, the point was made that the NCAA member schools seem to have reached a consensus on arguably their most contentious term—revenue distribution.

Thus, the NCAA cartel seems to have overcome the first of Stigler's challenges. Stigler claims that cheating represents the major threat to cartel stability. To understand how the NCAA overcomes Stigler's second challenge, it is important to understand how NCAA schools may stray from the cartel's rules. In a typical cartel, a firm may try to cheat the cartel by lowering the price to improve sales or lowering quality to decrease production costs. The NCAA members typically try to cheat the cartel in a different fashion: universities cheat to win football or men's basketball games. Winning conference titles, being invited to football bowl games, succeeding in March Madness, and being crowned national champion brings tremendous revenue, prestige, and media exposure. Therefore, the NCAA must police its collusive agents for trying to gain an unfair advantage over other cartel members.

Cartel behavior remains economically attractive as long as the expected cost of violating the agreement (rules violations) remains greater than the expected benefits from remaining in the cartel (additional revenue) (DeSchriver & Stotlar, 1996). With the establishment of the Committee on Infractions in 1951, the NCAA had a means of policing and punishing noncompliant members. Understand that this committee has no legal authority to either police or punish any university, yet the NCAA member schools voluntarily abide by NCAA rules, even when the punishment seems excessive. As a stark example consider the so-called death penalty imposed on Southern Methodist University in 1987 (Stahl, 2012).

Attorney Ian Ayres has argued that cartels can be identified by the pattern by which they punish alleged cartel members (Ayres, 1987). With that in mind, let's examine how the NCAA punishes its members. In other words, let's evaluate the rationale of the major infractions cited by the NCAA.

As table 3.1 demonstrates, the NCAA penalizes member schools most often for violations involving amateurism. Amateurism violations include outside compensation, inappropriate employment, improper accommodations, impermissible inducements and entertainment, travel expenses, and so on. Even though the NCAA owes its creation to safety concerns in college football a century ago, it now fails to police safety issues. Safety issues may include length/intensity of practice, equipment maintenance, water breaks, avoidance of hyperthermia, return-to-play guidelines after injury, and so on.

TABLE 3.1 NCAA Major Infraction Cases (March 5, 1990–July 21, 2012)

Safety	Academic	Recruiting	Amateurism
0	11	21	24

Source: NCAA (2013b).

Why Do Universities Obey NCAA Regulations?

Earlier in this chapter, it was brought out that the NCAA has no legal authority to regulate college sports. So why do universities capitulate to NCAA regulations? As already mentioned, the colleges benefit in multiple ways by the authority vested in the NCAA. It appears that there are five reasonable answers: (1) the NCAA organizes the cartel of college sports; (2) the NCAA obscures the school's academic mission with its athletic enterprises; (3) the NCAA employs a sophisticated and manipulative strategy that results in naïve, young athletes surrendering their financial rights in perpetuity for the benefit of universities; (4) the NCAA protects its member colleges from the medical consequences inherent to sports competition; and (5) the NCAA shields the universities from the absurdity of amateurism.

The Academic Experience of the College Athlete

For students who would have attended college even without an athletic scholarship, the athletic scholarship offers no added value, except if the athlete gained acceptance to a higher-tiered college because of his or her athletic talents (Taha, 2011). For students who would not have attended college without an athletic scholarship, the indirect scholarship value represents the difference between the present value of their lifetime earnings as college graduates and the present value of their lifetime earnings if they had not graduated from college (Taha, 2011). This value should be considered in the range of hundreds of thousands of dollars (Taha, 2011). For college athletes who do not graduate, there is a modest, at best, increase in lifetime earnings capacity (Taha, 2011).

This brings up the overwhelmingly important issue of graduation rates for athletes. In 2003, Division I FBS football programs had a graduation rate of 69.2 percent, where Division I-A basketball programs graduated 66.4 percent of their athletes (Taha, 2011). At the Big 12 school Oklahoma, the football graduation rate was calculated at 38 percent by the federal calculation and 47 percent by the NCAA calculation. (For transfer-out players and those who leave school for the pros, the federal calculation assesses them as nongraduates, where the NCAA does not) (Gregory, 2013).

These athletic scholarships do not come without costs to the students. College athletes typically have a lower grade point average and class rank than other college students. Football and men's basketball players have a history of academic underperformance compared with nonrevenue athletes and the student body (Taha, 2011). As would be expected, these revenue-sports athletes probably face greater time pressures and other distractions than the rest of the student body.

With widespread academic failure and fraud involving college athletes, for those who actually graduate, what does that diploma represent? If that parchment represents little or no real education, what happens to the NCAA position that an athletic scholarship is sufficient compensation (Knight Commission on Intercollegiate Athletics, 2012)? As Billy Hawkins, an associate professor and athlete mentor at the University of Georgia, puts it, "To get a degree is one thing, to be functional with that degree is totally different" (Ganim, 2014, p. 5).

Medical Consequences for College Athletes

In a variety of ways, the NCAA has limited the collegiate athletes' rights by way of the label "student-athlete." This became painfully obvious in the 1950s, when Ray Dennison died from a traumatic brain injury from college football. Ray's widow filed for worker's compensation death benefits (Branch, 2011). The case reached the Colorado Supreme Court, which ruled that colleges are "not in the football business" (Branch, 2011, p. 88). Since the college was not in the business of football, the college did not need to cover Mr. Dennison's death through worker's compensation. Walter Byers, former NCAA president, takes credit for coining the deliberately ambiguous term "student-athlete." When injured, the player is a student. When underperforming in the classroom, the player is an athlete.

Many college athletes suffer injuries from college sports, and many of these injuries linger after their college career ends. The NCAA requires universities to provide healthcare insurance during college participation but has not made clear standards for that coverage (O'Bannon, 2009). Each university can choose its own level of health insurance. Once the athlete leaves the college, the college has no responsibilities toward the athlete's ongoing healthcare.

Conclusion

The NCAA would do well to consider how the Olympics abolished the exploitative concept of amateurism. In 1978, President Jimmy Carter signed the bipartisan Amateur Sports Act, which ended Olympic amateurism (Branch, 2011). By 1986, the International Olympic Committee (IOC) had expunged the word "amateur" from its charter (Branch, 2011). The IOC simply lifted restrictions on Olympic competitors' commercial opportunities. In essence, the current Olympic model represents a restricted market model and has enjoyed tremendous success. The Olympics do not pay athletes; the IOC simply allows athletes to get paid (Hruby, 2012). Olympians can receive compensation from anyone, except the IOC, including corporations, personal donations, sponsorships, prize money, and even their home country. Despite much initial anguish about Olympic athletes being paid, the current IOC model represents a successful precedent for the professionalization of an amateur sports system (Branch, 2011). With the Olympic model translated into college sports, the universities would not pay their athletes; they would just let them pursue their commercial opportunities, such as endorsements, autograph signings, prize money, and so on (Nance-Nash, 2011).

Further, college athletes need a bill of rights. Stanley Eitzen (2000) proposed a bill of rights that included the following: (1) the right to transfer schools without penalty; (2) the right to a four-year scholarship guarantee; (3) the right to an open-ended scholarship until graduation if an athlete competes for a college for three or more years; (4) the right of athletes to be treated like other students—freedom of speech, privacy rights, fair redress of grievances, protection from physical/mental abuse; (5) the right to consult with agents; and (6) the right to endorsement revenue. I would add: (7) adequate health care; and (8) compensation for injuries with no statute of limitations.

Questions for Discussion

1. What is the legal definition of amateurism? Could amateurism in college sports exist without the NCAA?

2. Assume that the NCAA adopts the IOC's compensation rules. Explore any residual shortcomings regarding college athlete welfare.

3. Assume that college athletes formed unions and negotiated contracts with universities. Explain potential negative consequences. Consider Title IX and tax consequences.

References

"About the NAIA." (2016). NAIA. Retrieved from http://www.naia.org/ViewArticle.dbml?ATCLID=205323019

Ayres, I. (1987). How cartels punish: A structural theory of self-enforcing collusion. *Columbia Law Review, 87*, 295–325.

Barra, A. (2012, March 6). How the NCAA basketball cartel seized its power. *The Atlantic*. Retrieved from http://www.theatlantic.com/entertainment/archive/2012/03/how-the-ncaa-basketball-cartel-seized-its-power/254612/

Bergman, L. (2011). Money and march madness. PBS. Retrieved from http://www.pbs.org/wgbh/pages/frontline/money-and-march-madness/

Branch, T. (2011, October). The shame of college sports. *The Atlantic*, 80–110.

DeSchriver, T., & Stotlar, D. (1996). An economic analysis of cartel behavior within the NCAA. *Journal of Sport Management, 10*, 388–400.

Eitzen, S. (2000, September 1). Slaves of big-time college sports. *USA Today.*

Ganim, S. (2014, January 8). CNN.com. Some college athletes play like adults, read like 5th-graders. Retrieved from http://edition.cnn.com/2014/01/07/us/ncaa-athletes-reading-scores/

Gregory, S. (2013, September 16). A cut for college athletes. *Time,* 36–42.
Hruby, P. (2012, July 25). The Olympics show why college sports should give up on amateurism. *The Atlantic.* Retrieved from http://www.theatlantic.com/entertainment/archive/2012/07/the-olympics-show-why-college-sports-should-give-up-on-amateurism/260275/
Huma, R., & Staurowsky, E. J. (2012). The $6 billion heist: Robbing college athletes under the guise of amateurism. A report collaboratively produced by the National College Players Association and Drexel University Sport Management. Retrieved from http://www.ncpanow.org/news/articles/the-6-billion-heist-robbing-college-athletes-under-the-guise-of-amateurism
Igel, L., & Boland, R. (2011). National Collegiate Athletic Association. *Encyclopedia of Law and Higher Education.* Retrieved from http://sk.sagepub.com/reference/highereducation/n91.xml
Kahn, L. (2006). The economics of college sports: Cartel behavior vs. amateurism. IZA Discussion Paper No. 2186. Ithaca, NY: Cornell University Press.
Knight Commission on Intercollegiate Athletics. (2012). Retrieved from http://www.knightcommission.org
Koch, J. (1973). The troubled cartel: The NCAA. *Law and Contemporary Problems, 38*(1), 135–150.
Miller, A. (2013). NCAA Division I athletics: Amateurism and exploitation. *Sports Journal.* Retrieved from http://thesportjournal.org/article/ncaa-division-i-athletics-amateurism-and-exploitation/
Murray, K., & Burton, J. (2003). Senate Bill 193—Bill Analysis. Assembly Committee on Higher Education. *California State Senate Analysis,* prepared by Keith Nitta.
"The NAIA to NCAA." (2013). Retrieved from http://www.naiatoncaa.wordpress.com
Nance-Nash, S. (2011, September 13). NCAA rules trap many college athletes in poverty. *AOL.* Retrieved from http://www.dailyfinance.com/2011/09/13/ncaa-rules-trap-many—college-athletes-in-poverty/
NCAA. (2013a). Amateurism. Retrieved from http://www.ncaa.org/amateurism
NCAA. (2013b). NCAA rules violation. Retrieved from http://www.ncaa.org
NCAA. (2013c). Revenue. Retrieved from http://www.ncaa.org
NCAA. (2014a). 2012–13 Division I revenue distribution plan. Retrieved from http://www.ncaa.com
NCAA. (2014b). Eligibility Rules. Retrieved from http://www.ncaa.org
Nocera, J. (2011, December 30). The college sports cartel. *New York Times.* Retrieved from http://www.nytimes.com/2011/12/31/opinion/nocera-the-college-sports-cartel.html?r=0
O'Bannon, Edward, Jr. vs. National College Athletic Association and Collegiate Licensing Company. (2009). Class Action Complaint. US District Court Northern District of California.
Posner, R. (2011, April 3). Monopsony in college athletics. *The Becker-Posner Blog.* Retrieved from http://www.becker-posner-blog.com
Smith, C. (2012). March madness: A trip to the final four is worth $9.5 million. Forbes. Retrieved from https://www.forbes.com/sites/chrissmith/2012/03/14/march-madness-a-trip-to-the-final-four-is-worth-9-5-million/
Stahl, L. (2012, July 17). NCAA death penalty for SMU a blow for decades; Should Penn State suffer same fate? *Washington Post.* Retrieved from https://www.washingtonpost.com/blogs/she-the-people/post/ncaa-death-penalty-for-smu-a-blow-for-decades/2012/07/17/gJQA1t5pqW_blog.html
Stigler, G. (1964). A theory of oligopoly. *Journal of Political Economy, 72*(1), 44–61.
Taha, A. (2011). Are college athletes economically exploited? *Wake Forest Journal of Law & Policy,* 2(1), 69–94.
Wharton, D. (2013, June 20). O'Bannon vs. NCAA: Judge Weighing Class-Action Certification. *LA Times.* Retrieved from http://articles.latimes.com/2013/jun/20/sports/la-sp-obannon-vs-ncaa-20130620
Zola, W. (2013, February 11). The illusion of amateurism in college athletics. Huffington Post. Retrieved from http://www.huffingtonpost.com/warren-k-zola/college-athletes-pay-to-play_b_2663003.html

4

TODAY'S COLLEGE ATHLETE

Joy Gaston Gayles

Key Terms

- college athletes
- intercollegiate athletics
- higher education
- athletes on Division I campuses

When describing the experiences of athletes on Division I college campuses, most scholars compare athletes to nonathletes (Simons, Van Rheenen, & Covington, 1999; Watt & Moore, 2001). Such a comparison illuminates the unique ways in which participation in college sports impacts athletes and the additional responsibilities and requirements that must be managed for success in the classroom and on the field or court. In addition to taking classes, athletes must maintain academic eligibility requirements, take a full load of classes, make progress toward degree completion each year, practice, travel, compete, attend study hall, sustain injuries, and manage the psychological stress of winning and losing (Carodine, Almond, & Gratto, 2001). Although athletes make a conscious choice to endure these additional challenges, such experiences set them apart from their peers and require support from the university and athletic department in order achieve success both on the field and in the classroom.

Many of the ways in which the experiences of athletes are unique compared to their nonathlete peers are a result of the rules and regulations designed to govern and control college sports. The National Collegiate Athletic Association (NCAA), the athletic conference to which the institution belongs, and the college or university have regulations in place to which athletes must adhere in order to participate in college sports each year. The rules and regulations are designed to ensure that athletes make progress toward their degree and maintain a fair and equitable play across institutions within the NCAA.

College athletes who desire to compete in intercollegiate athletics must go through the NCAA Eligibility Center (formerly known as the NCAA Initial-Eligibility Clearing house). Initial eligibility requires that athletes graduate from high school and earn a minimum grade point average and test score based on a sliding scale. For example, under the current rules an athlete with a high school grade point average of 2.0 must have a SAT score of 1010 or a cumulative ACT score of 86. The relationship between grade point average and test score is inverted, such that lower grade point averages require higher test scores. In 2016 the sliding scale for initial eligibility will change for athletes at Division I institutions. In order to compete as a freshman in college, athletes will be required to earn a 2.3 grade point average in core courses. Further, athletes must successfully complete 10 of the 16 total required core courses before the start of their senior year of high school and 7 of the 10 courses must be in science, mathematics, and English. The sliding scale for test scores and GPA will increase. For example, a SAT score of 820 will require a grade point average of 2.5 in core courses. High school athletes who do not meet the initial eligibility standards cannot compete as a freshman. College athletes not in compliance will be allowed to practice and receive athletic grant-in-aid. If non-eligible athletes are successful in their first academic term, they may continue to practice during their freshman year of college.

Scholarship athletes are required to attend college full-time in order to participate. On most campuses this equates to taking 12 hours (four classes) per semester. To make sure students maintain 12 hours academic advisors often schedule athletes for 15 to 18 credit hours in the event that the student needs to drop a class in which he or she is performing poorly. In addition to taking a full load of classes, there are grade point average requirements that athletes must meet in order to participate each semester. In general, athletes cannot fall below a grade point average of 2.0.

College athletes are also unique because they have to balance the demands of academic requirements with practicing and competing in their sport. The NCAA mandates athletic departments to provide academic support and counseling services for athletes. Support services such as tutoring, supplemental instruction, computer labs, and course supplies must be provided to help athletes succeed in the classroom. In addition, NCAA rules state that athletes are not allowed to practice more than 20 hours per week; however, reports indicate that some athletes practice more than 40 hours per week on average, volunteering their time to review game tapes and condition for their sport (Wolverton, 2008).

Challenges for Athletes and Higher Education

The many rules and regulations, pressures, and scrutiny associated with intercollegiate athletics in higher education have created challenges for athletes and higher education institutions. Reports of scandals involving academic and social misconduct in intercollegiate athletics flood the media each year. The accusations and incidents have increased in severity over the years, and these scandals bring shame to the institution and spark distrust within the community. Some of the major challenges concerning athlete welfare include academic performance and graduation rates, balancing academic and athletic tasks, and the pay-for-play issue.

Academic Performance and Graduation Rates

The 1980s represents a period of increased concern about academic standards and performance for athletes. It was the first time that the NCAA enforced regulations for academic performance that were actually adhered to by member institutions. Proposition 48 and the Student Right to Know Act are two major reform efforts that set the foundation for academic standards.

STAKEHOLDER PERSPECTIVE

Pay-for-Play: A Moral Dilemma

Darin Moss is the director for compliance at Big Time University, USA. Big Time University is one of the top land-grant universities in the country with highly ranked athletic programs for the majority of the 14 sports offered. The basketball program has clinched two national championships in the past 7 years and is ranked number 1 in the country. Darin has worked in compliance for 10 years. He spent the first few years of his career working in compliance at the national collegiate athletic association before becoming the compliance director at Big time University. During his time at the NCAA he worked in investigations and is very familiar with the rules and regulations, infractions, and penalties associated with breaking the rules.

Working at Big Time University, Darin understands that students are under a great deal of pressure to manage their affairs both on and off the playing field. At the beginning of every academic year Darin and his staff meet with all athletes by sport to remind them of the rules and regulations associated with participating in intercollegiate athletics. Some of the major issues for athletes in high-profile sports are accepting gifts from agents, boosters, and others in the community. The NCAA is very strict concerning athletes accepting monetary gifts, making deals with agents, and academic misconduct.

The pay-for-play issue is one that Darin struggles with. On one hand, Big Time University generates large sums of revenue largely based on the athletic prowess of athletes. Yet athletes do not receive a direct share of the profit for their labor. Moreover, Darin knows that some of the most talented players come from poor backgrounds where the families of athletes in high-profile sports are depending on their loved one to "go pro." However, while the athletes are competing at the college level, they do not have enough money to cover daily living expenses, such as washing clothes, going to the movies, or buying a bus ticket home for the holidays.

The associated press recently interviewed Darin about this issue as Big Time University is currently under investigation for allegations of university basketball players accepting money from boosters. Darin Moss told the Associated Press that pay-for-play is a major issue plaguing college sports. As commercialism and revenue generation increase without consideration of the overall well-being of athletes, misconduct and scandals involving rule infractions will continue to escalate and burden higher education institutions.

NCAA member institutions have reported graduation rates since the mid-1980s under the Student Right to Know Act, which requires that higher education institutions make public graduation rate data as well as data on crime statistics so that students can make informed decisions about the institutions they desire to attend. The latest graduation rate data show that athletes graduate at higher rates compared to students in the general population (Christianson, 2012). In 2012 the NCAA reported that athletes who entered as freshmen during the 2004–2005 academic year graduated at a rate of 81%. The NCAA also reported that in 2012 athletes in football and men's basketball showed remarkable improvement compared to past years. Men's basketball players graduated at 74%, a 6-point increase from the previous entering class. Further, football players had a graduation rate of 70%, 1-point increase over the previous entering class. Moreover, across an 11-year period of data collection graduation rates for men's basketball increased 21 percentage points and graduation rates for football players increased 7 percentage points.

Scholars and critics have questioned why the graduation rate data reported by the NCAA are so high (Southall, Eckard, Nagel, & Hale, 2012). One of the major reasons why the data vary so widely is because the NCAA and the federal government use different metric systems. The NCAA developed the Graduation Success Rate (GSR) to better account for transfer students who leave the institution in good standing. Thus, outgoing transfer students in good standing are included in the receiving institutions cohort of athletes. The current GSR is based on four cohorts of entering classes from 2002 to 2006. The GSR reported by the NCAA is usually about 20 percentage points higher than the rate reported by the federal government, which excludes transfer students from the calculation (Steinbach, 2012). Using the Federal Graduation Rate, athletes who entered in 2005 graduated at a rate of 65%, two percentage points higher than students in the general population did. Another reason why the GSR is higher than the Federal Graduation Rate is that for the first time Ivy League institutions were included in the calculations. It is important to note that Ivy League institutions are not like other Division I institutions because they do not award athletic scholarships.

Without probing any further, the fact that graduation rates have increased, particularly for high-profile sports, is good news. However, further examination of graduation data unmasks major differences in academic performance and successful degree completion. For example, disaggregating graduation rates by race and ethnicity shows major disparities. According to the GSR, African American athletes graduated at a rate of 54%. Although this represents an increase of 19% over time, the rate still lags behind students in the general population. More alarming is that African American males graduated at a rate of 49%—an increase of 16 points over time. However, like African American females this rate lags behind the average rate for all African American athletes and students in the general population. African American female athletes, however, are faring well graduating at a rate of 64%, which is on par with the average graduation for athletes in the general student population.

Balancing Academics and Athletics

Perhaps one of the most challenging and stressful tasks faced by athletes is the act of balancing academic, athletics, and social demands (Adler & Adler, 1991; Comeaux & Harrison, 2011; Gaston-Gayles, 2004; Simons, Van Rheenen, & Covington, 1999). On most days athletes wake up early, take a full day of classes, attend practice, eat dinner, and then go to study hall. By the time study hall is over late in the evening it is time to rest and prepare to do it all over again the next day. Such a rigid schedule leaves limited time for social activities and in some cases not enough time to meet with professors during office hours and tutors for supplemental instruction. Moreover, balancing academic and athletic demands can be even more strenuous for athletes who enter college academically underprepared.

Scholars have studied the challenges athletes face balancing academic and athletic roles and responsibilities. Adler and Adler (1991) conducted one of the first studies on the topic using ethnographic techniques to study the basketball team at a major Division I institution. Overall they found that the male basketball players in the study had high aspirations toward academic performance in college; however, the demands of participating in their sport led to overinvolvement in athletics as early as the first and second semester of their college career. Adler and Adler coined the term *role engulfment* to characterize athletes who became overinvolved with athletic demands and as a result devoted little time to academic and social experiences during college.

A major problem resulting from overinvolvement in athletics is isolation from the general student body. Critics have argued that athletes form a separate subculture on college campuses that isolates them from the student body and impacts the extent to which they benefit from the college experience in ways similar to their peers (Bowen & Levin, 2003; Shulman & Bowen, 2001). Parham's (1993) study on the experiences of athletes supports that they have difficulty balancing academic and athletic tasks and experience social isolation from spending so much time in the athletic domain. The study also found that athletes experience mental and emotional stress from dealing with the pressures of winning and losing and managing relationships among competing groups, such as coaches, friends, and family. Parham concluded that the demands of balancing so many stressors make the athlete population vulnerable to other issues, such as lower gains in learning and personal development.

Other studies have examined the issue of balancing academic and athletic demands using motivation theory. It is quite natural for athletes to enter college highly motivated in the athletic domain because the university recruits and awards scholarships based on athletic talent. The problem is when students enter the university without the same level of motivation in the academic domain. Lack of academic motivation seems to be most problematic for high-profile athletes (Gaston-Gayles, 2004; Simons, Van Rheenen, & Covington, 1999). Gaston-Gayles (2004) developed a scale to measure athletes' motivation toward sports and academics and found that what mattered most in terms of academic performance was the extent to which athletes were motivated academically. Having high aspirations to excel in the athletic domain did not influence academic performance; however, lack of academic motivation, regardless of athletic motivation, had a negative influence on academics.

Other studies have examined motivation using self-worth theory to understand differences in motivation for the student athlete population. Simons, Van Rheenen, and Covington (1999) examined achievement motivation for athletes using self-worth theory and found that most athletes in revenue sports were failure avoiders—motivated to achieve success in one domain while avoiding failure in another. Moreover, failure avoiders are characterized by attitudes and behaviors that result in low academic performance such as use of self-handicapping excuses, low academic self-worth, higher problem levels in reading and studying, and less intrinsic motivation.

When athletes place too much emphasis in the athletic domain and become isolated from the student body, the question is raised as to whether athletes benefit from the college experience similar to their nonathlete peers. The idea that athletes make up a separate subculture on college campuses leads to discussion about possible negative consequences of participating in college sports. Gayles and Hu (2009) examined the athlete experience using national data from the NCAA and found that athletes interacted with peers other than athletes more commonly than any other form of engagement measured in the study. However, athletes participated in student organizations least frequently. In addition, interacting with peers other than teammates was one of the most influential factors in outcomes such as personal self-concept and learning and communication skills. A unique finding in this study, however, was that these effects were more beneficial for athletes in low-profile or Olympic sports. More investigation is needed to understand what factors matter relative to cognitive and affective gains for athletes in high-profile sports.

Pay-for-Play

The debate over whether to compensate athletes for their participation in college sports is a growing area of concern for intercollegiate athletics and higher education. College athletes, particularly those who participate in revenue sports such as football and men's basketball, generate large sums of revenue for athletic departments; yet athletes do not receive any share of the profit from the revenue they help generate. Further, athletic departments generate revenue from merchandise sales using the number and image of high-profile athletes.

Commercialism associated with college sports is a growing problem that institutions will have to address in the near future. As commercialism increases in the form of television contracts, ticket sales, high-salary coaches, and advertising endorsements, so does the pressure to produce winning teams and generate revenue. Over the years, cases of academic and social misconduct have increased in frequency and severity. Further, the commercialized values of intercollegiate athletics run contrary to the goals and values of higher education institutions. Institutions of higher education will need to figure out the proper role and function of intercollegiate athletics in higher education and take steps to align the values and goals of educating students to the goals and values associated with participation in college sports.

CASE STUDY

Pay-for-Play

The pay-for-play issue is predicated on the question of whether athletes should receive monetary compensation for their participation in college sports. The commercialism associated with college sports has increased exponentially over the years and institutions generate millions of dollars annually from television contracts, ticket sales, tournaments, and advertising deals. At the heart of the pay-for-play issue is the tension between the fact that athletic departments generate large sums of revenue and the individuals responsible for generating the revenue do not receive a direct share of the profit. In fact, athletes represent the only stakeholders who do not receive a direct share of the profit.

Some have argued that college athletes do receive payment in the form of an athletic scholarship. However, others have questioned if $40,000 to $50,000 over a total of 4 years is equivalent to the billions of dollars generated annually by athletic departments. Moreover, if athletes in high-profile sports are not successfully graduating from college, then is the promise of earning a college degree enough to compensate athletes for their labor?

Institutions of higher education adhere to the principle of amateurism as it allows for a peculiar institution such as college sports to exist within higher education institutions (Thelin, 2012). Compensating athletes directly would go against the values and principles of higher education and would change the face of college sports as we know it. Questions about how much athletes should be paid, should all athletes receive the same amount, should all athletes be paid or just athletes in revenue-producing sports are some of the questions that will have to be addressed if such a policy were enacted.

The NCAA recognizes the academic, financial, and social pressures faced by college athletes but remains strictly against compensating athletes for participation in the college sports. The collegiate model dates back to the 1950s and implies that athletes are also students (not employees of the institution). The NCAA recently passed legislation for institutions to award athletes up to $2,000 over the cost of attendance. However, this legislation was put on hold because athletic departments complained that they did not have enough revenue to do so. Further athletes are allowed to work no more than 20 hours per week and cannot be compensated more than $2,000 beyond the cost of attendance. Although this would allow athletes to earn additional money for daily living expenses, working a part-time job further complicates the issue of balancing academic and athletic demands.

About 300 athletes participating in high-profile sports across several Division I institutions recently filed a law suit against the NCAA for rights and royalties associated with marketing jerseys with players' names and numbers on them. College athletes feel that they should benefit from advertising and merchandise sales that use their names and numbers. The lawsuit indicates that they want direct compensation for and rights to merchandise sales.

The NCAA has taken a firm stance against pay-for-play and has held true to the amateur status of college sports. A few reform efforts that address the pay-for-play issue have been approved, but the NCAA has made clear that the measures taken are not a form of pay-for-play. In the 1990s the NCAA allowed athletes to work no more than 20 hours per week and earn no more than $2,000 above the cost of tuition. In 2011 the NCAA also approved a rule allowing athletic departments to add up to $2,000 above the cost of tuition to athletic grant-in-aid for athletes in an effort to close the gap between tuition and fees and the full cost of attendance. Because of complaints from athletic departments across the country, the NCAA has since tabled the rule until a solution is reached concerning how athletic departments can afford to increase scholarships for athletes. The following questions remain:

Should athletes be compensated beyond athletic grant-in-aid, and what does this mean for intercollegiate athletics on college campuses?

Conclusion

Although there are many challenges and problems with college sports on college campuses, intercollegiate athletics serves a unique purpose that should not be overlooked. If governed and controlled properly, intercollegiate athletics can serve as a bridge that connects the university to the community, provide opportunities for students to receive a quality education and develop character, and unite the campus community around a common goal. Reform agendas led by groups such as the Knight Commission on Intercollegiate Athletics and The Drake Group call for better alignment between the values and goals and intercollegiate athletics and institutions of higher education. For example, a recent Knight Commission Report (2010) entitled *Restoring the Balance* calls for greater transparency concerning spending in intercollegiate athletics, putting into place practices that lead to making academics a priority, maintaining the amateur status of college sports, and treating athletes as students first. At the heart of all reform efforts should be the welfare of the student athlete. Policy recommendations and rule changes must consider what is in the best interest of students and how can we better educate and support the athlete population in ways that support the mission of higher education institutions.

Questions for Discussion

1. What are some of the major issues facing intercollegiate athletics in American higher education today?
2. Do you think that athletes at Division I institutions should be paid for their participation in intercollegiate athletics? Why or why not?
3. What are the pros and cons for institutions of higher education concerning paying athletes for participating in intercollegiate athletics?

References

Adler, P. A., & Adler, P. (1991). *Backboards and blackboards: College athletes and role engulfment.* New York: Columbia University Press.

Bowen, W. G., & Levin, S. A. (2003). *Reclaiming the game: College sports and educational values.* Princeton, NJ: Princeton University Press.

Carodine, K., Almond, K. F., & Gratto, K. K. (2001). College student athlete success both in and out of the classroom. In M. F. Howard-Hamilton & S. K. Watts (Eds.), Student services for athletes, *New Direction for Student Services*, 93, 19–33. San Francisco: Jossey-Bass.

Christianson, E. (2012, October 25). DI men's basketball, FBS football graduation rates highest ever. *NCAA News.*

Comeaux, E., & Harrison, C. K. (2011). A conceptual model of academic success for student-athletes. *Educational Researcher,* 40, 235–245.

Gaston-Gayles, J. (2004). Examining academic and athletic motivation among student athletes at a Division I university. *Journal of College Student Development,* 45(1), 75–83.

Gayles, J. G., & Hu, S. (2009). The influence of student engagement and sport participation on college outcomes among Division I student athletes. *Journal of Higher Education,* 80, 315–333.

Knight Commission on Intercollegiate Athletics. (2010). *Restoring the balance: Dollars, values, and the future of college sports.* Miami, FL: Author.

Parham, W. (1993). The intercollegiate athlete: A 1990s profile. *Counseling Psychologist,* 21, 411–429.

Shulman, J. L., & Bowen, W. G. (2001). *The game of life: College sports and educational values.* Princeton, NJ: Princeton University Press.

Simons, H. D., Van Rheenen, D., & Covington, M. V. (1999). Noncognitive predictors of student-athletes' academic performance. *Journal of College Student Development,* 40, 151–162.

Southall, R. M., Eckard, E. W., Nagel, M. S., & Hale, J. M. (2012). *Adjusted graduation gap report: NCAA Division-I football.* Chapel Hill, NC: College Sport Research Institute.

Steinbach, P. (2012). Record NCAA graduation rates don't tell the whole story. Retrieved from http://www.athleticbusiness.com/Governing-Bodies/record-ncaa-graduation-rates-don-t-tell-the-whole-story.html

Thelin, J. R. (2012). College athletics: Continuity and change over four centuries. In G. S. McClellan, C. King, & D. L. Rockey, *The handbook of college athletics and recreation administration* (pp. 3–20). San Francisco: Jossey-Bass.

Watt, S. K., & Moore, J. L. (2001). Who are student athletes? In M. F. Howard-Hamilton & S. K. Watts (Eds.), Student services for athletes, *New directions for student services*, 93, 7–18. San Francisco: Jossey-Bass.

Wolverton, B. (2008). Athletes' hours renew debate over college sports. *Chronicle of Higher Education,* 54(20), A1.

FURTHER READING

Could “Fair Pay to Play Act” Pave Way Toward End of Amateurism in Collegiate Athletics?

Michael McCann

If you have a digital edition of this book, please click on the link below to access the article:

https://sports.yahoo.com/could-apos-fair-pay-play-162941230.html

If you have a print edition of this book, please use your cell phone to scan the QR code below to access the article:

Zion Williamson Injury Wearing Nike Shoe Rips Through the Business of Basketball

CBS News

If you have a digital edition of this book, please click on the link below to access the article:

https://www.cbsnews.com/news/zion-williamson-injury-in-nike-shoe-rips-through-the-business-of-basketball/

If you have a print edition of this book, please use your cell phone to scan the QR code below to access the article:

Jim Thorpe's Olympic Gold Medals Restored

New York Times

If you have a digital edition of this book, please click on the link below to access the article:

https://www.nytimes.com/1982/10/14/sports/jim-thorpe-s-olympic-medals-are-restored.html

If you have a print edition of this book, please use your cell phone to scan the QR code below to access the article:

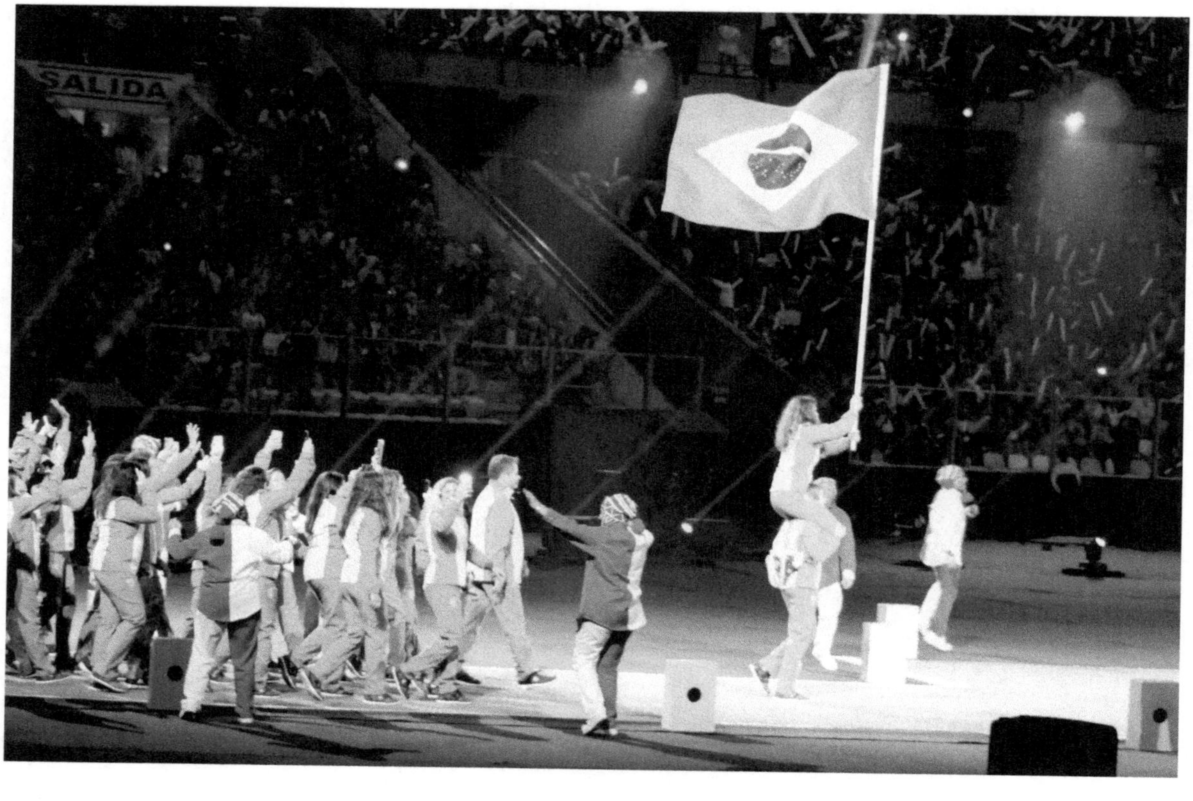
SALIDA

CHAPTER 3

POLITICS AND NATIONALISM IN SPORT

O'er the land of the free and the home of the brave!" Boisterous cheers immediately follow the final words of the US national anthem at sporting events. These symbols of nationhood, nationalism, and pride—the American flag and anthem—are used in the ceremony and tradition that is part of American **sporting nationalism**. At baseball games from coast to coast and encompassing professional, amateur, and club teams, this ceremony evolved after September 11, 2001, to include "God Bless America" and almost replace "Take Me Out to the Ballgame." In the twentieth-century world, sport and nationalism combine to exemplify a desire for homogeneity that includes members of a social world who are patriotic to the State and excludes any outlier that appears to disrespect the militant ceremony that exists during a sporting event.

The problem with sporting nationalism is the conflation of **patriotism** with **nationalism**. These are two completely different terms. Take a moment and attempt to differentiate between the two. Students usually do not have trouble answering what patriotism is. Simply stated, it is a love for a country. Nationalism is much different. While nationalists can say they love their country, they desire **homogeneity** within their group. Homogeneity can exclude people from being accepted into the nation or, in this case, the social world of sport. For example, African American athletes who make a political statement before a sporting event are excluded. One might argue that the dominant group believes this to be disrespectful. However, the dominant white group at these events has not experienced **systemic racism**. In other words, many cannot understand the plight of being black in America. Another way to examine these two terms is by answering the following question: Can you be patriotic to another nation or national team than the one from your home country?

The answer is, simply, "yes." As defined earlier, patriotism is a feeling of love for a country and does not necessitate the acceptance of the dominant group in that society. For example, during the summer of 2019, I attended the Pan American Games in Lima, Peru. During events with Team USA athletes, I wore my USA shirt, my friends raised a flag in the stands, and we supported our national team. When Team USA was not competing, I often cheered for Mexico because of my Mexican heritage. Finally, when neither team competed, I supported the local team of athletes from Peru. Mexican and Peruvian fans did not accept me as part of their homogeneous group, but they appreciated my patriotic support of their athletes at an international sporting event.

Sporting nationalism and society have clashed in the twenty-first century. Football and baseball are no longer merely games, but spaces that define and contest national identity. During the summer and fall of 2016, athletes used this space to contest national identity and bring awareness to the social inequality that exists in US society. It is this playing field that has become a contested space for something much more than a game. In this land of the free, these athletes and fans are standing up to racial injustice. In doing so, some have opposed the ceremonial playing of the national anthem by a peaceful protest of kneeling. For the dominant group of sport and society, this was seen as unpatriotic. Dominant narratives revealed there is a privilege in sport that precludes athletes of color from making any statement that is not in line with the dominant group in control of sport and society.

5

POLITICS AND GOVERNMENT IN SPORTS TELEVISION

Dennis Deninger

> A sporting system is the by-product of society and its political system, and it is just boyhood dreaming to suppose you can ever take politics out of sport.
>
> (Peter Hain, Member of British Parliament)

TABLE 5.1 The Rundown

- Sports and political symbolism.
- Sports as a forum for politics.
- The event as a political statement.
- Berlin 1936 and Olympic boycotts.
- The event as a political stage.
- Mexico City 1968 and Munich 1972.
- Sports stars as political icons.
- Economics makes sports political.
- Public vs. private funding for stadiums.
- NCAA College Football and the Supreme Court.
- The Federal Communications Commission.
- Media ownership limitations.
- Public access to television programming.
- Must-carry and retransmission consent.
- The congressional connection.

If there were a sports utopia, the vast majority of fans would want it to be a place of festival and spectacle where all games were contests of skill and will, matching the best athletes and teams in competitions that would, with each renewal, reach new heights and create ever more amazing highlights for us all to cheer and enjoy. In sports utopia politics and government would play no role whatsoever. But as each of us knows all too well, there is no such place.

Sports and Political Symbolism

Games and matches are more than simply competitions; they are events that play a role in the construction and representation of local, regional, and national identities. The quest for victory and the unwillingness to settle for anything less is paramount in sports, and in politics. Winning tells all challengers that your city, region, or nation is better than theirs. It sets the highest standards, works the hardest to reach its goals, will endure all struggles and overcome all obstacles to prevail. For much of the world, and for millions of Americans, gridiron football represents the United States. Success is built on superior strength, teamwork, and the ability to impose one's will by any means necessary on the opposition. The symbolism of baseball as the original "national pastime" is tied up in the values upon which the country was founded, where boys and girls played on open fields and pastures, and, regardless of an individual's humble beginnings, working hard and striving to excel, would reap the rewards of success.

The power of symbolism is not lost on politicians. Nor is the ability to simultaneously reach a vast audience of potential voters. President William Howard Taft started a tradition that has connected

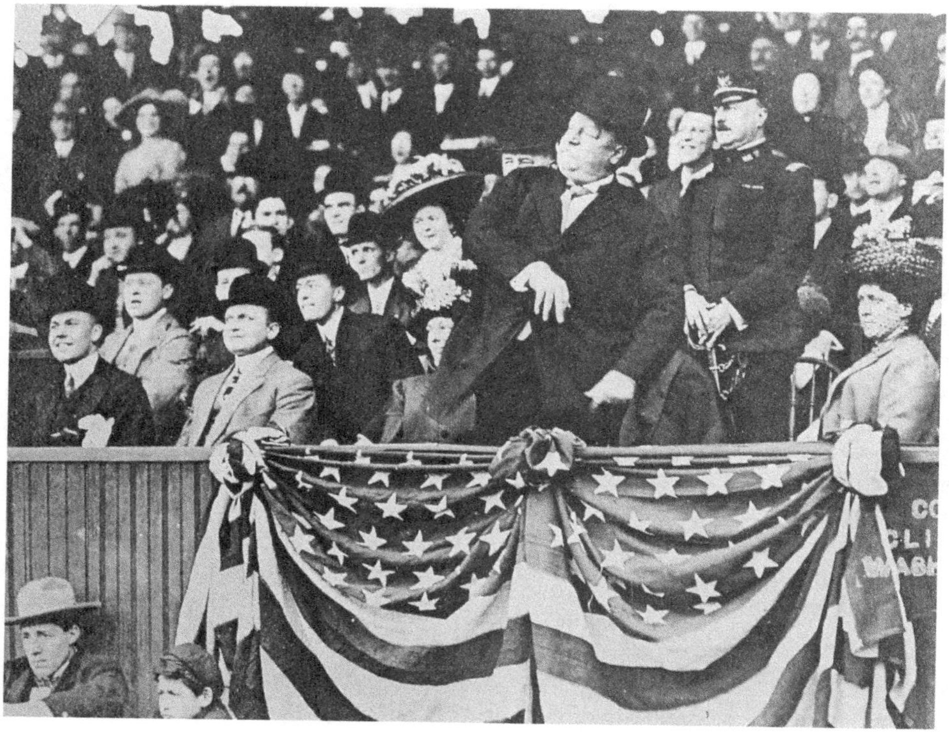

FIGURE 5.1 President William Howard Taft started a tradition when he threw out the first ball to open the 1912 baseball season

Source: reprinted with permission of Getty Images

politics and sports since 1912: throwing out the ceremonial "first ball" of the baseball season. From their seat in the stands, Taft and successive presidents presented a smiling, positive image as men of the people who enjoyed taking in a game just as much as the average guy. The symbolism changed when presidents stepped out of the stands and onto the field to make the "first pitch" from the mound. Now the president is "one of the players," a man of action standing shoulder to shoulder with elite athletes on ground where only they, and a select few who receive special permission, are allowed to tread. Sitting in the stands was fine for newspaper photos; pitching from the mound makes better television.

Sports as a Forum for Politics

The first pitch is symbolic and largely devoid of any political message beyond that of a leader openly sharing his or her love for the sports that the nation holds close to its heart. However, any gathering with thousands of spectators in the audience and millions watching on television can be used as a political forum by individuals or groups who will exploit the captive audience to make their stands known. There are three broad categories to examine.

The Event as a Political Statement

Throughout the 20th century and into the 21st there are numerous examples of sports events that by virtue of their very existence, timing, and competitors have become political statements. The very fact that the Olympic Games were held in Berlin in 1936 made a political statement even before sprinter Jesse Owens, an African-American, won the first of his four gold medals. In 1931, two years before Adolf Hitler rose to power, the International Olympic Committee (IOC) had selected Berlin over Barcelona to host the games. When it became evident that Hitler's Third Reich was an oppressive dictatorship that trampled the rights and endangered the lives of anyone who was not a member of the white "Aryan" race, there was an international outcry and demands that the games be moved out of Germany.

The president of the American Olympic Committee in 1933 was Avery Brundage. His initial reaction to news that Jewish athletes in Germany were being persecuted and would not be allowed to compete was to say that, "The very foundation of the modern Olympic revival will be undermined if individual countries are allowed to restrict participation by reason of class, creed, or race." However, after the Germans invited Brundage to see for himself in a carefully orchestrated visit to the country in 1934, he became a staunch advocate in favor of sending the American team to compete in Berlin. His message to anyone who believed that sending a team would be an endorsement of Hitler's hateful policies was, "The Olympic Games belong to the athletes and not to the politicians."

The boycott movement fell apart in December of 1935, after the Amateur Athletic Union (AAU) voted in favor of American participation. Hitler and his Nazi Party got their international stage upon which to demonstrate the "natural supremacy" they claimed. The German team did win the largest number of medals in Berlin: thirty-three gold, twenty-six silver, and thirty bronze for a total of eighty-nine, but it was Jesse Owens' world records and four gold medals that made the most powerful political statement: Hitler's racial convictions were wrong.

The staging of the Olympics in Moscow in 1980 was seen as a political statement by those who opposed the Soviet invasion of Afghanistan in 1979. A total of sixty-seven nations refused to send their teams to Moscow, joining a boycott led by US President Jimmy Carter. The number of nations that did participate was eighty, the smallest field for a summer Olympiad since the 1956 games in Melbourne,

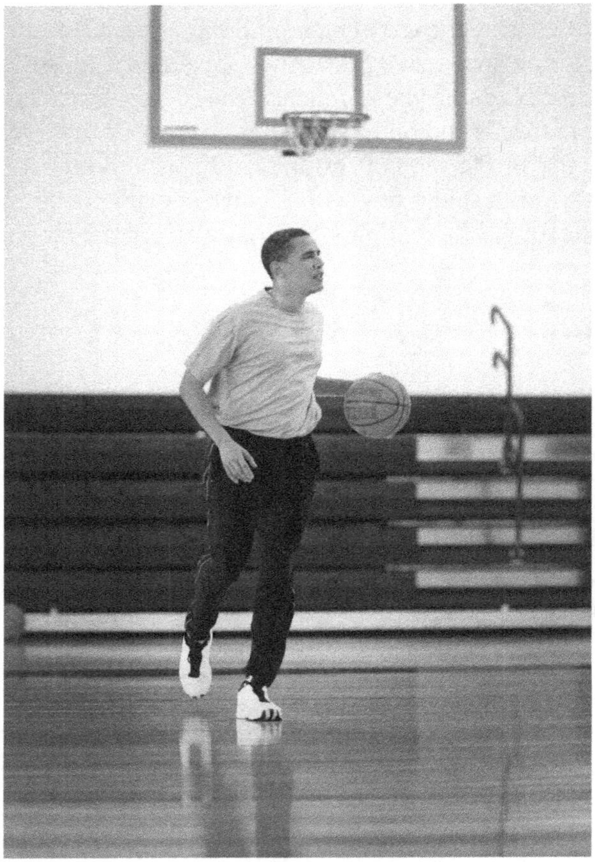

FIGURE 5.2 President Barack Obama playing basketball presents the image of a fit and active leader, connecting him to younger generations

Source: reprinted with permission of Getty Images

Australia. NBC had purchased the rights to televise the 1980 Summer Games in 1974, long before the Afghanistan invasion or subsequent boycott. The $72.3 million in rights that NBC paid, along with all other expenditures made by the network in preparation for the telecasts from Moscow, was lost. No American team meant there would be no American television coverage.

Every international sporting event held before 1994 that excluded the Republic of South Africa can be interpreted as a political statement in opposition to that nation's apartheid policy that separated the races into a hierarchy with whites at the top. That was the year in which South Africa held its first democratic elections open to all races. Following the election of Nelson Mandela as president, teams from South Africa again were welcomed at international competitions.

The Event as a Political Stage

The larger the audience for a sporting event, the more the reward outweighs the risk to use it as a stage upon which to make a political statement. The world was watching on October 16, 1968, when

American sprinters Tommie Smith and John Carlos used the Olympic medal stand in Mexico City to make a controversial statement about racial repression in the United States. In the months leading up to the Olympics, America was in turmoil. Dr. Martin Luther King, Jr. and Robert F. Kennedy had both been assassinated. Riots in American cities had led to recriminations and heightened racial tension. A sociologist at San Jose State University in California, Dr. Harry Edwards, established the Olympic Project for Human Rights and attempted to organize a boycott of the games by African-American athletes.

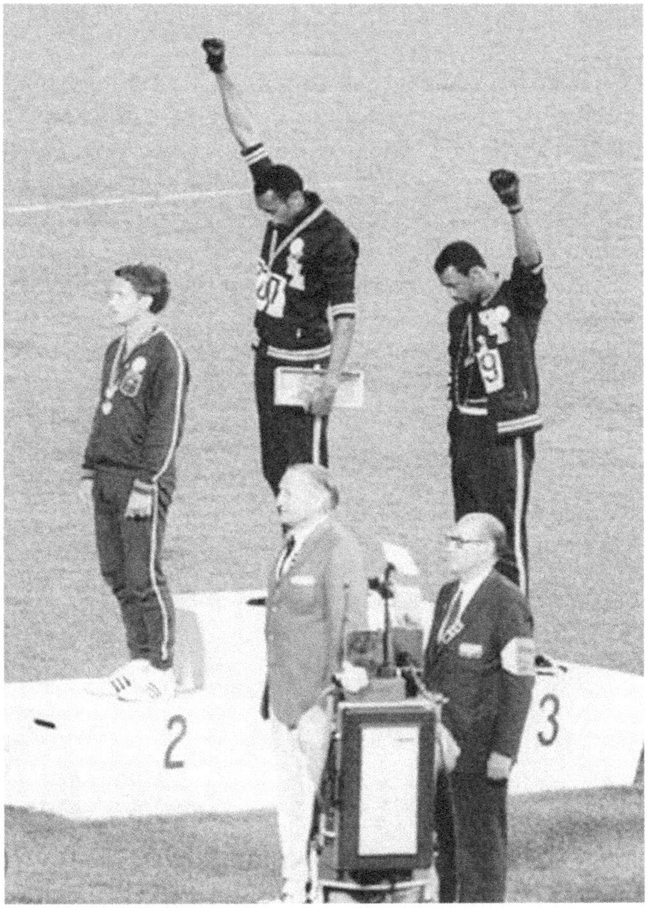

FIGURE 5.3 After Tommie Smith won gold and John Carlos took the bronze in the 200-meter dash at the 1968 Summer Olympics in Mexico City, they raised gloved fists to make a political statement about racial conditions at home in the United States. Australian Peter Norman won the silver. All three men wore badges showing their support for the Olympic Project for Human Rights

The boycott did not occur, but Smith and Carlos felt compelled to make a silent statement in Mexico City to show their solidarity with blacks who they saw as being oppressed back home. Tommie Smith won the 200-meter dash in a then world record 19.83 seconds at the 1968 Summer Games, and John Carlos finished third. Both men had trained at San Jose State.

When they walked into the stadium to receive their medals they shed their shoes to portray the poverty that African-Americans had endured. Smith wore a black scarf and Carlos a beaded necklace that they later explained represented their black pride and memorialized "those individuals that were lynched, or killed, and that no one said a prayer for, that were hung and tarred. It was for those thrown off the side of the boats in the Middle Passage."

When the "Star Spangled Banner" began to play, Americans watching on ABC and a global audience saw Smith and Carlos, with their medals around their necks and Olympic Project for Human Rights badges on their chests, each raise a black-gloved fist. "We are black and we are proud of being black," said Carlos after the demonstration. "Black America will understand what we did tonight." The IOC did not understand, reacting sternly and immediately to what it saw as an inappropriate insertion of domestic political issues into the Games. The IOC chairman was Avery Brundage, who thirty-two years earlier had supported American participation in the Berlin Olympics. "If these boys are serious," he said, "they're making a very bad mistake. If they're not serious and are using the Olympic Games for publicity purposes, we don't like it."

Smith and Carlos were immediately evicted from the Olympic village, sent home, and banned from all future international competition. They each suffered economically and personally for decades for what heavyweight boxing champion Muhammad Ali later called "the most courageous act of the 20th century."

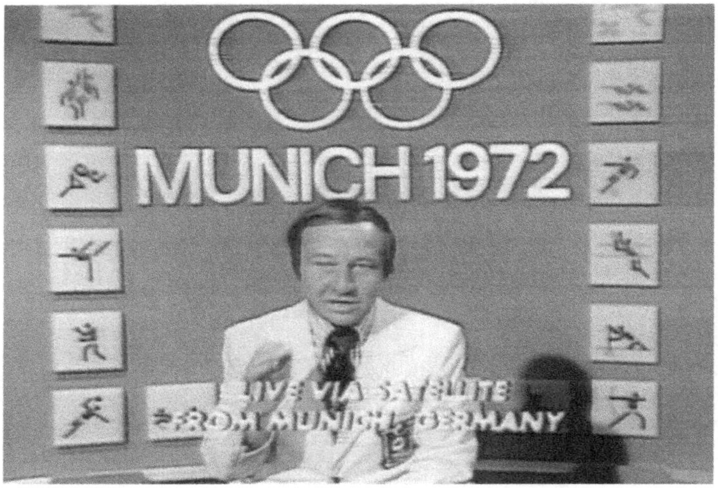

FIGURE 5.4 Jim McKay reported for ABC Sports from the 1972 Summer Olympic Games in Munich and anchored coverage of the terrorist attack that resulted in the deaths of eleven members of the Israeli Olympic delegation

Source: reprinted with permission of Getty Images

A tragic attempt to use the Olympics as a stage for political coercion was at the 1972 Summer Games in Munich. Germany had not hosted an Olympics since the Berlin games in 1936, and its goal was to show how the nation had changed since the end of the Third Reich and World War II. Palestinian terrorists from the "Black September" movement dashed those hopes when they invaded the Olympic village, killed two members of the Israeli team and took nine others hostage. The terrorists demanded the release of 234 Palestinians and other prisoners in Israeli jails as well as freedom for the two German founders of the violent Baader-Meinhof group, Andreas Baader and Ulrike Meinhof.

Americans watched in horrified disbelief as Jim McKay anchored ABC's coverage. When the eighteen-hour standoff ended in a hail of gunfire that left all the hostages dead aboard a helicopter at the Fürstenfeldbruck NATO airbase, they heard him say in utter sadness, "They're gone. They're all gone."

The Munich massacre forever changed international athletic events and their television coverage, pushing the security of participants and spectators to the forefront. The selection of host nations is now viewed through the lens of geopolitics for potential targeting by factions who see an opportunity to put their ideologies and demands on a stage to be seen by a worldwide television audience. And the screening, credentialing, and access for media to venues and athletes were tightened to prevent infiltration by elements that might seek cover for their extremist motives by masquerading as members of the press.

Sports Stars as Political Icons

The athletes we see on television are themselves icons for a broad range of political constituencies. They represent who we are: people who grew up in our city, state, or nation, members of our ethnic, social, or affinity groups as varied as fellow alumni from the college we attended, children who grew up in poor families, who had blue-collar dads, people who have come through divorce or recovered from serious injury, or who volunteer in their hometowns. We celebrate the athletes' superior skill, their determination, stamina, strength, resourcefulness, and fair play, the qualities we value most in ourselves *and* in our elected representatives.

Dozens of athletes have parlayed cheers into votes by convincing constituents that the leadership and positive attributes they demonstrated in their sports careers could be successfully applied to government when coupled with their education and civic interests and/or experience. Some notable examples:

- Bill Bradley—New York Knicks forward, then US Senator from New Jersey for eighteen years.
- Steve Largent—Record-setting NFL receiver, served eight years as Congressman from Oklahoma.
- J.C. Watts—University of Oklahoma quarterback, who also served eight years in Congress representing Oklahoma.
- Jim Bunning—Hall of Fame Major League pitcher who threw no-hitters in both leagues, elected to Congress and then to two terms in the US Senate representing Kentucky.
- Jack Kemp—Buffalo Bills quarterback, and then congressman from Buffalo, secretary of Housing and Urban Development for President Ronald Reagan, and Republican nominee for vice-president in 1992.
- Dave Bing—Basketball Hall of Famer who was an All-American at Syracuse and then a perennial NBA all-star with the Detroit Pistons; he was elected mayor of Detroit in 2009.
- Kevin Johnson—NBA All-Star guard who was elected in 2008 as the first African-American mayor of Sacramento, California, eight years after he had retired from play.

Economics Makes Sports Political

Nothing stirs as much political interest and ire as how elected representatives spend the tax dollars that government collects. Symbolism may get some candidates elected. How they spend the public's money can get them voted out of office. When tax dollars are spent to stage sports events or to build and maintain venues, government and sports organizations become partners. As a result, the actions, decisions, and statements made by each partner take on considerable political weight. These partnerships can be volatile due to the fact that government is subject to the shifting mood of the public come Election Day each year. Officials who support sports partnerships or new stadium building projects can quickly be replaced by combative antagonists who will raise questions about how every public dollar is being spent. Media coverage of such debates merges news with sports, and suddenly the game is not the "only thing."

Recent history is replete with examples. The hundreds of millions of dollars in tax-free financing that was provided for the new Yankee Stadium became a campaign issue in the New York City mayoral election of 2009. The debate over what percentage the public should pay, if any, for the construction of a new football stadium for the Minnesota Vikings was an issue in the 2010 election for governor of Minnesota. The Securities and Exchange Commission (SEC) subpoenaed documents to investigate if any federal securities laws were violated in connection with the public financing of Miami's new retractable-roof baseball stadium built for the Marlins. The overwhelming proportion of publicly financed sports venues, compared with the very few that have been built exclusively with private funds, has turned tax subsidies for sports into a political issue almost everywhere there are professional franchises.

TABLE 5.2 Public Financing of Stadiums and Arenas

NFL	Eleven stadiums built with 100% taxpayer financing: Atlanta, Buffalo, Green Bay, Kansas City, New Orleans, Oakland, San Diego, San Francisco, St. Louis, Tampa Bay, Tennessee
	Three stadiums built with 0% taxpayer financing: Carolina, New England, New York (Meadowlands)
MLB	Seven stadiums built with 100% taxpayer financing: Anaheim, Atlanta, Chicago White Sox, Kansas City, Oakland, Tampa Bay, Washington
	Four stadiums built with 0% public financing: Boston, Chicago Cubs, Florida, Los Angeles Dodgers

Source: National Sports Law Institute Sports Facility Reports

The economics of sports and the extent of its availability to the public on commercial television have also led to government intervention, leaving organizers and leagues with less than the total control they enjoyed in the days before TV. Any action that limits or restricts commerce in the United States is bound to be challenged in court. The billions of dollars that are spent on television rights and advertising each year most certainly qualify sports as "commerce," and as a result the courts have had an impact on what is seen and how it is delivered.

Perhaps no court ruling has had a greater effect on the availability of sports content on American television than the decision handed down by the US Supreme Court in 1984 in a case brought by the Universities of Oklahoma and Georgia, representing the College Football Association (CFA), against the National Collegiate Athletic Association, the NCAA. Beginning in 1951, and continuing through a succession of contracts with NBC, CBS, and ABC, the NCAA had tightly controlled how many college football games would be televised per weekend and per season. The original fear shared by the NCAA and its member universities was that games on TV would diminish the number of fans attending in person. So the first contract limited NBC to a total of twelve Saturday afternoon telecasts during the college football season, and no school could be featured more than once.

The restrictions were loosened over the years as the popularity of college football on television raised the sport's profile and attendance. But, in 1981, the NCAA contract with ABC still limited the appearances of any team to no more than six over the course of two seasons. The newly formed CFA, which represented the Division I schools with major football programs, signed a separate deal with NBC that year which would dramatically increase television exposure, and with it the rights fees, for these universities. In response, the NCAA announced in September of 1981 that it would take disciplinary action against any CFA member that complied with the NBC contract.

That's when Oklahoma, Georgia, and their fellow CFA universities filed a complaint in Federal District Court charging that the NCAA had been violating the Sherman Antitrust Act by placing anti-competitive limitations on how many games could be sold to television networks, and the price that could be charged for that content.

The case went all the way to the US Supreme Court, which ruled in 1984 in favor of the CFA, opening the floodgates to allow the hundreds of games that are now televised each year and for which the universities are compensated at the highest rates the market will bear. In his majority decision Justice John Paul Stevens wrote, "the finding that many more games would be televised in a free market than under the NCAA plan is a compelling demonstration that the plan's controls do not serve any legitimate precompetitive purpose." The judicial branch of government gave more fans more games and made college football a bigger sport with far more revenue than the NCAA on its own may have ever achieved.

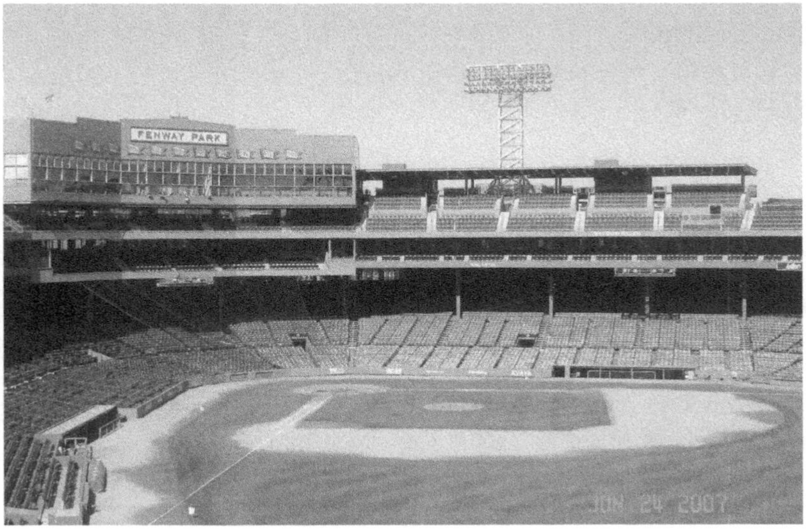

FIGURE 5.5 Fenway Park in Boston, which opened on April 20, 1912, is one of only four current Major League Baseball stadiums that were built with no public financing

The Federal Communications Commission

Before there was sports television there was a Federal Communications Commission (FCC). The agency was established by the Communications Act of 1934 to regulate interstate and international communications in the fifty states, the District of Columbia, and US possessions. At the time, those communications included just radio and telegraph, but with advancements in technology the scope of the FCC's regulation has been broadened to encompass television, satellite, cable, wireless, and broadband.

The airwaves used to transmit broadcast and data signals are a public resource that, just like the air we breathe, cannot be owned by any individual or organization, corporate or otherwise. The spectrum of airwaves has no borders that would allow for local, regional, or state regulation, so it fell to the federal government to make the decisions as to how the airwaves would be used, by whom, and for what purposes. The fact that today there are media that communicate exclusively via fiber optic or coaxial cable, or other devices that do not go "over the air," has not given them license to operate in an unregulated environment.

The areas of FCC oversight that relate most directly to sports television are:

- Media ownership.
- Public access to television programming.
- "Must-carry" and retransmission consent.

Media Ownership

The number of frequencies available for broadcasting is not unlimited, so the FCC early on instituted a licensing application procedure by which it approves the allocation of space on the broadcast spectrum to only those companies or individuals who meet or exceed a set of federal standards. The granting of broadcast licenses is never in perpetuity, but rather they are reviewed every five years, or more frequently if judged necessary by the FCC, to ensure that all standards are being met.

As the regulator of communications for a democratic nation, the FCC has from its beginning included as an important part of its mission a guarantee to the public that no one corporation, no matter how powerful, will ever be able to control all the messages that any American receives via television, satellite, cable, wireless, broadband, or any future medium not yet invented. The FCC's stated goal is to protect the public interest by fostering competition, localism, and diversity. It enforces a set of media ownership rules and restrictions that it reviews and adjusts every four years to ensure that there will be a multitude of "independent voices" accessible to all Americans.

The current rules prohibit any merger among the top-four broadcast networks in the United States: ABC, CBS, NBC, and FOX. There are no limits on the number of television stations that any one company can own; however, collectively no media owner is allowed to control stations that would reach a market universe larger than 39 percent of the total US population. If one entity owns a television station in New York City, Chicago, and Los Angeles, its total market universe is approximately 10 percent of all the TV homes in the United States. It would be allowed to own or buy more stations, but only until its universe as a group hit 39 percent. (The 39 percent figure was a compromise in 2003 when the FCC had approved a change in the ownership limit from 35 percent to 45 percent of the population. Congress voted to keep the limit at 35 percent. A compromise brokered after a threatened veto by then President George W. Bush set 39 percent as the mark.)

The FCC also governs how many television and radio stations any company can control in one designated market area (DMA). Multiple ownership is allowed for up to two TV stations and six radio stations in large DMAs, as long as the FCC can verify that there are at least twenty individually owned "independent voices" in that metropolitan area.

The impact on sports television of these regulations is that there will always be competition for broadcast rights, local teams and events will have equal opportunities for coverage even if they are not owned by or in partnership with a dominant media company, and, when controversies arise, a multitude of reports and opinions can share the airwaves.

Public Access to Television Programming

The FCC "is committed to fostering a strong and independent broadcast media that provides Americans with multiple and diverse sources of news, public affairs and entertainment programming," said FCC Chairman Julius Genachowski in May of 2010 when the latest four-year review of broadcast ownership rules began. Access to television sports is a major part of that "entertainment programming." That's why it is highly unlikely that the Super Bowl will ever move to a cable channel exclusively: anyone who didn't subscribe to a service that distributed that channel would be denied access to the game. That would not be tolerated by either the FCC or the senators and representatives whose constituents live in the small percentage of homes (less than 10 percent) that still get their TV signals over the air.

A succession of public access disputes over sports programming have been brought to the FCC over the past several years, notably a discrimination complaint lodged in 2006 by the NFL Network against Comcast. The NFL claimed that Comcast had unfairly placed its network on a pricey digital sports tier, which had only 2 million subscribers, while sports networks owned by Comcast including Versus and the Golf Channel were made available to more viewers on one of its more popular tier offerings. In October of 2008 the FCC ruled in favor of the NFL, and in May of 2009 Comcast moved NFL Network to the same tier as its owned networks, making it accessible to approximately 10 million homes.

Just a few months later Comcast and its networks were back in the FCC's public access sights when the company announced plans in December of 2009 to acquire controlling interest of NBC Universal from General Electric. The FCC and the Justice Department did grant approval for the takeover in January 2011, but not before clearly stipulating that the combined Comcast NBC Universal had to allow rival cable and broadband distributors reasonable access to each of the programming networks that it owned. That would prevent the conglomerate, if it ever chose to do so, from making any of its networks exclusive to Comcast customers only.

The FCC also put in place conditions requiring Comcast to negotiate fairly with rival programmers, the networks that it does not own, to give them an equal opportunity to deliver their content to Comcast subscribers. The combination of NBC Sports with Versus and the Golf Channel gives Comcast a formidable sports presence and puts the company in a stronger bargaining position when its contracts with ESPN come up for renewal.

The FCC had previously adopted rules that forbade cable companies that own programming channels from refusing to allow competing multi-channel video programming distributors, such as AT&T and Verizon, to offer those channels. Comcast and Cablevision had challenged those rules, but the US Court of Appeals for the District of Columbia Circuit decided the case in the FCC's favor in March of 2010. The result is more public access to more content including sports. Comcast, and all other multi-channel distributors that own regional sports networks, must make their content, including hundreds of live games, available at market prices to services like U-Verse and Fios with which they compete for subscription customers.

Must-Carry and Retransmission Consent

The FCC first adopted "must-carry" rules in 1972 responding to the fears of local television station owners that they would lose audience and advertising dollars if people could get entertainment, news, and sports from a cable running directly into their homes as an alternative to their over-the-air signals. (See Chapter 12 for more on the economic implications of "must-carry" and retransmission regulations.)

Federal courts found the must-carry rules to be a restriction of the First Amendment right of free speech following challenges in the 1980s by several cable operators and by Turner Broadcasting. Congress stepped in and passed the Communications Act of 1992, which still required cable companies to carry local commercial and public stations, but allowed them to drop redundant signals if, for example, there were two college stations within the fifty-mile radius that both carried the same PBS programming. Two years later the FCC gave stations a choice of maintaining their must-carry status with the local cable systems, or be carried under a new regulation that required the cable operator to obtain "retransmission consent." The retransmission consent rules gave strong local network affiliates and independent stations increased power to negotiate their terms of carriage, including channel preference, with the cable company.

Paying for content from broadcasters that had always been free did not sit well with multi-system operators like Cablevision, who in October of 2010 chose to drop FOX from its channel lineup rather than pay the monthly per home fee that the network had demanded. The public relations battle lines in this and in similar disputes are almost always about the sports that viewers would miss if no agreement were reached. In fact 3 million Cablevision homes did miss a New York Giants game and the first two games of the 2010 World Series on FOX because of the dispute. A settlement was agreed to and FOX returned to the Cablevision lineup just before the first pitch of World Series game three.

Issues that affect millions of people inexorably spawn proposed legislative remedies from representatives who are either truly concerned about the services provided to the citizenry, or anxious to win votes from disgruntled constituents, or both. Less than a week after the Cablevision homes in New York, New Jersey, Connecticut, and part of Philadelphia lost FOX in the fall of 2010, Senator John Kerry of Massachusetts sent draft legislation to the FCC chairman that would protect consumers during retransmission consent disputes. If millions more viewers are affected by similar service interruptions in the future, and especially if live sports programming is blacked out, it will surprise no one if this bill or one like it starts to gain momentum on Capitol Hill.

The Congressional Connection

The level of congressional interest and intervention in sports television issues has grown in direct proportion to the industry's growth in audience and income, as would be the case with any expanding sector of the economy. A major milestone was the Sports Broadcasting Act of 1961, which we discussed in Chapter 4. It allowed leagues of individually owned teams in multiple states to act as single entities in negotiating broadcast rights with television networks, without fear of being found in violation of any federal antitrust statutes.

As cable television reached into the majority of American homes in the late 1980s and early 1990s, and live sports coverage began to migrate to ESPN, TBS, and other networks that were not available free over the air, legislation was proposed by a number of representatives on Capitol Hill to limit the "pay-per-view siphoning from free TV." The FCC had adopted rules in 1975 to restrict the programming that cable or subscription TV services could offer as a means of protecting broadcast stations, but these "anti-siphoning" regulations were struck down as invalid, arbitrary, and capricious in 1978 by the US Circuit Court of Appeals in the case of *HBO vs. FCC*.

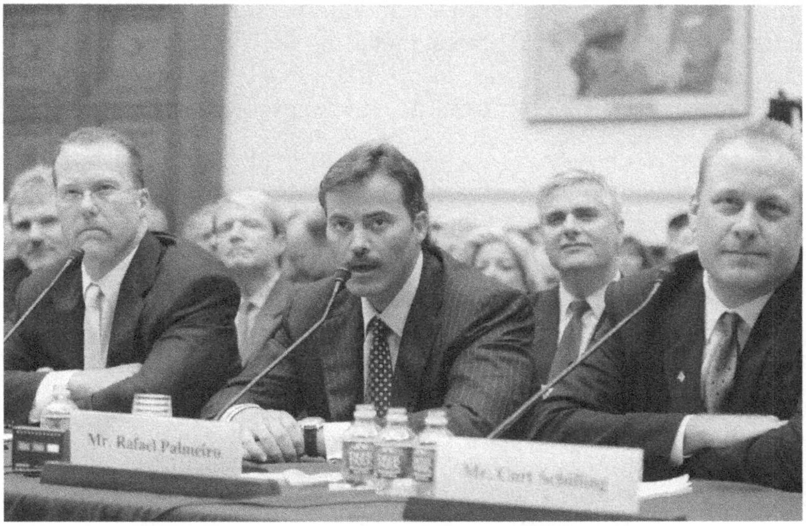

FIGURE 5.6 The House Committee on Oversight and Government Reform heard testimony in 2005 from Major League Baseball players, left to right: Mark McGwire, Rafael Palmeiro, and Curt Schilling

Source: reprinted with permission of Getty Images

That ruling did not however halt the efforts by some representatives to win congressional approval of laws that would impose restrictions on cable sports programming. None succeeded. The cable industry was able to demonstrate that, despite the fact that hundreds of hours of sports were being shown exclusively on cable stations, the volume of sports programming on broadcast networks had increased, not declined.

More people paying more attention to sports, and consuming more of it on television, has had the effect of bringing a far wider range of issues before Congress for discussion if not resolution. At the epicenter of the sports debate in Washington, DC, has been the House Committee on Oversight and Government Reform. In 2005, the committee held hearings on the use of steroids in baseball that included testimony from, among others, former Baltimore Orioles slugger Rafael Palmeiro, who waved his finger in his strident denial, and Mark McGwire, who hit seventy home runs for the St Louis Cardinals in 1998, but famously told the congressmen that he was not there "to talk about the past."

The Committee on Oversight picked up the mantle again in 2008 following the December 2007 release of the Mitchell Report that the commissioner of baseball had commissioned to investigate the illegal use of performance-enhancing substances. The star witnesses were Roger Clemens, who won 354 games in his twenty-four seasons as a Major League pitcher, and his former trainer, Brian McNamee, who claimed that he had administered banned substances to Clemens with the pitcher's knowledge and approval.

Neither of these sets of hearings resulted in the passage of federal legislation to impose governmental jurisdiction over the testing of athletes for any substances, but it is noteworthy that the proceedings were carried live on television and generated national publicity. It is unlikely that television would have paid attention if the House Committee on Oversight and Government Reform had strictly limited itself to its list of legislative responsibilities as set forth in House Rule X, clause 1:

- Federal civil service, including intergovernmental personnel; and the status of officers and employees of the United States, including their compensation, classification, and retirement.
- Municipal affairs of the District of Columbia in general (other than appropriations).
  - Federal paperwork reduction.
  - Government management and accounting measures generally.
  - Holidays and celebrations.
  - Overall economy, efficiency, and management of government operations and activities, including federal procurement.
  - National archives.
  - Population and demography generally, including the Census.
  - Postal service generally, including transportation of the mails.
  - Public information and records.
  - Relationship of the federal government to the states and municipalities.
  - Reorganizations in the executive branch of the government.

The Committee uses as justification for its investigations and involvement that part of its overall charge that calls for it to review and study on a continuing basis "any conditions or circumstances that may indicate the necessity or desirability of enacting new or additional legislation addressing subjects within its jurisdiction (whether or not a bill or resolution has been introduced with respect thereto)."

High-profile sports that attract millions of television viewers, which are played by athletes who compete at the risk of personal injury to themselves and others, who become national celebrities with multi-million dollar contracts and are emulated by young people across the country, in an industry with an annual economic impact in the billions will always come under the scrutiny of government and elected representatives. There could be no other reasonable expectation. Nor is it likely that politicians will miss many opportunities to increase public awareness of issues they deem important to the public welfare, which at the same time increase awareness of themselves.

Summary

The ideal long clung to by the IOC and lifelong sports fans that politics should play no role whatsoever in sport is antiquated and unrealistic. It may have been possible in the era before television when sports were neither a stage nor an economic powerhouse, but not now. The innocence is gone forever, but the symbolism of sport remains in its celebration of athletes as icons representing their nations, regions, racial, ethnic, and affinity groups, and people who share the same personal history.

Sporting events that draw the attention of millions are often used as forums for politics, in the very fact that they are staged in a certain city or country, or that they include or exclude certain competitors. With the guarantee of national or international television coverage, sports is also seen as a political stage from which controversial positions can be espoused, and, in the case of extremists, burned into the public consciousness through acts of terrorism like the Munich Olympics invasion of 1972.

The vast amounts of money involved in sports, television, and the construction of venues naturally invites government oversight and involvement. The leagues and teams that use public funding for a new stadium or arena, or to stage a major event, automatically find themselves as partners with the governmental bodies that oversee the distribution of tax revenue. These partnerships can abruptly change depending upon whether supportive government representatives get re-elected or replaced by opponents of the project at hand.

The FCC exercises authority over the ownership of all electronic media, public access to programming, and the retransmission of television signals by any video distributor. Each of these areas has an impact on how Americans receive their sports on TV, and on the business of sports television.

Congress steps in when issues arise that require a change in the law, or when representatives believe that an investigation or public hearing is necessary to increase national awareness or focus the spotlight on conditions that exist within sports that they want to see changed. Any spillover from the glare of television coverage that might brighten a politician's chances for re-election is a welcomed side-effect.

Discussion Topics/Assignments

1. Research one or more of these Olympic Games and discuss how the events were used as either a political statement or as a stage for political reasons: the 1936 Berlin Games, the 1968 Mexico City Games, or the 1972 Munich Games. How has what happened at these events changed sporting events and their coverage on television?

2. Do a study of the stadiums or arenas where your favorite teams play to determine how they were financed. How has the use of public funding, or the lack of it, affected how the team does business in the community?

3. Study the 1984 US Supreme Court ruling that changed how college football is distributed on television in the United States. Compare the number of games and individual team exposure before the ruling to after.

4. How have different committees such as the House Committee on Oversight and Government Reform or the House Judiciary Committee investigated sports issues? What legislation or changes have resulted?

5. Examine the disputes between cable systems and broadcasters that have resulted in the suspension of service to customers. An example is the Cablevision dispute with FOX in 2010. How has sports been used as a negotiating tool in each dispute?

6

MATTERS OF LIFE AND DEATH

RACISM, PATRIOTISM, AND POLICING IN *ALL AMERICAN BOYS*

Luke Rodesiler

On September 22, 2017 (C-SPAN), the President of the United States publicly disparaged professional football players who, by taking a knee during the playing of the national anthem at games, peacefully protested police violence against people of color. In the weeks and months that followed, athletes kneeling to protest police violence sparked wide-ranging conversations about racism, patriotism, and policing. And such conversations were not limited to the adults in the room. High school students joined the conversation (Armbrester, 2017), as did their elementary counterparts (Strauss, 2018). The phenomenon is one example of sports culture captivating students' interests and providing familiar ground for students to explore sociopolitical issues some might deem beyond their reach in other contexts. The study of select sports-related young adult literature stands to provide additional opportunities for students to examine such issues.

At first glance, sports culture might appear beyond the scope of the middle school language arts classroom. A closer look suggests otherwise. For example, scholars have suggested sports culture as a site of research and inquiry (Wilhelm, 2016), advanced the study of sports figures to understand myth creation (Gahan, 2014), and encouraged the writing of sports-based fiction to build empathy and understanding (Nobis, 2016). Moreover, scholars have recommended using well-crafted sports columns as mentor texts (Gallagher, 2011, p. 64) and documented educators tapping students' knowledge of sports culture to teach writing (Smagorinsky, Johannessen, Kahn, & McCann, 2010, p. 115). In these ways and more, sports culture can support traditional instructional goals in the language arts classroom.

But sports culture can provide avenues for promoting critical literacy practices too. By positioning students to examine how texts advance or disrupt power relations that fuel injustices and inequities, teachers can foster critical literacy (Janks, 2014; Morrell, 2005). Teachers can incorporate in the language arts curriculum a variety of sports-related texts to support such aims. For example, scholars have advocated studying sports-related movies to disrupt racial

Luke Rodesiler, "Matters of Life and Death: Racism, Patriotism, and Policing in All American Boys," *Voices From the Middle*, vol. 26, no. 2, pp. 20-24.

stereotypes (Garland, 2016), described interrogating racist mascots and logos in professional and amateur athletics (Rodesiler & Premont, 2018), and promoted studying sports-related music and film to teach critical media literacy (Fabrizi & Ford, 2014). As these examples indicate, the range of viable sports-related texts for classroom use is wide.

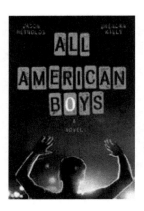

Teachers can also advance critical literacy by facilitating the purposeful and intentional study of sports-related literature. For instance, scholars have encouraged critically examining microaggressions and bullying behaviors in sports-related fiction (Sieben, 2016), suggested exploring how authorship informs meaning and identity in athletes' memoirs (Skardal, 2016), and recommended interrogating sports-related young adult literature through ideological lenses of cultural pluralism and assimilation (Gonzales, 2016). Such approaches give teachers opportunities to engage students in critical conversations at the intersection of sport and society. Among possible conversations, few—if any—are more pressing today than those that critically address racism and policing. For too many people, those conversations are matters of life and death. Fortunately, such conversations can begin with the study of *All American Boys* (Reynolds & Kiely, 2015).

The Novel

Suggested for readers aged 12 to 18 (Kirkus Reviews, 2015), and perhaps best suited for students in eighth grade or beyond, *All American Boys* is narrated by Rashad, a teen artist and ROTC member, and Quinn, a White teen on the school's basketball team. Their worlds collide when Quinn stumbles upon Officer Paul Galluzzo, his father figure, beating Rashad. The officer mistakenly believes Rashad assaulted a woman while stealing from a convenience store. The White policeman's assault of the Black teen in baggy clothing propels this compelling narrative. Rashad must come to terms with inadvertently stirring a growing movement and a clash between his socially conscious brother and his no-nonsense father. Meanwhile, Quinn struggles to make sense of the assault, the privileges he has known, and his complicity in the racism splintering his team and community.

Reframing the Conversation

All American Boys was published in September 2015, almost a year before Colin Kaepernick, former quarterback of the National Football League's San Francisco 49ers, began kneeling during the national anthem to protest police violence against people of color. Still, many read the novel today with their understandings of police violence and athletes' protests framed by the increased attention the president's disparaging words brought to the issue. In many instances, media coverage has presented athletes' protests as "anthem protests." Such phrasing is problematic, for it could be read by casual observers as though athletes are unpatriotically protesting the national anthem. That would be a gross misconception that dismisses the intended target of the protests: police violence against people of color.

To reframe the conversation before beginning the novel, teachers might help students recognize the media's misplaced focus by presenting headlines from various outlets and asking students what they notice about how the protests are represented. Take, for example, the following headlines:

- "Athletes, Activists Spar on Kneeling National Anthem Protests" (Tatum, 2017)
- "Texas Teens Kicked Off Football Team for Anthem Protest" (Miller, 2017)
- "National Anthem Protests Sidelined by Ambiguity" (Branch, 2018)

Teachers can prompt a critical reading of such headlines with questions like the following: Considering these headlines, what seems to be the target of the athletes' protests? What makes you think so? What potential ramifications stem from representing athletes' protests in this way? How might you rewrite the headlines to more accurately represent these protests?

After disrupting how athletes' protests are commonly represented, teachers can reaffirm the focus of the protests by presenting statistics about police violence (e.g., Black people constituted 25 percent of those killed by police in 2017 but just 13 percent of the national population (Mapping Police Violence, 2018)) and/or images of Black men killed by police officers in recent years, such as Philando Castile, Freddie Gray, Samuel DuBose, and so many more. For students who are removed from such harsh realities, reframing the conversation stands to establish the weight of issues raised in *All American Boys*.

Discussing Sociopolitical Issues

Reading *All American Boys* presents ample opportunities for students to discuss urgent sociopolitical issues and ways to improve our world in the face of those challenges. Consider, for example, the following possibilities.

Connections from readwritethink

Books about sports can capture the excitement of the big game, but the best sports books do something more. They depict teens living complex lives where involvement in sports is part of a larger coming of age process. Tune in to hear about works of sports fiction and nonfiction that explore issues of identity and belonging, courage and equal rights, and changes over time in American history and culture.

Lisa Storm Fink
www.ReadWriteThink.org
http://bit.ly/1WiGH43

Police Violence

The first chapter closes with Rashad sharing an unsettling thought as sirens near: "My brain exploded into a million thoughts and only one thought at the same time—please don't kill me" (p. 23). Teachers can help students contextualize events in the novel by offering prompts like the following: Given recent history across the United States, why might Rashad find himself pleading for his life in this circumstance? How, if at all, do you see factors such as race, sex, gender, and culture contributing to the events that culminated in Officer Galluzzo assaulting Rashad?

Racism

Talking with his friend Jill, Quinn declares, "I'm not racist!" In response, Jill describes forms racism can take: "Not like KKK racist. I don't think most people think they're racist. But every time something like this happens, you could, like you said, say, 'Not my problem.' You could say, 'It's a one-time thing.' *Every time* it happened." Jill eventually concludes, "I think it's all racism" (p. 184). With questions like the following, teachers might prompt students to consider the range of racism Jill described: What forms does racism take in the novel? In our daily lives? What actions might we take to combat the discreet and overt racism Jill described?

Athletes as Activists

Eventually, Coach Carney mandates that basketball players not attend any protests, lumping activism in with partying as distractions players must avoid (p. 224). Recalling that specific passage, teachers might invite students to weigh athletes' roles in the fight for social justice by posing questions like the following: Should athletes—amateurs like Quinn or professionals like Colin Kaepernick—concern themselves with activism? Why or why not? At this point in the novel, how might Quinn answer that question?

Protests and Patriotism

During the protest, Quinn explains: " ... I wondered if anybody thought what we were doing was unpatriotic. It was weird. Thinking that the protest was somehow un-American. That was bullshit. This was very American, goddamn *All-American*" (p. 294). To help students make connections between Quinn's words and real-world criticisms lobbed at protesting athletes, teachers can facilitate discussion with prompts like this: The president has condemned athletes who protest, contending that they disrespect our country by kneeling during the national anthem, yet Quinn argues that protesting is "very American." What makes protesting a patriotic act? Whose position—Quinn's or the president's—do you align with? Why?

These passages and prompts offer just a sampling of the opportunities for important discussions available as students read *All American Boys* before further exploring and promoting social justice.

Exploring and Promoting Social Justice

After students have read and discussed *All American Boys*, teachers can invite them to explore further the amalgam of sociopolitical issues and sports culture. Post-reading activities might include the following, each of which culminates in students sharing final products with audiences beyond the teacher.

Conducting and Publishing Inquiry Projects

Inquiry projects are often marked by students' extended focus on a meaningful issue they chose to investigate with a small group of classmates (Daniels & Zemelman, 2014, p. 260). To extend the exploration of issues related to *All American Boys*, relevant inquiry projects could involve the following:

- Researching incidents of police violence (i.e., locally, regionally, or nationally)
- Interrogating media representations of athletes who, like Quinn, have protested police violence against people of color (e.g., Colin Kaepernick, Eric Reid, Michael Bennett)
- Studying judicial rulings about students' right to protest
- Investigating local reactions to athletes protesting police violence
- Examining other historical sports-related protests (e.g., the Black 14, the Black Power salute at the 1968 Olympics, the 1980 Olympics boycott)
- Exploring the lives of athletes who embraced activism throughout history (e.g., Billie Jean King; Brendon Ayanbadejo; Muhammad Ali).

Once projects are complete, students can go public with the outcomes of their inquiries to promote social justice. This might include students publishing findings on a class website or blog; posting findings in the classroom or a high-traffic area within the school; presenting findings for an audience of their peers; or disseminating their research through classroom publication.

Drawing and Publishing Political Cartoons

In the novel, Rashad describes his friend Carlos's graffiti masterworks, and Carlos puts those art skills to use by spreading the tag "RASHAD IS ABSENT AGAIN TODAY" on their school sidewalk, a unifying statement against police violence (p. 197). Encouraging tagging tends to be frowned upon, but teachers can help students appreciate using art to promote social justice. And sharing the power of political cartoons is a logical start.

Following a gallery walk to examine how cartoonists have commented on police violence, actions athletes have taken in protest, and the president's response, teachers can provide lessons to support students in designing, drawing, and publishing original political cartoons. For instance, teachers might present mentor texts (Figures 1 and 2) to help students discern and consider the unique tools cartoonists use to craft social commentaries, including symbols, labels, and exaggerated elements. After crafting original political cartoons that address issues related to *All American Boys*, students could publish their social commentaries in a class anthology, post them online, or plaster them around the classroom, school, or greater community. Inviting students to share their cartoons positions them to project their voices and contribute to advancing social justice.

Conclusion

As Rashad and Quinn discovered in *All American Boys*, justice and understanding do not flourish in silence. Rather, they require open dialogue and the raising of voices willing to speak truth to power. Instead of discouraging students from talking about racism and police violence, as Coach Carney and other adults in Quinn's life did, teachers can create opportunities for students to engage critically with texts that address such grave matters. In the language arts classroom, teachers can incorporate thought-provoking texts, including those from sports culture, to begin critical discussions and inspire among students the courage shown by protestors—real and fictional, athletes or otherwise—who oppose racism, police violence, and other abuses of power.

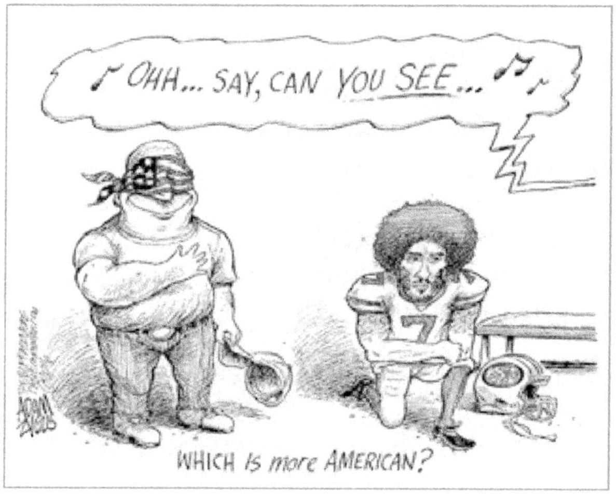

FIGURE 6.1 Political cartoon addressing athletes' protests of police violence

Darkow, J. (2016, September 21). *Why Kaepernick kneels.* [Cartoon]. Retrieved from https://www.cagle.com/john-darkow/2016/09/why-kaepernick-kneels

Davies, M. (2016, August 31). *America's not great.* [Cartoon]. Retrieved from http://www.gocomics.com/mattdavies/2016/08/31

Hall, E. (2017, August 31). *Rights.* [Cartoon]. Retrieved from http://editorialcartoonists.com/cartoon/display.cfm/153821

Margulies, J. (2016, September 5). *Colin Kaepernick.* [Cartoon]. Retrieved from https://www.cagle.com/jimmy-margulies/2016/09/colin-kaepernick-2

Necessary, K. (2017, September 25). *Taking a stand by kneeling.* [Cartoon]. Retrieved from https://www.wcpo.com/news/cartoons/editorial-cartoon-taking-a-stand-by-kneeling

Priggee, M. (2017, October 16). *Protest.* [Cartoon]. Retrieved from http://globegazette.com

Sheneman, D. (2016, September 21). *That's offensive!* [Cartoon]. Retrieved from http://www.gocomics.com/drewsheneman/2016/09/21

Zyglis, A. (2016, September 6). *Which is more American?* [Cartoon]. Retrieved from http://thecontributor.com/graphics/which-more-american

FIGURE 6.2 Suggested mentor texts for a study of political cartoons

References

Armbrester, S. (2017, December 1). I am a cheerleader, and here's why I take a knee. *National Public Radio*. Retrieved from https://www.npr.org/2017/12/01/567845804/i-am-a-cheerleader-heres-why-i-take-a-knee

Branch, J. (2018, January 1). National anthem protests sidelined by ambiguity. *The New York Times*. Retrieved from https://www.nytimes.com/2018/01/01/sports/nfl-national-anthem-protests.html

C-SPAN. President Trump remarks at Senator Strange campaign rally. 44:42–47:48 Retrieved from https://www.c-span.org/video/?434480-1/president-trump-campaigns-alabama-senator-luther-strange&start=2729

Daniels, H., & Zemelman, S. (2014). *Subjects matter: Exceeding standards through powerful content-area reading* (2nd ed.). Portsmouth, NH: Heinemann.

Fabrizi, M. A., & Ford, R. D. (2014). Sports stories and critical media literacy. *English Journal*, *104*(1), 42–47.

Gahan, C. M. (2014). The highlight with a thousand faces: Sports and our yearning for hero and myth. *English Journal*, *104*(1), 37–41.

Gallagher, K. (2011). *Write like this: Teaching real-world writing through modeling and mentor texts*. Portland, ME: Stenhouse.

Garland, K. (2016). Exploring racial stereotypes through sports-related film. In A. Brown & L. Rodesiler (Eds.), *Developing contemporary literacies through sports: A guide for the English classroom* (pp. 167–172). Urbana, IL: National Council of Teachers of English.

Gonzales, K. (2016). Beneath the surface: Ideologies of multicultural sports literature. In A. Brown & L. Rodesiler (Eds.), *Developing contemporary literacies through sports: A guide for the English classroom* (pp. 11–16). Urbana, IL: National Council of Teachers of English.

Janks, H. (2014). Critical literacy's ongoing importance for education. *Journal of Adolescent & Adult Literacy*, *57*(5), 349–356.

Kirkus Reviews. (2015, August 1). [Review of the book *All American boys*, by Jason Reynolds and Brendan Kiely]. Retrieved from https://www.kirkusreviews.com/book-reviews/jason-reynolds/all-american-boys

Mapping Police Violence. (2018). Retrieved from https://mapping policeviolence.org

Miller, J. R. (2017, October 2). Texas teens kicked off football team for anthem protest. *New York Post*. Retrieved from https://nypost.com/2017/10/02/texas-teens-kicked-off-football-team-for-anthem-protest

Morrell, E. (2005). Critical English education. *English Education*, *37*(4), 312–321.

Nobis, M. (2016). Writing sports fiction to build empathy and understanding. In A. Brown & L. Rodesiler (Eds.), *Developing contemporary literacies through sports: A guide for the English classroom* (pp. 67–72). Urbana, IL: National Council of Teachers of English.

Reynolds, J., & Kiely, B. (2015). *All American boys*. New York, NY: Caitlyn Dlouhy/Atheneum.

Rodesiler, L., & Premont, D. (2018). On second thought: Teaching for social justice through sports culture. *English Journal*, *107*(6), 82–88.

Serwer, A. (2017, September 23). Trump's war of words with Black athletes. *The Atlantic*. Retrieved from https://www.theatlantic.com/politics/archive/2017/09/trump-urges-nfl-owners-to-fire-players-who-protest/540897

Sieben, N. (2016). Teaching writing hope for a just society. *The English Record*, *67*(1), 99–121.

Skardal, R. (2016). Power, authorship, and identity in texts by and about high-profile athletes. In A. Brown & L. Rodesiler (Eds.), *Developing contemporary literacies through sports: A guide for the English classroom* (pp. 55–59). Urbana, IL: National Council of Teachers of English.

Smagorinsky, P., Johannessen, L. R., Kahn, E. A., & McCann, T. M. (2010). *The dynamics of writing instruction: A structured process approach for middle and high school*. Portsmouth, NH: Heinemann.

Strauss, V. (2018, January 26). Students write about NFL anthem protests: "Just because we are fourth graders doesn't mean we don't think about serious things." *The Washington Post.* Retrieved from https://www.washingtonpost.com

Tatum, S. (2017, September 28). Athletes, activists spar on kneeling National Anthem protests. *CNN.* Retrieved from http://www.cnn.com

Wilhelm, J. (2016). Inquiring minds learn to research, read, and write. In A. Brown & L. Rodesiler (Eds.), *Developing contemporary literacies through sports: A guide for the English classroom* (pp. 98–100). Urbana, IL: National Council of Teachers of English.

FURTHER READING

Things We'd Change in Sports: It's Time to Stop Playing the National Anthem at Sporting Events

Nancy Armour

If you have a digital edition of this book, please click on the link below to access the article:

https://www.usatoday.com/story/sports/columnist/nancy-armour/2019/03/14/national-anthem-star-spangled-banner-sports/2979056002/

If you have a print edition of this book, please use your cell phone to scan the QR code below to access the article:

Veterans Speak Out Against the Militarization of Sports

Howard Bryant

If you have a digital edition of this book, please click on the link below to access the article:

https://www.wbur.org/onlyagame/2018/07/20/military-sports-astore-francona

If you have a print edition of this book, please use your cell phone to scan the QR code below to access the article:

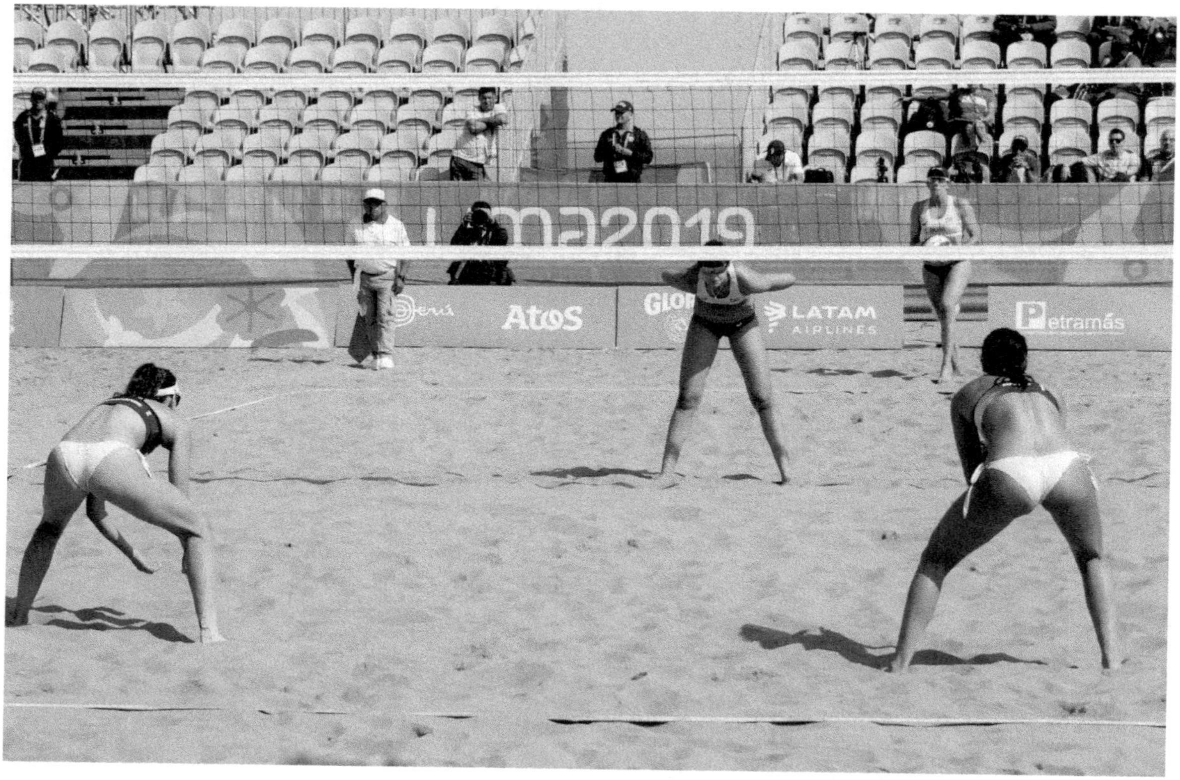
Atos
LATAM
AIRLINES
Petramás

CHAPTER 4
MEDIA AND SPORT

The sports media reproduces the on-field and off-field activities that an audience finally sees. I experienced this at the 2019 Pan American Games in Lima, Peru. I brought a United States flag to the Greco-Roman wrestling competition. When I returned home, I watched the events I attended. In every US broadcast I could be spotted on the screen. You did not have to strain to find me; I was always a full-screen image with the announcer continuously pointing out fans from the United States. However, in reality, I only spotted one other set of US fans at the wrestling competition, and they were the parents of a wrestler. The reproduction of the live event was manipulated to suggest heavy support for Team USA. When we watch live sports, there are dozens of cameras that the producer switches between. The producer identifies particular images that align with the current social, cultural, or political trends in sport at the time and then narrates the story that the audience receives. **Reproduction of sports** by the media attempts to tell the story that is the most exciting, controversial, or focuses on highly emotive topics prevalent in sport at that time. Moreover, the media is drawn to injuries and accidents, like the example in the QR code Further Reading section of this chapter: "Here's why we need to stop watching video of Auburn gymnast Samantha Cerio's injury." When critically examining sports media, look closely at the following questions. Why do the producers identify certain people on and off the field during a televised sporting event? What happens when the sports media is dominated by one ethnic/racial group? Or, as has been the case for nearly all of the twentieth century and much of the twenty-first century, what happens when the dominant group of media producers and sports writers are men? You can replace "men" with "Christian," heterosexual," or "former athletes" and see that there might be a specific motivation behind the reproduction of sports in the media. Media narratives about women in sport have been distorted for decades and focused on **non-sport issues** like their personal lives, **appropriate femininity** and sexuality when discussing their identity as a mother rather than an athlete, and the **sexualization** of women in sport as seen in the introductory image of this chapter. Sports media and broadcast have long focused on trivializing women in sport rather than celebrating athleticism.

The increase in social media has led to increased tension with social issues in sport because anyone can broadcast an opinion. While social media can be dangerous because of cyberbullying, false narratives, and disparaging comments, many athletes have commented that they prefer their Twitter and Instagram accounts over the sports media. They believe they can take some of the power away from media institutions and sportswriters; they have control of what they want fans and followers to know. They also have the opportunity to address or correct a negative story about them or a false narrative spread through social media.

7

THE SOCIAL AND CULTURAL IMPACT OF TELEVISED SPORT

Dennis Deninger

> The media is a primary site for the construction and constitution of identities, collective and individual, rather than merely a secondary reflection of already formed identities.
>
> (Ben Carrington, Ph.D., University of Texas Dept. of Sociology)

TABLE 7.1 The Rundown

- The impact of sports on personal identity.
  - What we wear.
  - What we consume.
  - What we do.
  - What we say.
- The passion for sports drives behavior.
- The portrayal of women in TV sports.
- "The Battle of the Sexes."
- Women sportscasters.
- The impact of television sports on racial attitudes.
- Minorities assume leadership positions.
- The black quarterback.
- Muhammad Ali.
- The race and gender report card.
- Althea Gibson and the impact of TV coverage.

In the same way that sports is part of the identity of nations it is also integral to how millions of Americans define themselves. Consider the people you know, or simply look in the mirror, to see the evidence of how the mass distribution of sports in the United States and around the world has affected what people wear, the food and drink we consume, the words and phrases we use in daily speech, how we spend our leisure time, and our attitudes about race and gender.

The Impact of Sports on Personal Identity

What We Wear

It is difficult for most people alive today to remember a time when sports apparel and footwear were worn only by athletes and did not constitute such a large percentage of an average person's wardrobe or closet. Look back at photographs or film of sporting events from the 1940s, 50s, or 60s and take a close look at the crowds. In the summer they wore shirts and blouses, many men with ties and felt hats, and in the winter you see overcoats and jackets. But you don't see the proliferation of team jerseys and caps proudly proclaiming one's team loyalty that fill the stands at games in the 21st century. The transition from fans who dressed like average people to fans who dressed like their favorite athletes, or in the colors of their favorite teams, is concurrent with the expansion of sports on television in the years since 1970.

Michael Jordan's role in the growth of Nike presents an excellent example of how sports on television and the marketing of sports celebrities has changed how Americans identify themselves through their choice of clothing. In fiscal 1984, the year that Nike signed an endorsement deal with Jordan as he was leaving the University of North Carolina, the company had total revenues of $919,806,000. Jordan led the NBA in scoring in his first season with the Chicago Bulls and again in the 1986–87 season. Nike sales went over the $1 billion mark for the first time in 1986, and another crucial milestone came in 1987. That's when ESPN's cable penetration exceeded 50 percent of American homes, putting Michael Jordan's amazing highlights in front of a growing national audience every night on *SportsCenter*. Jordan won the first of his five NBA Most Valuable Player (MVP) awards at the conclusion of the 1987–88 season just as Nike introduced its "Just Do It" advertising campaign. The company's sales hit $1.7 billion in fiscal 1989, an increase of more than 70 percent in the five years following their signing of Michael Jordan.

By 2003, the year in which he played his last NBA game, then as a member of the Washington Wizards, Nike's annual revenue had reached $10.7 billion, which translates to millions of Americans wearing Nike sneakers and athletic gear, "just doing it" dressed like their favorite professional athlete. If the NBA's exposure on television had remained limited to one or two games per weekend on the broadcast networks, and video from every Bulls game was not being featured on a nightly basis, it is safe to conclude that Jordan's impact on consumer behavior and on Nike's sales would have been geometrically smaller.

What We Consume

The impact that Michael Jordan had on behavior went beyond what Americans put on their feet and on their backs, to what they put in their stomachs. Gatorade signed Michael Jordan as its brand spokesman in 1991 and launched its "Be Like Mike" advertising campaign. He led the Bulls to their first NBA Championship that season, winning awards as the NBA regular season and finals MVP, and Gatorade sales increased faster than the rest of the soft-drink industry. The product got plenty of television air time with its bright orange coolers and green cups visible on the sidelines at basketball and football games. Gatorade was what the viewing public saw the best athletes use to keep themselves hydrated, so it became a more popular choice among active young people and adults who had the same kind of thirst that could be satisfied with a beverage offering the same beneficial effects.

The pattern repeats itself over and over with products from energy bars to golf clubs and baseball caps. Each of us makes a social statement about ourselves through the products we use and wear, and for millions the decision to buy those products is made as a way to emulate the star athletes we see on television.

What We Do

Gatorade became part of how Americans in communities large and small celebrate championships at all levels of sport as the result of what they saw after New York Giants games in the 1985 and 1986 seasons. During the week of practice leading up to a nationally televised New York Giants vs. Washington Redskins game on October 20, 1985, New York Giants coach Bill Parcells had been riding his nose tackle Jim Burt, telling him that his opponent on the Redskins line, Jeff Bostic, was going to "eat him up" on Sunday. Burt was infuriated and when the Giants won 17–3, he took his revenge with a cooler full of Gatorade. "I was the only one who had the guts to do it without knowing what his reaction was going to be," Burt told Darren Rovell for his book about the Gatorade brand, *First in Thirst.*

Jim Burt and teammate Harry Carson continued the Gatorade showers the following season, turning them into a ritual after every Giants victory. That season New York went 14–2 in the regular season and won the NFC title for a trip to the Rose Bowl in Pasadena for Super Bowl XXI. With a huge national audience watching, Parcells got doused again as the Giants beat the Denver Broncos 39–20, and, with zero marketing effort on the part of Gatorade, the tradition of American victory celebrations was changed forever.

A footnote to the story is that one year before Jim Burt soaked Bill Parcells, Chicago Bears coach Mike Ditka was actually the recipient of the NFL's first Gatorade shower. On November 25, 1984, after the Bears beat the Vikings 34–3 in Minnesota, linemen Steve McMichael and Dan Hampton were the culprits. But they didn't repeat the prank, and it didn't happen in front of a massive Super Bowl audience.

The sports that Americans watch on television directly affect the pursuits we choose for our leisure hours when the set is turned off. From an early age, the events and stars that children see on television can influence the decisions they make about what sports they will pursue, which in countless instances are decisions that will change the course of their lives. One need only check the enrollment figures for local gymnastics schools after each Summer Olympics is televised to prove this hypothesis. And participation in a sport as a child is one of the primary factors determining fan allegiances as adults.

TABLE 7.2 US high school sports participation, 2010–11

Boys' Sports	Participants	Girls' Sports	Participants
1. Football (eleven-man)	1,108,441	1. Track & field	535,672
2. Track & field (indoor + outdoor)	649,591	2. Basketball	438,933
3. Basketball	545,844	3. Volleyball	409,332
4. Baseball	471,025	4. Softball (Fast Pitch and Slow Pitch combined)	400,974
5. Soccer	398,351	5. Soccer	361,556
6. Wrestling	273,732	6. Cross-country	204,653
7. Cross-country	246,948	7. Tennis	182,074
8. Tennis	161,367	8. Swimming & diving	160,881
9. Golf	156,866	9. Competitive spirit	96,718
10. Swimming & diving	133,900	10. Lacrosse	74,927

Source: National Federation of High School Associations 2010–11 High School Athletics Participation Survey

The hours each week that more than 30 million fantasy sports players spend drafting and trading players, managing their teams and doing research on the internet, is time they would spend doing something else if it weren't for sports on television. It is possible to play fantasy exclusively online using statistics, analysis, and projections, but scouting players and tracking their performances in live games is a large part of the appeal. Research done for the Fantasy Sports Trade Association (FSTA) projects that 19 percent of American males and 8 percent of females over the age of twelve play at least one fantasy sport. Fantasy football is the runaway favorite with over 60 percent of all players owning at least one team. Fantasy baseball is a distant second with just under 20 percent participation. The FSTA research done by Ipsos Public Affairs includes demographic profiles showing that fantasy players are more likely to be college educated than not, and are also more likely to be employed full-time than the general public.

What We Say

If you did not watch sports on television, would you speak a different language? To answer that question think about how often you use words or phrases from sports as metaphors or short-hand to make your listener quickly understand your point. The English language is filled with "sports-speak," which is nothing new. In *Romeo and Juliet*, Shakespeare wrote this line for Juliet when she was contemplating suicide: "A bloody knife shall play the umpire." It may not be new, but its prevalence and acceptance into common discourse are largely attributable to what is said on television.

What has also become all too common across the country is trash talking. In professional leagues, talking "trash" is a means toward sharpening the competitive edge over an adult opponent by finding and exploiting a sore spot or sensitivity. But it has been mimicked by children who watch TV and know how being cruel to others can reduce rivals to tears, which in turn may offer a better chance for victory. Incidents such as the October 2008 pee-wee football game in Pittsburgh's Mon River League, where parents had to pull the teams off the field because of fears that the trash-talking would lead to something dangerous, became so prevalent that many youth sports associations now include "no trash talking" clauses in their player/parent and coaches codes of ethics.

TABLE 7.3 "Sports speak" How many of these expressions do you use in conversation?

1. Touch base with.	15. "Three strikes" law.	30. Slam dunk.
2. Monday morning quarterback.	16. Strike out.	31. Take your best shot.
	17. Pass the baton.	32. Drop the ball.
3. Screwball.	18. Touch and go.	33. Time out.
4. Out in left field.	19. Hit full stride.	34. Kick off.
5. Step up to the plate.	20. Put on a full press.	35. Throw a curveball.
6. Get to first base.	21. Heavy hitters.	36. Hail Mary.
7. Reach the goal line.	22. One on one.	37. Punt.
8. Heading for home.	23. Sticky wicket.	38. Jump the gun.
9. Double play.	24. Beat to the punch.	39. Go for the gold.
10. "Pinch hit for me."	25. The home stretch.	40. Make a pit stop.
11. "Go to bat" for me.	26. Game on!	41. Behind the eight-ball.
12. Up to par.	27. Batting 1.000.	42. Down for the count.
13. Extra innings.	28. Knock it out of the park.	43. Hit it out of the park.
14. Overtime.	29. Knockout blow.	44. "She's out of your league."

The Passion for Sports Drives Behavior

Perhaps nothing defines an individual better than his or her passions, the independent choices one makes in life. Octagon, the world's largest sponsorship consulting firm, started conducting studies in 2005 to better understand what drives different people to be passionate about different sports in ten different countries around the globe. Octagon's researchers, led by senior vice president for insights and strategy, Simon Wardle, who created the Passion Drivers® concept, interviewed thousands of sports fans and identified twelve separate factors that explain why people love sports. Almost all have sociological implications as they describe patterns of human behavior.

Octagon's Passion Drivers research, which went to version 3.0 in 2011, is sold to advertising, marketing, and media clients. Here is an overview of the motivating factors with none of Octagon's proprietary statistical analysis as to which are more or less important in any specific country or for any particular sport.

- *Active appreciation*—this is based on personal participation in the sport of which you are now a fan. You played the game in the backyard, with friends, or participate at any recreational or competitive level.
- *Love of the game*—you have loved the sport since childhood, more than likely attending or watching on television with a parent or siblings as you grew up.
- *Team devotion*—loyalty to your college team, to your regional favorite, or simply to a team for which you developed an obsession. Television has made it possible for these loyalties and obsessions to develop regardless of geography, such as the little boy in Connecticut who grows up loving the Cincinnati Bengals because he fixated on the team's orange and black tiger-striped helmets when he was three years old.
- *Player affinity*—fans draw human connections with, or identify with, players. A generation of baseball fans grew up in the 1950s and '60s idolizing Mickey Mantle and Willie Mays. In the 1980s and '90s Michael Jordan assumed the "affinity throne," but the player with whom

a fan makes a connection need not be famous. Your choice of heroes can help explain who you are.

- *Talk and socializing*—sports fosters social interaction within peer groups and across generations and across gender and ethnic bounds. It creates conversation and connects the fan with friends and strangers alike.
- *All consuming*—a special event like March Madness or an annual event like the Super Bowl draws fans in because of its overwhelming social and media presence, regardless of whether they follow the sport during its regular season. One gets swept up in the tide of excitement and emotion that surrounds the game.
- *Nostalgia*—history and personal memories of bygone teams or players can be powerful motivators. Looking back fondly to connect special memories to the present works to keep the love of that sport alive for a lifetime.
- *Player excitement*—there are certain players in sport whose talent, ability, or superior performance command admiration. *SportsCenter* highlights of emphatic dunks, improbable catches or runbacks, amazing shots from tennis courts or golf courses can fuel this player excitement.
- *Gloating*—there are those who enjoy reveling in the agony of others, who need to feel superior. Think of the heated competitions among fantasy football players, or gamblers who have to announce their winnings (read: superior skill and judgment) to all their Facebook friends or co-workers.
- *Personal indulgence*—for their personal entertainment many fans are willing to make sacrifices, because the time they set aside to watch their favorite sport or the resources they commit to buying that season ticket is the one special thing they do for themselves. This may include some overt selfishness, but the indulgence is part of what defines who these individuals are in life.
- *Sense of belonging*—it's important for many fans to identify themselves as "part of the tribe," like "Red Sox Nation." There is a comfort in gathering with other like-minded individuals at games or in front of the television. It provides a social sense of connection: dressing, talking, and thinking like other tribe members helps people figure out how they fit into their social structure.
- *TV/media preference*—some fans make their choices based on consumption preferences. If they have established a connection or a bond with ESPN, or NBC, or any network or website as a credible source with congenial or entertaining talent, they may choose to watch more games or consume more video product from these media "friends."

Everyone's personality is shaped to some degree by the passions, sports-related or not, which are developed over a lifetime. Television coverage of sports plays a role in all of the motivational forces listed above with the only exception possibly being "active appreciation," and clearly the choices made by young people as to which sport to play are very often influenced by the games or athletes they see on TV at an early age.

The Portrayal of Women in TV Sports

Televised sport has played an important role in changing the dominant ideas about gender in American society. Our cultural understanding of femininity has been radically altered by images of women with athletic skill, muscles, and endurance. In the America of the mid-20th century the individual sports that required grace, glamour, and self-sacrifice such as figure skating, tennis, golf, or gymnastics were seen as most suitable for women. Sports that demanded strength, stamina, and speed, any team sport involving contact and any sport such as auto racing that came with a degree of risk, were traditionally the domain of males only.

The version of basketball that was designed specifically for women one year after Dr. James Naismith published his original rules of the game in 1891 divided the court into three sections to limit the amount of running and exertion required of female players. In 1938 the three sections were reduced to two, with six players per team. Three players per team were restricted to each half of the court so that only three of the six ever got the chance to score a basket. The other three were full-time defenders at the opposite end of the floor. Girls were only allowed three dribbles per possession and "no snatching or batting the ball away from a player" was permitted. Basketball for women was meant to be a form of exercise that promoted socialization and cooperation, not strenuous competition. Full-court, five-on-five women's basketball was not officially sanctioned until 1971, but six-on-six basketball was widely played until 1993 at high schools in a few Midwestern states, most notably Iowa.

Women had experimented with and adapted most every sport by the end of the 20th century. The competition that they relished, coupled with the strength and endurance they built, represented a form of female empowerment to a society that for generations had accepted male domination as the natural order. To many men and women alike the changes were a threat to their pre-conceived notions of the ideal woman and mother. A female athlete with muscles did not fit what had been the cultural template, and neither did a woman who dared challenge a man on the field of play.

One of the true pioneers of gender equity did just that in 1973, and because of Billie Jean King barriers began to fall and previously unimagined opportunities began to open for women in sports. Her tennis match against former Wimbledon champion Bobby Riggs was called "the Battle of the Sexes," and it aired live from the Houston Astrodome in prime time on ABC television on September 23, 1973.

Riggs had won Wimbledon in 1939, but by 1973 he was a 55-year-old hustler hoping to get publicity and make a few bucks challenging the women professional tennis players of the era. He goaded them with "male chauvinist pig" rhetoric about how a woman's place was in the home "barefoot and pregnant" and how no woman athlete could beat a skilled man regardless of his age. Riggs' favorite T-shirt bore the acronym "WORMS" for a fictitious "World Organization for the Retention of Male Supremacy." Margaret Court took the bait and played Riggs on Mother's Day, 1973. The Australian star was twenty-five years younger than her opponent and had won seventeen grand slam singles titles, including all four majors in 1970, but she lost 6–2, 6–1 to Riggs in just fifty-seven minutes in a match in San Diego that aired on CBS.

Billie Jean King had resisted Riggs' taunts, but when she learned that Margaret Court had lost she resolved to play him so that her campaign for equal prize money for women players on the tennis tour would not be jeopardized for years to come. She was twenty-nine and had won the Wimbledon singles and doubles titles in 1973. In her career, Billie Jean King won a total of thirty-nine grand slam singles and doubles tournaments, but no victory would have a more momentous impact than "the Battle of the Sexes."

She arrived at the Astrodome court on a gold litter carried by four muscular men dressed as Roman slaves. Riggs, wearing a satin "Sugar Daddy" jacket for his hastily signed candy sponsor, was wheeled out to the court on a rickshaw pulled by sexily attired models he called "Bobby's Bosom Buddies." Howard Cosell, ABC's provocative commentator from *Monday Night Football* and virtually every Muhammad Ali boxing match, added his dramatic observations to heighten the sense of theater.

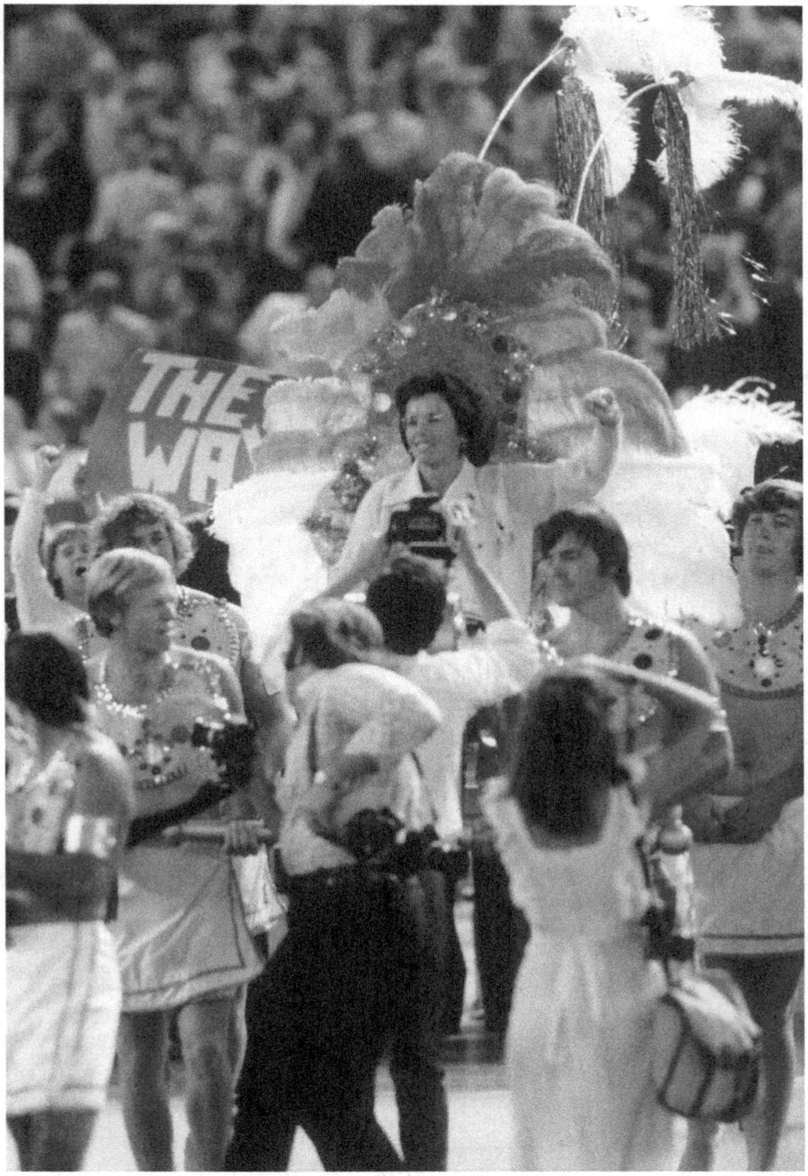

FIGURE 7.1 "The Battle of the Sexes" tennis match in 1973 was a media spectacle. Billie Jean King's victory over Bobby Riggs had a lasting impact on the image of women in American sport and society

Source: reprinted with permission of Getty Images

Before a worldwide television audience estimated at 50 million, Billie Jean King out-hustled Bobby Riggs, winning 6–4, 6–3, 6–3, and in so doing "she convinced skeptics that a female athlete can survive pressure-filled situations and that men are as susceptible to nerves as women," wrote Neil Amdur of the *New York Times*. Martina Navratilova later said of King, "She was a crusader fighting a battle for all of us. She was carrying the flag; it was all right to be a jock." *Life* Magazine named Billie Jean King one of the "100 Most Important Americans of the 20th Century." She was the only female athlete on the list.

Billie Jean King helped change how young women thought about themselves and how men thought about women. The role of sportscaster, which had been monopolized by men, was also beginning to change. Donna de Varona had been seen nationally reporting on *ABC's Wide World of Sports* and the network's Olympic telecasts, but, when Phyllis George debuted in 1975 as the co-host of *The NFL Today* on CBS alongside Brent Musburger and Irv Cross, the male-only domination of major team sports commentary in the United States started to crumble.

Phyllis George had toured the country as Miss America 1971, and she had impressed media executives with her personality, poise, and intelligence during her television guest appearances. She brought far more than a pretty face to the interviews, feature stories, and on-set reports that she did on CBS. Phyllis George added character and depth to story lines, often getting athletes to open up and show their personal side because of her comfortable humanity. Girls who loved sports but who were never going to achieve the international athletic success of Billie Jean King now had role models in George and de Varona, who via their visibility on television served as trailblazers in the process of redefining women in American culture.

The Impact of Television Sports on Racial Attitudes

When the dramatic series *I Spy* premiered on NBC in the fall of 1965, Bill Cosby became the first African-American to have a starring role in a weekly television program in the United States. Up to that point the only minority stars that Americans saw on TV with any regularity were professional athletes such as Willie Mays of the San Francisco Giants, Bill Russell of the Boston Celtics, or heavyweight boxing champion Muhammad Ali. Their representation in the media helped the process of broadening and improving the understanding of diversity and race in this country.

Americans who grew up in the 1950s, as television penetration was exploding from less than 10 percent of homes at the beginning of the decade to nearly nine out of ten homes by 1960, came of age recognizing that people of different races played for the same teams. In 1946 the unwritten color ban in the NFL was broken when the Cleveland Rams moved to Los Angeles, and, as part of their lease agreement for the publicly owned Los Angeles Coliseum, agreed to add UCLA stars Kenny Washington and Woody Strode to their roster. The following year Jackie Robinson broke Major League Baseball's color barrier that had excluded players of color since 1889. The NBA's first black players made their debuts in 1950: Earl Lloyd for the Washington Capitols followed by Chuck Cooper of the Celtics and Nat Clifton of the New York Knicks. Their presence by no means implied that professional sports was a space devoid of racial discrimination, but it did begin to build a sense among those who saw them play in person and on television that players from diverse backgrounds would be selected based on merit and that their contributions to team success were valuable. The fan bases for teams and sports expanded to include more minorities in the decades since these pioneers made their mark. These increasingly diverse crowds and television audiences collectively cheering for victories and championships have helped bring people of all colors together.

Minorities Assume Leadership Positions

The opportunities for minorities in the major sports however were limited for years to the role of "performer." The presence of African-Americans or Hispanics on the playing field and their absence from any leadership positions such as coach, manager, captain, or quarterback reinforced a racial hierarchy that always put whites in charge. At its core, racism is about domination, one group exerting its control over others. As long as the leadership positions were "whites-only," sport in America was not a true meritocracy and therefore retained the vestiges of racism. This hierarchy was reaffirmed every time a television camera showed a quarterback calling signals or cut to the sidelines or dugout to show the managers and coaches, all of whom were white.

The athletic skill of minority players in the NFL had become inarguably evident in the years since the integration of the league began in 1946, but there was a perception among many white fans in America that they did not possess the combination of intellect and leadership required to be a quarterback. In 1953, the Chicago Bears had just two African-Americans on their roster; one was a rookie from Michigan State named Willie Thrower. On October 18, 1953, he entered the Bears' game against the San Francisco 49ers in relief of starter George Blanda. He threw eight passes, completing three before Blanda returned. Willie Thrower was the first black quarterback to play in the NFL since the league's color barrier fell, but his name is largely forgotten because those eight passes were the only ones he was ever allowed to throw in his career.

The first black quarterback to start a game in professional football was Marlin Briscoe, who took the first snap for the Denver Broncos in the fourth game of the 1968 season vs. the Cincinnati Bengals. He faltered in the first half and was replaced by Steve Tensi. The first African-American to start a season at quarterback for an NFL team was Joe Gilliam, Jr., who led the Pittsburgh Steelers for the first six games of the 1974 season. He too struggled and was replaced as the starter in game seven that year by Terry Bradshaw, who went on to win four Super Bowls with the Steelers and was elected to the Football Hall of Fame. The stumbles made by these early pioneers gave those who still believed in the old racial hierarchy what they saw as justification for their prejudice. The process of burying forever the myth that blacks couldn't succeed at quarterback gained momentum when Doug Williams quarterbacked the Washington Redskins to victory and was named the MVP of Super Bowl XXII before a television audience of millions in January of 1988.

The responsibilities and decision-making skills required to lead a team on the field are not insignificant, but they pale in comparison to those of a coach or manager. Bill Russell was the cornerstone for the Boston Celtics during their run of nine NBA championships in the ten years from 1956–66. He was named the team's player-coach for the 1966–67 season, succeeding the legendary Red Auerbach who was retiring. Russell thus became the first African-American to coach a team in any of the major American sports. He served as player-coach for three years and stepped aside after having led the Celtics to eleven NBA titles in his thirteen seasons. Russell was named the NBA's MVP five times and is a member of the Naismith Basketball Hall of Fame.

Major League Baseball's first black manager was perennial all-star Frank Robinson, who took the helm with the Cleveland Indians in 1974, just as his Hall of Fame playing career was coming to an end. The first minority head coach in the NFL was Hispanic. Tom Flores was promoted from assistant coach to head coach of the Oakland Raiders in 1979, and he proceeded to lead the silver and black to championships in Super Bowls XV and XVIII. When Flores retired in 1988 he was succeeded by Art Shell, making Shell the league's first African-American head coach.

As diversity spread from the player level to management, the identity of minorities in sport and throughout society underwent a reconstruction as America watched on television. A milestone came quietly in early 2007 when the coaches of the two teams in Super Bowl XLI were both African-American: Tony Dungy of the Indianapolis Colts and Lovie Smith of the Chicago Bears. These two men at the pinnacle of their sport were the leaders of men from many different ethnic backgrounds. They were the bosses. And at the conclusion of that 2006 regular season, 60 years after the NFL had begun to integrate, Dungy and Smith would be judged by the overwhelming majority of fans based on the quality of their work and their won-lost records, not the color of their skin.

Changing Perceptions

No one in the history of sport since the advent of television challenged racism more boldly than Muhammad Ali. Born Cassius Clay in Louisville, Kentucky, he won a gold medal as the Olympic light heavyweight champion at the Rome games in 1960. He was eighteen years old. At twenty-two he won the world heavyweight championship by knocking out Sonny Liston and announced to the world that he "must be the greatest." Shortly after the fight Ali made another announcement: that he had joined the Nation of Islam and was changing his name, first to Cassius X, then to Muhammad Ali. "I know where I'm going," he said, "and I know the truth and I don't have to be what you want me to be. I'm free to be what I want."

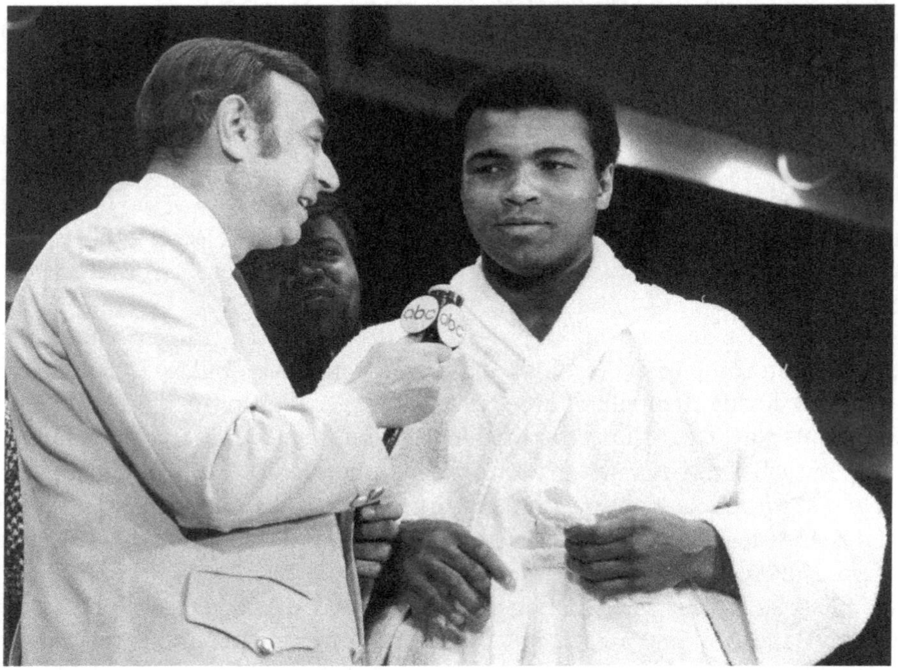

FIGURE 7.2 Muhammad Ali in one of his many interviews with Howard Cosell of ABC Sports

Source: reprinted with permission of Getty Images

Ali was stripped of his title in 1967 after he refused induction into the military on the grounds that he was a conscientious objector whose religion forbade taking up arms against others. Ali won his case against the US Justice Department three years later when the US Supreme Court found in his favor, but those were three years in which he had been unable to pursue his livelihood and compete in the ring. He regained his world title in 1974 by defeating then-champion George Foreman in "the Rumble in the Jungle" in Kinshasa, Zaire, which is now known as the Democratic Republic of the Congo. Ali would retire from boxing in 1981 having won the heavyweight championship three separate times.

Muhammad Ali's arrival on the sports scene was a watershed event. His impact on the sports media was immense because he was never afraid to speak, he looked confidently into the camera, he was controversial and quotable, never subservient. Ali dashed any semblance of racial hierarchy. He held his own and traded barbs over the course of several interviews with ABC's Howard Cosell, a man who had many more years of education than Ali, but no greater command of the language or understanding of the world around him. Muhammad Ali would not be dominated; his words and actions transmitted into homes across the country and around the world shook those who had complacently perpetuated the two-tier society that put whites on the top and everyone else beneath.

If sport is indeed going to completely shed the inequities of the past, there is still catching up to be done. Calling the plays on the field and calling the shots from the sideline or bench are one beachhead. Calling the games on television is quite another. The representation of minorities in the announce booth and the studio lags far behind their numbers on the field or court. Every year the University of Central Florida's Institute for Diversity and Ethics in Sports does a "race and gender report card" for each of the major sports in the US. The 2011 survey showed that, while 78 percent of the players in the NBA were African-American, only 17 percent of the radio and television talent covering the games were black. Seventy-two percent of NBA broadcasters that year were white. There was an even greater discrepancy in the NFL where 67 percent of the players but only 8 percent of the radio and television commentators and reporters were African-American. Seventy-nine percent of all broadcasters covering the NFL at the local and national level were white in 2011.

The argument is not that in order to achieve racial equity the ratio of minority broadcasters to players in any sport needs to be one-to-one. A case could in fact be made for the desirability of a one-to-one ethnic ratio not between players and sportscasters, but instead between the make-up of each sport's fan base and the sportscasters who serve those fans. Using that premise, if 79 percent of all NFL fans were white, then the same percentage of white NFL broadcasters would be equitable. What the argument is about is the end of racial discrimination and the accurate portrayal of minorities and women as equal partners in society, capable of achievement to the fullest extent of their talents and deserving of the opportunity to reach their goals.

One final point that demonstrates the power of television in molding our perceptions of sports reality: if you were to ask any group of adults, "Who was the first African-American to win a grand slam tennis title?" the answer you would undoubtedly hear most often is "Arthur Ashe." Ashe, a member of the International Tennis Hall of Fame, won the US Open in 1968 and the Wimbledon men's singles title in 1975. Both events were televised nationally. The first African-American to win a grand slam was actually Althea Gibson, the Wimbledon and US Open women's singles champion in both 1957 and 1958, but those tournaments were not on television. Althea Gibson was a pioneer, a remarkable athlete who, when her tennis playing days were over, became the first African-American to join the Ladies Professional Golf Association, and she too is a Hall of Famer. But her achievements made less of a lasting impact because what she did was not seen on TV.

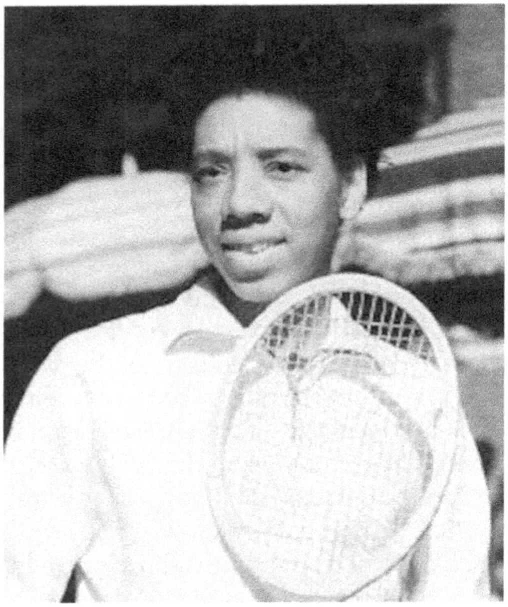

FIGURE 7.3 Althea Gibson was the first African-American to win a major tennis title. She was the Wimbledon and US Open women's singles champion in 1957 and 1958

Source: courtesy Notable Biographies

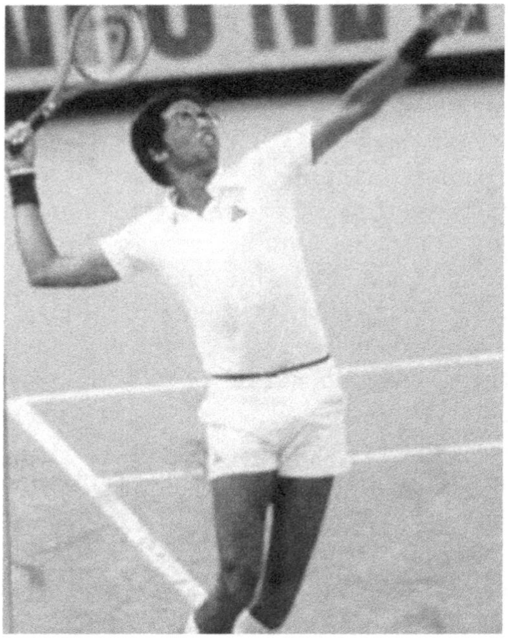

FIGURE 7.4 Arthur Ashe won the US Open men's singles in 1968, eleven years after Althea Gibson's first grand slam championship. But Ashe's victory had far greater impact because it was televised nationwide and Gibson's was not

Source: courtesy Hickok Sports

Summary

The passion for sports and its proliferation on television affect millions of people's personal decisions and preferences as to how they spend their time, the products they consume, the words and phrases they use, how they perceive themselves, and how they perceive and interact with others. Sports television has helped American society change by providing a platform upon which racial hierarchies and gender stereotypes could be challenged and overthrown, where personal initiative, skill, and determination could overcome every obstacle, even racial discrimination. The recognition that people of color were deserving of and capable of success in sports leadership positions, and their ascension to those jobs in increasing numbers, has been a major step forward in the drive for racial equity that began with the integration of player rosters in the 1940s and 1950s.

This is not to say that sport has become race-neutral or that racism and stereotyping don't still exist, or that work does not still need to be done to reach equitable participation at all levels. In fact the representation of African-Americans in the professional basketball and football games seen on television has created a false stereotype among minority youth who perceive sports as providing a vast potential for their personal upward mobility, when in fact the number of jobs as a "pro athlete" is infinitesimal compared with the work force as a whole.

Media coverage of sports has helped Americans understand the issues of race and gender, allowing them to construct collective and individual identities that reflect the growth of diversity and the higher standards for performance and competition that are its direct result. Television magnifies reality and at its best exposes inequities in sport, thus accelerating social and cultural change.

Discussion Topics/Assignments

1. Do a self-assessment. How has your perception of the opposite gender and of races other than your own been influenced by the sports you see on television?

2. Research how the color barriers were broken in any of the sports you play or follow. Who took the initiative? What was the effect on the players, the team, and/or league in the first year of integration? What role did the media play?

3. Select a female pioneer from a traditionally male sport and write a profile that includes the obstacles and stereotypes she had to overcome, what level of support she received from the public and from within her sport, and the impact she made for other women who followed. Example: Janet Guthrie, who was the first woman ever to drive in the Indianapolis 500.

4. Do a tally of every member of a minority group who has ever served as head coach or manager in any of the major sports leagues. What trends can you identify? Has there been steady growth? Any reversals? Which sport has hired the fewest minority team leaders?

5. Find videos online of Muhammad Ali from the 1960s and 1970s. Compare his demeanor with that of other African-American celebrity athletes of the era. Discuss how Ali forced Americans to perceive blacks differently. How effective do you think his interviews with Howard Cosell were in changing perceptions of race?

6. Compare the careers of Althea Gibson and Arthur Ashe. How did Gibson open doors for Ashe? How did winning his first major title on television increase the impact that Ashe had in sport and society in the years afterward?

Bibliography

Fantasy Sports Trade Association. "Fantasy Sports Participation Sets All-Time Record, Grows Past 32 Million Players," press release, June 10, 2011.

Rovell, Darren. *First in Thirst: How Gatorade Turned the Science of Sweat into a Cultural Phenomenon*, AMACOM Books, 2006.

8

THE EFFECT OF SOCIAL MEDIA ON THE 2012 LONDON OLYMPICS

Andy Miah

Social Media as Generators of News

Outside of the new configuration of journalists' roles and relationships, there is also evidence of how content generated for social media exposes gaps within our media culture, particularly around the generation of news. The Olympic Games have demonstrated this at moments when a concern about the professional media has gained attention through its proliferation within social media. For example, on the night of the opening ceremony of the 2012 London Games, the hashtag #NBCfail began to trend on Twitter as a result of criticisms of NBC's live television coverage, a narrative that continued throughout the Olympic and Paralympic Games (Carter 2012). The criticism was focused on the lack of live coverage, the failure to broadcast aspects of the ceremony, and the interruption of content by commercials. In response to this, the British journalist Guy Adams tweeted the email address of the president of NBC Olympics and invited people to send their complaints directly to him. As a result, Adams was temporarily suspended from Twitter for breaching its guidelines, which provoked further debate about whether this person's email was private or not and whether Twitter should be involved in policing such incidents at all. Yet the more interesting point here is that it shows how original news stories are generated within social-media platforms and how a Twitter hashtag can quickly become an influential force within the news agenda. The #NBCfail period is a good indication of how user-generated content can shape the news agenda and of how what happens in social media has come to influence the creation of news. Yet there must be some strategic value in NBC's approach, as the same story was repeated in 2016 at Rio, where it was criticized for the volume of commercials in the Olympic Games Opening Ceremony.

Bibliography

Carter, Chelsea J. 2012. "Viewers Outraged after NBC Cuts Away from Olympics Closing Ceremony." http://www.cnn.com/2012/08/13/sport/olympics-nbc-fail/

FURTHER READING

Here's Why We Need to Stop Watching Video of Auburn Gymnast Samantha Cerio's Injury

Bill Goodykoontz

If you have a digital edition of this book, please click on the link below to access the article:

https://www.azcentral.com/story/entertainment/media/2019/04/12/why-we-shouldnt-share-video-auburn-gymnast-samantha-cerios-injury/3448200002/

If you have a print edition of this book, please use your cell phone to scan the QR code below to access the article:

Caroline Gleich Fights Back Against Cyber Harassment

Kate Siber

If you have a digital edition of this book, please click on the link below to access the article:

https://www.outsideonline.com/2247211/caroline-gleich-fights-back-against-cyber-harassment

If you have a print edition of this book, please use your cell phone to scan the QR code below to access the article:

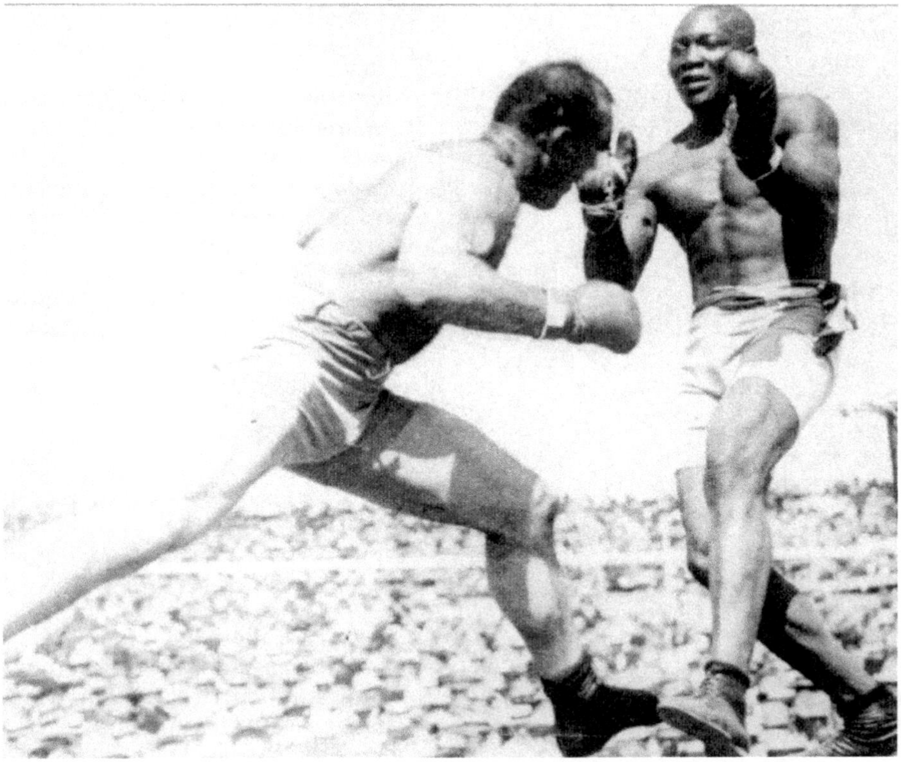

CHAPTER 5

RACE AND RACISM IN SPORT AND SOCIETY

Three nights after the opening ceremony of the 2016 Olympic Games, the awards ceremony at the women's gymnastics team final became a social media topic of concern. The team from the United States won the gold medal, and Gabby Douglas, an African American female team member, inadvertently disrupted this nationalistic discourse. Douglas, a 2012 Olympic gold medalist, helped the team to a second consecutive team gold medal. During the medal ceremony, Douglas stood with her teammates, sang along to the national anthem, but with her hands at her side. Immediately, social media posts unleashed an avalanche of criticism that the athlete was dishonoring the Stars and Stripes. August 9, 2016, was the second anniversary of the death of Michael Brown, shot and killed by a Ferguson, Missouri, police officer. Brown's death and multiple other deaths of unarmed black men by white police officers was the impetus behind the **Black Lives Matter** movement. As Douglas stood on the podium of the medal ceremony, social media bullies began to speculate her motivation behind not placing her hand on her heart. Anonymous strangers on Twitter like @ReallyRick of Nashville, Tennessee, posted, "Just because you didn't make the all-around finals doesn't mean you have to be a disrespectful ***** Gabby Douglas!" Numerous posts criticized the twenty-year-old African American athlete's attitude, her lack of excitement while watching teammates perform, and her hair. Read more about this in the QR code "Further Reading" section of this chapter: "Rio 2016: Gabby Douglas's Olympic Experience Fits the Pattern of How We Treat Black Female Athletes."

Was all of the animosity from critics stemming from Douglas not placing her hand over her heart? Not exactly. One week later, US track and field shot putters Ryan Crouser and Joe Kovacs won the gold and silver medals, respectively. During their medal ceremony, neither athlete placed his hand over his heart. Social media lacked any condemnation of these two athletes and their "refusal" to honor the national anthem. **White privilege**, and possibly being a man in the world of sport, protected them from ridicule, leaving the dominant audience to believe there must have been some acceptable reason for their inaction. White privilege is often unrecognizable because the person on the receiving end goes through their daily activities without disruption. For a person of color, disruptions occur when questioned how they got involved in a sport like swimming, which has mostly white athletes in the United States. This disruption to their daily life may occur when scrutinized by security while walking through a high-end department store. And for Douglas, it occurred when she failed to put her hand over her heart, similar to Crouser and Kovacs. Systemic racism that exists in many social institutions led to the condemnation of Douglas through cyberbullying and exposed a privilege that existed on the medal stand for white athletes.

Following the conclusion of the Olympic Games in August 2016, sports fans turned their attention to the National Football League. Awaiting them was Colin Kaepernick, who had decided that racial injustice in the United States needed more attention. In a symbolic move, Kaepernick refused to stand up for the national anthem. His purpose was to bring attention to the racial injustice that befalls African Americans, specifically for police disproportionately targeting African Americans, and the racial profiling that led to the death of these victims. Other black athletes followed Kaepernick's lead. Three University of Nebraska football players protested racial injustice in the United States by kneeling during the anthem before a September 24, 2016, football game against Northwestern University in Evanston, Illinois. Senior linebacker Michael Rose-Ivey, DaiShon Neal, and Mohamed Barry peacefully protested antiblack violence by taking a knee. Their actions ignited a firestorm of racist comments and death threats by University of Nebraska fans and a member of the university Board of Regents. Rose-Ivey publicly addressed the fans on September 20, 2016, with an impassioned statement about his experience following that game. He concluded with remarks about the Nebraska community and their threats: "Another [fan] believed that since we didn't stand for the Anthem that we should be hung before the Anthem for the next game. These are actual statements we received from fans."[1]

Rather than address the racist comments made by students and fans, and instead of acknowledging the death threats these young men received, one of the first questions Board of Regents member Hal Daub asked was if these were "scholarship" athletes. This line of questioning demonstrates his belief that he has the power to remove them from the team for not following the dominant sports ideological script associated with the national anthem. When powerful men in sport or society overlook racism in the name of 100 percent Americanism, they give credibility to hateful speech and help people rationalize **racism** and **discrimination** while simultaneously ignoring greater society's criticism of their hate speech. The argument for 100 percent Americanism was an argument that generated support for Jim Jeffries, a white boxer, over Jack Johnson, a black boxer; both featured in the image. Jeffries had a nickname, "the Great White Hope," because white society in the United States needed him to reclaim the World Championship Boxing title from Johnson. On July 4, 1910, Johnson defeated Jeffries, and race riots broke out across the country. Chapter 5 examines the social problem of racism in sport and society.

Figure Credit

Fig. 5.1: Source: https://commons.wikimedia.org/wiki/File:Jeffries_Johnson.jpg.

1 Andrew Joseph, "Nebraska Regent Wants Football Players Kicked Off the Team for Anthem Protests," *USA Today*, September 27, 2016, http://ftw.usatoday.com/2016/09/nebraska-regent-football-anthem-protest-michael-rose-ivey

9

INTRODUCTION TO "BEFORE JACKIE ROBINSON:

THE TRANSCENDENT ROLE OF BLACK SPORTING PIONEERS"

Gerald R. Gems

Introduction

Before Jackie Robinson is a cooperative effort to recover a significant part of the past. It attempts to fill a significant hole in the literature of our American history. Why does that matter? Our personal histories make us who we are as individuals, and our collective histories provide us with a national identity as Americans. One of the characteristics of American culture that differentiates it from so many others in the world is the influence of race in American history. The genre of "new biography" that has emerged in the twenty-first century places greater emphasis on "the socially contested nature of identity constructions, so that it treats biography as acts of identity politics in the social struggles of a time," a method that allows "social groups to reach an understanding about who they are and who they want to be."[1] This volume makes a distinct attempt to incorporate the factors of race and race politics over a transitional period in American history that eventually transformed the nature of American society and American history.

The choice of subjects provides a sense of chronological change and the incremental transition in race relations in American culture over approximately a half century. Sports provided a very visible means of that process. While many Americans might be familiar with Jack Johnson, Joe Louis, and Jesse Owens, all of whom operated on an international stage, we chose to examine the lives of no less important athletic pioneers, once well known but increasingly forgotten, who pushed the social boundaries on other levels in their quest to dismantle racism.

Slavery commenced with some of the earliest colonial settlers in 1619 and held a central role in the American economy and society for the next 250 years. The Civil War, which pitted Americans

1 Volker Depcat, "The Challenges of Biography: European-American Reflections," *Bulletin of the German Historical Institute* 55 (Fall 2014): 39–48 (quote, 46–47).

and even families against one another, is attributed to the enslavement of African Americans. It cost more than six hundred thousand American lives, the greatest disaster in the history of the nation.

With the end of the Civil War and the reorganization of the defeated Confederate states, a period known as Reconstruction, the undertaking offered hope and promise to the newly liberated slaves. That optimistic expectation proved illusory and temporary. When the presidential election of 1876 resulted in a stalemate, the two political parties reached an agreement that gave the presidency to the Republican candidate, Rutherford B. Hayes, but allowed the Democrats to resume their previous control of the southern states. Restrictive suffrage qualifications, complete disenfranchisement, Jim Crow segregation laws, and the sharecropping system quickly returned blacks to a state of peonage, reinforced by widespread lynchings, the ramifications of which still beset the American society today.

A former slave, Booker T. Washington, founded the Tuskegee Institute in Alabama in 1881; it taught vocational skills and provided black teachers for the segregated schools. Rather than social equality Washington preached the acquisition of skills for the workplace. His accommodationist and non-threatening philosophy won him support from white leaders and recognition as the top black spokesperson of the late nineteenth century. Under such guidance athletes found some limited opportunity in the dominant white culture—but not equality. Blacks faced continual denigration and stereotyping and were often depicted as cartoonish minstrels or Sambo figures in the white media, incapable of full inclusion in the white mainstream society.

Jockeys such as Isaac Murphy, Willie Sims, and Jimmy Winkfield won numerous Kentucky Derby races from 1884 to 1902 and earned considerable sums for their skills, but they were only the employees of wealthy owners who garnered the larger prizes and national acclaim. The black jockeys also suffered the resentment of their white competitors. The jockeys, however, fared better than other athletes. Moses Fleetwood Walker reached the zenith of professional baseball as a catcher for the Toledo team in the American Association in 1884, but white opponents refused to participate in games against him, causing the management to release him and relegating him to the minor leagues thereafter. The white crusade to oust black players from the top echelons of professional baseball continued relentlessly for the remainder of the century. In the South, blacks were completely segregated from interracial competitions in team sports by custom and by law. Any who violated the southern social norms risked beatings, incarceration, and lynching. In the northern states some black football players won recognition for their abilities as individuals who contributed to team success, but they regularly faced the ire of white opponents who sought to injure them. Still William Henry Lewis won All-American honors at Harvard in 1892 and 1893 and eventually rose to the position of assistant U.S. attorney general in Boston, where a local barber had refused to cut his hair.[2] Such black achievements and successes were virtually excluded from presentation at the 1893 World's Fair in Chicago, dubbed the "White City" by the media.[3]

Lewis's ascendance represented a black invasion of the white power structure, but his talents overcame prejudice. Other northern blacks began to test white assumptions of superiority in other forms of sport. Like in horse racing, blacks were expected to serve wealthier golfers as caddies in an employer-employee relationship. When John Shippen, who had learned to play golf as a caddie for whites, entered the sacrosanct U.S. Open in 1896, the other entrants arranged a boycott. Only the courageous efforts of U. S. Golf Association (USGA) president Theodore Havemeyer, who supported

2 Gerald R. Gems, Linda J. Borish, and Gertrud Pfister, *Sports in American History: From Colonization to Globalization* (Champaign IL: Human Kinetics, 2008), 144, 207, 211; Gerald R. Gems, *For Pride, Profit, and Patriarchy: Football and the Incorporation of American Cultural Values* (Lanham MD: Scarecrow Press, 2000), 114.

3 See Ida B. Wells, "The Reasons Why the Colored American Is Not in the Columbian World Exposition," in *Black Writing from Chicago: In the World, Not of It?*, ed. Richard R. Guzman (Carbondale: Southern Illinois University Press, 2006), 20–28.

Shippen, saved the tournament. Shippen represented a challenge to the white concept of the self-made man, presumably reserved for white males. A loss to a nonwhite could damage the perception of white racial superiority, a basic tenet of the racist society that upheld white privilege. Shippen continued to challenge white hegemony, entering the tournament repeatedly in 1899, 1900, 1902, and 1913. The USGA would eventually adopt a whites-only policy. Such exclusionary tactics resulted in black golfers forming their own parallel organization, and Shippen became a golf instructor, eventually employed at Shady Rest Golf and Country Club, a black enterprise established in Scotch Plains, New Jersey, in 1921. He had made a formidable statement in the quest for equality but had little to show for it, dying in poverty and largely forgotten at the age of eighty-nine in 1968.[4]

Cyclist Major Taylor personified another such provocation as his abilities clearly surpassed that of his white opponents as he set numerous world records in head to head competition and won the world championship by 1899. His success fostered the animosity of white cyclists and their collusion to hinder his efforts forced him to seek his fortune abroad, where he earned as much as $10,000 annually. Such physical prowess offered one means of social mobility when other avenues were denied.[5]

Such head-to-head individual competitions challenged the dominant Social Darwinian beliefs in white superiority. Boxers had already confronted that awareness by the late nineteenth century. White perceptions of blacks as physically inferior, weak-willed, cowardly, lacking in toughness and personal discipline, and unable to withstand a stomach punch enabled black fighters to enter the professional ring. White audiences expected to see and enjoyed watching black boxers being pummeled by white opponents. White men organized "battle royals" in which black youth were thrown in a ring, sometimes blindfolded, to fight until the last one standing was awarded with cheers or coins. At the professional level John L. Sullivan, who held the heavyweight championship from 1882 to 1892, instituted a ban on black challengers to ensure that the symbolic title of physical supremacy remained in white hands.

In 1891 Peter Jackson, the top black heavyweight of the era, fought Jim Corbett to a draw after sixty rounds, negating the belief in blacks' limited endurance. The next year Corbett defeated John L. Sullivan to gain the championship, but he never gave Jackson a rematch. On the same program in which Corbett defeated Sullivan, known as the Carnival of Champions, George Dixon thoroughly thrashed Jack Skelly, a white fighter, to claim the featherweight championship. A day after the mauling an editorial appeared in the *New Orleans Times-Democrat* that objected to the interracial bout: "We of the South who know the fallacy and danger of this doctrine of race equality, who are opposed to placing the negro [*sic*] on any terms of equality, who have insisted on a separation of the races in church, hotel, car, saloon and theatre; who believe that the law ought to step in and forever forbid the idea of equality by making marriages between them illegal, are heartily opposed to any arrangement encouraging this equality, which gives negroes false ideas and dangerous beliefs."[6] The color line was enforced in the South thereafter and given legal sanction in the Supreme Court decision in the case of *Plessy v. Ferguson* in 1896, the unsuccessful suit of a New Orleans mulatto who had refused to take a segregated seat in a railway car.

Black boxers might compete at the lower weight classes because the heavyweight title symbolized the top tier of physical superiority, and in 1902 Joe Gans became the first black fighter acknowledged as a world champion when he captured the lightweight crown. In 1906 he added the welterweight title, and his forty-two-round war with Oscar "Battling" Nelson was considered to be the "fight of the century" and elicited the highest purse for a boxing match up to that date. A black newspaper claimed

4 http://johnshippen.net/john-shippen-biography.html (accessed July 27, 2013).

5 Andrew Ritchie, *Major Taylor: The Fastest Bicycle Rider in the World* (San Francisco: Van der Plas/Cycle Publishing, 2010).

6 Colleen Aycock and Mark Scott, eds., *The First Black Boxing Champions: Essays on Fighters of the 1800s to the 1920s* (Jefferson NC: McFarland, 2011), 32–59; *New Orleans Times-Democrat*, September 8, 1892, 4.

that Gans enjoyed more celebrity than Booker T. Washington, yet Gans suffered bankruptcy and an early death. His success proved to be ephemeral.[7]

By that time W. E. B. Du Bois, a Harvard PhD, had assumed a more militant stance in opposition to Booker T. Washington's accommodationism. Du Bois declared that blacks need not acquiesce because a "talented tenth" of their number could compete equally with whites on a level playing field. In Chicago a young multisport star, Sam Ransom, proved that assertion in the high school ranks. He was accorded unbiased recognition by the more liberal Chicago media but did not receive a remuneration in the form of college scholarships offered to his white teammates. In 1903 Dubois asserted that "submission to civic inferiority ... is bound to sap the manhood of any race in the long run."[8] Ransom would assume a more deliberate engagement in American citizenship and fight for greater rights and recognition of blacks throughout the remainder of his life.

Shortly after Ransom's athletic triumphs, Jack Johnson, king of the black heavyweights, destroyed the myth of white supremacy. When champion Jim Jeffries retired from the ring undefeated, Tommy Burns emerged as the new titleholder, and he embarked on a global tour to maximize the profit of his title. Jack Johnson followed him to Australia, where Burns was coerced to fight Johnson for a magnificent sum. It proved to be a gross mismatch as Johnson toyed with Burns before ending his short reign. As the world champion, Johnson refused to give other top black boxers a shot at his title, so Joe Jeannette, Sam Langford, Sam McVea, and others traveled to Europe to gain fame and fortune, as did many black musicians and the celebrated dancer Josephine Baker in later years.

Johnson proceeded to outrage whites by his flamboyant lifestyle, liaisons and eventual marriages to white women, and the fact that a series of "white hopes" could not dislodge him from his position atop the heavyweight ranks. On July 4, 1910, the previously undefeated Jeffries even came out of retirement to restore the laurels to the white race, but he too tasted an ignominious defeat at the hands of Johnson. Johnson's victory fostered race riots throughout America, a measure of whites' vitriolic backlash at their comeuppance. Films of the fight were banned, and the U.S. government got further involved by charging Johnson with a violation of the Mann Act, involving the transportation of women across state lines for illegal purposes, and Johnson became a fugitive. Despite Johnson's dominance of the heavyweight ranks, or perhaps because of it, D. W. Griffith's popular 1915 movie, *The Birth of a Nation*, continued to portray black men as primitive, oversexed, and immoral savages, less than worthy of full citizenship. Johnson lost the title to Jess Willard in Havana, Cuba, in 1915 (Johnson claimed that he threw the fight), and upon his return to the United States in 1920 he served a year in prison and was never permitted to fight for the championship again.[9]

While the federal government persecuted and prosecuted Johnson, the United States portrayed itself more liberally and democratically in the pluralistic representation of the 1912 Olympic team, which featured the black sprinter Howard Drew, the Hawaiian swimmer Duke Kahanamoku, and Native American Jim Thorpe. Drew became known as "the world's fastest human." Kahanamoku garnered six medals as an Olympian from 1912 to 1932, and Thorpe was dubbed the greatest athlete in the world after winning both the pentathlon and the decathlon, but neither blacks, Hawaiians, nor Native Americans were accorded the full rights of citizenship.[10]

---

7 Colleen Aycock and Mark Scott, *Joe Gans: A Biography of the First African American World Boxing Champion* (Jefferson NC: McFarland, 2008).

8 Du Bois cited in Martin Summers, *Manliness and Its Discontents: The Black Middle Class and the Transformation of Masculinity, 1900–1930* (Chapel Hill: University of North Carolina Press, 2004), 4.

9 Randy Roberts, *Papa Jack: Jack Johnson and the Era of White Hopes* (New York: Free Press, 1983); Theresa Runstedtler, *Jack Johnson: Rebel Sojourner, Boxing in the Shadow of the Global Color Line* (Berkeley: University of California Press, 2012).

10 Debra A. Henderson, "Howard Drew," in *African Americans in Sports*, ed. David K. Wiggins (Armonk NY: M. E. Sharpe, 2004), 88.

After the turn of the century more southern blacks, like Jack Johnson, who was born in Galveston, Texas, migrated northward for opportunities unavailable in the South and in search of a better life. Between 1915 and 1970 an estimated six million southern blacks sought refuge outside that region. Many traveled to northern cities, where they vied with millions of mostly European immigrants for more plentiful and better-paying jobs. The multitudes of European groups often segregated themselves in urban neighborhoods with countrymen whose language and culture they understood, a choice that allowed for a more gradual assimilation into American culture. Southern black migrants had less choice in their accommodations, as white realtors and property owners conspired to prevent black home ownership in their areas, resulting in the ghettoization of blacks within major cities. Within such neglected communities blacks were forced to largely develop their own resources and institutions. Employers and religious groups, such as the YMCA, even built separate sport and recreational facilities to maintain such exclusion lest blacks and poor whites fraternize in their leisure pursuits and possibly unite in labor unions to oppose their bosses.[11]

Sol Butler, the son of a former slave, emerged as a track star during the World War I years, but the carnage derailed the Olympic Games in 1916. Butler set a new American record in the long jump as a soldier at the Inter-Allied Games, a military Olympics held in Paris in the wake of the war. In the 1920 Games he was injured and unable to capitalize on his athletic fame. Thereafter he managed to make a living as a football and basketball star, a sportswriter, and in movie roles. He parlayed his athletic abilities into coaching positions in Chicago within the black community, helping black youth to develop their athletic talents as his life became more closely intertwined with the popular culture. As is true for many black men today, violence permeated urban neighborhoods and dreams went unfulfilled, and Butler eventually lost his life in a bar shootout.[12]

Violence against blacks continued after the war in the form of race riots and lynchings as returning white and black veterans and hosts of ethnic immigrants competed for jobs. Chicago suffered a major race riot in 1919, ignited when black youth wandered across the dividing line that segregated their separate sections of a public beach. The resultant bloodshed lasted for a week, cost thirty-eight lives and more than five hundred injuries, left more than one thousand homeless, and required the intervention of the National Guard to quell the violence. Rube Foster, another Texas transplant, had moved to Chicago as a pro baseball player—and even partnered with a white co-owner of a team—before acquiring his own baseball club. Foster's early success as an entrepreneur signaled the possibilities of life in the more liberal northern cities, but the continued influx of southern blacks threatened the job security of working-class whites. In the wake of the race riot Foster decided to initiate the Negro National League, as black players were still barred from the white Major League teams. The venture proved so successful that a second pro circuit, the Eastern Colored League, appeared in 1923. Foster provided talented black athletes with a stage to display their skills in a "public ritual of performance" that allowed them to establish their newfound sense of masculinity.[13] Other black entrepreneurs found in baseball another means to engage in the popular culture. Some of them merged their baseball enterprises with the numbers racket, a form of the poor man's lottery in black neighborhoods, where residents constructed an alternative economy to meet their needs.

When Bessie Coleman could not meet her psychological, emotional, and occupational needs, she left the country voluntarily because American flight instructors refused to teach her to fly a plane. She found such tutelage in France and returned as the first black female pilot, extending the perceived

11 Isabel Wilkerson, *The Warmth of Other Suns: The Epic Story of America's Great Migration* (New York: Random House, 2010), 9.
12 James E. Odenkirk, "Sol Butler," in Wiggins, *African Americans in Sports*, 55.
13 Summers, *Manliness and Its Discontents*, 4.

limits of feminine possibilities. Coleman pushed both racial and gender boundaries, attempting daring feats in barnstorming air shows and exhibitions until such deeds took her life in 1926. Coleman's escape to Paris in response to the impediments she faced in the United States was not atypical. The French capital had served as a refuge for African Americans since the late nineteenth century.

Henry O. Tanner, a black art student, left the United States in 1891 to study in Rome but became so enchanted with the City of Lights that he stayed in Paris. "At no time was he made to feel unwanted or inferior because of his color, which had not always been so in Philadelphia," where he had studied at the Pennsylvania Academy of the Fine Arts.[14] Peter Jackson, the heavyweight boxer, soon followed Tanner to Paris, and a bevy of black fighters popularized boxing in France after the turn of the century. An American writer claimed, "They earn more in a week there than they used to in many months over here."[15] Jack Johnson, as a fugitive from American prosecutors, also resided in Paris, where he mixed boxing with theatrical performances and became a local celebrity until World War I interrupted his interlude. The French had seemingly obtained a fascination with the black body that paved the way for a multitude of African American jazz age entertainers during the 1920s.[16]

The 1920s are considered the first Golden Age of sport in the United States, as the new technology of the radio, motion pictures, and extensive media coverage of athletic stars brought celebrity, fame, and heroization to champions. The era also produced a black renaissance in sports, literature, art, and music, centered in New York's Harlem and Chicago's Bronzeville neighborhoods, where athletes often carried the banner of racial dignity. Such developments promoted black pride and drew attention to African American culture, accomplishments, and abilities, but these did not gain full acceptance in the dominant white mainstream culture. In New York Marcus Garvey preached black nationalism and black enterprise and team owners subscribed to the latter. As it had with Jack Johnson, the federal government perceived Garvey as a threat. He was incarcerated in 1925 and deported to his native Jamaica two years later.

After Johnson's loss of the championship white successors instituted a color ban on black heavyweights. Harry Wills remained a top contender during Jack Dempsey's reign as champion but never got a shot at the crown despite compiling a record of 68-9-3 with fifty-four knockouts and living an abstemious lifestyle. Wills had also defeated Willie Meehan, a boxer who had only lost once to Dempsey in four fights.[17] At the lower weights Tiger Flowers became the first black to capture the middleweight title in 1926. Flowers lived in a large house in Atlanta, ostentatiously but spotlessly as a church deacon and a philanthropist. He proved acceptable to whites as one "who knew his place" and did not assert the recalcitrant attitude of northern blacks. Flowers's career, however, proved short-lived as he died the following year as a result of surgery around his eyes to remove scar tissue caused by boxing.[18] The same could not be said of Francisco Guilledo, a Filipino who assumed the ring name of Pancho Villa, the revolutionary Mexican bandit who had terrorized the American Southwest during World War I. Villa had learned to box from the American soldiers who still occupied his island country since the Spanish-American War of 1898. After defeating the best of the Americans in Manila, he traveled to the

---

14 David McCullough, *The Greater Journey: Americans in Paris* (New York: Simon and Schuster, 2011), 428.

15 Rudolph Fisher, "The Caucasian Storms Harlem," in *Voices from the Harlem Renaissance*, ed. Nathan Irvin Huggins (New York: Oxford University Press, 1995), 74–82 (quote, 80). See also Gwendolyn Bennett, "Wedding Day," 191–97, in the same collection, for the story of Paul Watson, an African American boxer-musician who also resided in Paris.

16 Runstedtler, *Jack Johnson*, 150, 164–95.

17 http://boxrec.com/search.php?status=all&cat=boxer&first_name=Harry&last_name=Wills&submit=Go&pageID=3 (accessed November 24, 2013); Dennis Gildea, "Harry Wills," in Wiggins, *African Americans in Sports*, 408–9. Wills's record does not include another 19-1-3 record with five more knockouts during the World War I era, when sportswriters rendered the decisions as boxing was officially banned in most states.

18 Andrew M. Kaye, *The Pussycat of Prizefighting: Tiger Flowers and the Politics of Black Celebrity* (Athens: University of Georgia Press, 2004).

United States, where he won the world flyweight championship and antagonized whites as a smaller version of Jack Johnson. He dressed lavishly, spent his money extravagantly, and cavorted with a bevy of white women, followed by his large entourage. Like other people of color, he was racialized by sportswriters, who rationalized his speed and consequent wins over white opponents as the works of an inhuman demon. He, too, died after a short reign of two years due to blood poisoning after surgery for infected teeth in 1925. His wife claimed his death amounted to a murder, and Filipinos considered it a national tragedy. When his body was returned to the Philippines for burial, one hundred thousand mourners attended his funeral.[19]

Both Jack Johnson and Pancho Villa had become enamored of the vibrant nightlife then permeating urban centers as musicians from the South brought ragtime music and then jazz and the blues to northern climes in their migrations. Chicago became a center for the music and recording industry, and Jack Johnson opened an early black and tan cabaret there where upper-class whites drawn to the new genre went "slumming" with black entertainers and dancers to experience a sensuality absent in their own lives. The musical attractions provided other venues for entrepreneurs as black youth and Filipinos flocked to nightclubs and dance halls in search of excitement deemed immoral by white puritans.[20]

Black athletes also had close ties with the music industry as musicians, singers, talent scouts, and booking agents. Paul Robeson, Fritz Pollard, and Jay Mayo "Ink" Williams gained their initial fame on the football field because civic rivalries that spawned incessant gambling required the best athletes and profit and pride superseded race. Within that competitive environment Pollard became the first black quarterback and the first black head coach in the nascent NFL due to his athletic skills, and he recruited other blacks for his ventures. Robeson joined Pollard on the gridiron but would gain greater stature as a singer, actor, and civil rights activist before being chased out of the United States due to his political convictions. Pollard too turned to the music industry and other ventures, as all blacks were weeded out of the NFL after the 1933 season through the efforts of George Marshall, owner of the Washington franchise. But Pollard's son would contribute to the Americans' rejection of Aryan supremacy at the Nazi Olympics of 1936 when he became a bronze medalist in the 110-meter hurdles race.[21]

Basketball provided more opportunities for athletes to make a living during the 1920s as a burgeoning professional circuit and interracial challenge matches offered income during the winter months. Not only black southerners but also more than 140,000 Caribbean migrants traveled to the United States between 1899 and 1937. Bob Douglas, born in St. Kitts (one of the British Virgin Islands), traveled to New York, where he organized a fully professional unit in 1923 known as the Renaissance Five, a reference to the Renaissance Ballroom, from which they emanated. Sport merged with other elements of the popular culture as intermissions at the popular dance halls featured basketball games, and the Renaissance moniker served to market the dance hall as well as the basketball team. The Rens not only prospered, but they also beat the white professional teams and won the first national pro tournament in 1939. Like the boxing victories of Joe Louis, such successes instilled and maintained black pride and a sense of self-worth.[22]

19 Gerald R. Gems, *The Athletic Crusade: Sport and American Cultural Imperialism* (Lincoln: University of Nebraska Press, 2006), 61–62.

20 Summers, *Manliness and Its Discontents*, 173–75; Kevern Verney, *African Americans and U.S. Popular Culture* (London: Routledge, 2003), 26–30; Chad Heap, *Slumming: Sexual and Racial Encounters in American Nightlife, 1885–1940* (Chicago: University of Chicago Press, 2009); Paul G. Cressey, *Taxi-Dance Hall: A Sociological Study in Commercialized Recreation and City Life* (Chicago: University of Chicago Press, 1932).

21 John M. Carroll, *Fritz Pollard: Pioneer in Racial Advancement* (Urbana: University of Illinois Press, 1992); Martin Bauml Duberman, *Paul Robeson: A Biography* (New York: Ballantine Books, 1989).

22 Summers, *Manliness and Its Discontents*, 4.

A similar undertaking occurred in Chicago, where the Savoy Five played at the Savoy Ballroom but soon began barnstorming as the Harlem Globetrotters. They assumed the reference to the New York neighborhood as a tribute to its national influence in black life. Both black teams employed a distinctive style of play, executing sharp, crisp passes; dexterous dribbling; and a fast pace in an entertaining style that sometimes baffled white opponents and spectators. Two of the early Globetrotters' players, Tommy Brookins and Harold "Killer" Johnson, became more deeply involved in the music industry and other more nefarious ventures within the popular culture. Johnson earned his nickname for his deadly shooting skills with a basketball before turning to entertainment management and club ownership. Brookins claimed that he had been swindled out of ownership of the team by booking agent Abe Saperstein, a claim that caused his departure to Europe, where he began his music career. He later owned a Chicago nightclub and retired to St. Maarten in the Caribbean. The Globetrotters would win the second professional basketball tournament in 1940 before achieving international fame as comedic entertainers.[23]

Black female basketball teams also proliferated during the interwar years, sponsored by churches and businesses. Isadore Channels starred for the Olivet Baptist Church team and then joined the famed Roamers, who played interracial matches with white women. Members of such teams crossed both social and economic classes, exhibiting the more cooperative nature of society within the black communities. Another barnstorming team, the Philadelphia Tribunes, featured Ora Washington. Both she and Channels were multisport stars. When blacks were banned from the national white tennis association, they formed their own, the American Tennis Association, in 1916. Channels dominated the national championship during the 1920s, winning four individual titles and one doubles crown. Washington followed suit as the dominant player in the 1930s. Blacks could not play in the USLTA tournament until 1948, and stars such as Althea Gibson and Arthur Ashe then rose to prominence, but pioneers such as Channels and Washington sparked the early interest in tennis in black communities. Such women operated within a complex amalgamation of religious, gender, and class relations that pushed the boundaries of femininity long before Venus and Serena Williams transformed the sport of tennis.

Black male athletes such as Eddie Tolan and Ralph Metcalfe became more conspicuous as members of the U.S. Olympic teams in the 1930s, and the heroics of Jesse Owens in the 1936 Games in Berlin undermined Hitler's assertions of Aryan supremacy. Tidye Pickett, the first African American female to make an American Olympic team, did not enjoy such celebrity but rather endured racist harassment and ostracism in 1932. She persevered to return in 1936, only to suffer another tragic setback before becoming a successful educator in relative obscurity. Pickett's educational attainments defied the stereotype of blacks' mental ineptitude.

While black participation in contact sports such as boxing increased during the 1930s, such activities were associated with the lower classes. French sociologist Pierre Bourdieu claimed that one's upbringing within a particular social class determined one's worldview and lifestyle, but the segregated black communities of urban America harbored residents of all classes, from the homeless to millionaires, exposing inhabitants to a greater variety of cultural possibilities. Blacks aspired to greater socioeconomic mobility but found resistance when they tried to contest with whites in the more genteel sports of tennis and golf. As was the case with tennis, blacks had to form their own professional golf circuit, the United Golfers Association (UGA), because the PGA refused to recognize them until 1961.[24]

Teddy Rhodes, like John Shippen, taught himself to play golf as a caddie, and he dominated the UGA, winning more than 150 tournaments, although the prize money paled in comparison to the white

23 http://www.pbs.org/wnet/finding-your-roots/stories/famous-relatives/mu-ancestor-tommy-brookins (accessed July 27, 2013).

24 Pierre Bourdieu, *Outline of a Theory of Practice* (Cambridge: Cambridge University Press, 1972).

PGA circuit. Rhodes became the personal golf tutor of boxing champion Joe Louis, who also sponsored Rhodes on the black golf circuit. Rhodes and two other golfers sued the PGA for its segregation practices, and he managed to play in the 1948 U.S. Open, still fighting the same battles John Shippen had fought a half century earlier. Illness forced Rhodes's retirement, but he continued to instruct the young black golfers who finally won entry into the PGA in the 1960s, a civil rights progression that eventually produced Tiger Woods. The case of Teddy Rhodes clearly indicated that Jackie Robinson's entry into Major League Baseball, though monumental in its significance, had not produced wholesale racial acceptance in American society. A more extensive civil rights movement and an athletic revolution led by Muhammad Ali and other courageous black athletes remained to accomplish that task.

This book concentrates on popular culture, and more specifically sport, as one aspect of American history during the later years of the nineteenth century and the first half of the twentieth century, with the aim to recover the stories of individuals who helped to change the course of the nation. It consciously avoids the stories of more well-known athletes whose lives are chronicled in full-length biographies. It does so within the framework of popular culture in the form of music and sport, which allowed African Americans a measure of opportunity. Even as slaves they were permitted—even expected—to entertain whites. Popular culture allowed them to do so but also provided avenues for greater independence, personal expression, and slow societal change. While many people are aware of the accomplishments and influence of athletes such as Jack Johnson, Joe Louis, Jesse Owens, Jackie Robinson, and Muhammad Ali, such luminaries of the black sporting experience did not emerge spontaneously. Their rise was part of a gradual evolution in social and power relations in American culture over the course of a half century (ca. 1890–1940s). The freedom of speech and religion that eventually exonerated and allowed for the heroization of Muhammad Ali was built upon the stoicism of Jackie Robinson, who endured the pressures of racism to prove that whites and blacks could cooperate seven years before the United States Supreme Court struck down the separate-but-equal doctrine that endorsed segregation in the *Brown v. Board of Education* case in 1954. Robinson's sacrifices were made possible by the gradual but temporary acceptance of black athletes as national heroes. Both Jesse Owens and Joe Louis personified American ideals and democratic values when the nation needed their physical prowess to destroy the Nazi myth of Aryan supremacy in the 1930s, but once both men had accomplished their task, they were relegated to their former status of second-class citizens. Both suffered bankruptcy, and Louis died a pauper.

This book addresses the stories and hardships endured by those pioneers who paved the way for Jackie Robinson and Muhammad Ali to bring about social change. They too contributed much to the larger story of our collective history by their heroic confrontations with the entrenched racism of their times to bring about the incremental changes that allowed for Jackie Robinson to make his historic breakthrough. They did so by courageously crossing racial, social, political, economic, and cultural boundaries in an expression of human agency in the confrontation of a repressive white domination. Their arduous efforts resulted in a richer, better, and more inclusive American culture. The book follows a chronological order to provide for historical contextualization and to analyze the gradual progress, and at times remission, of the cultural flow. Historian Renee Romano has asserted that "Once a past no longer proves useful, it recedes into the pages of books and archives rather than circulating in the broader culture."[25] This work attempts to rescue the meaningful lives of a handful of athletic pioneers from the dustbin of history and reclaim their significance. It addresses, to some degree, the incomplete story of the nation and the historical amnesia that afflicts many of its inhabitants.

25 Renee Romano, "Beyond 'Self-Congratulatory Celebration': Complicating Civil Rights Anniversaries," *American Historian* (November 2014): 29–32 (quote, 30).

10

INTRODUCTION TO A SPECTACULAR LEAP

BLACK WOMEN ATHLETES IN TWENTIETH-CENTURY AMERICA

Jennifer H. Lansbury

Introduction

A misty rain fell on the spectators gathered at Wembley Stadium in London, England, but the crowd was still strong at 60,000. It was the final day of track and field competition for the XIV Olympiad. Dusk was quickly approaching, but the women's high jump competition was still underway. Two athletes remained, an American by the name of Alice Coachman and the British, hometown favorite, Dorothy Tyler. With an Olympic gold medal on the line, both athletes seemed content to remain all night, if necessary, as they continued to match each other at height after height. But then at 5′6½″, neither one cleared the bar. The audience waited in the darkening drizzle while the judges conferred to determine who would be crowned the new Olympic champion. Finally, the judges ruled that one of the two athletes had indeed edged out the other through fewer missed attempts on previous heights. Alice Coachman had just become the first African American woman to win an Olympic gold medal. Her leap of 5′6⅛″ on that August evening in 1948 set new Olympic and American records for the women's high jump. The win culminated a virtually unparalleled ten-year career in which she amassed an athletic record of thirty-six track and field national championships—twenty-six individual and ten team titles. From 1939, when she first won the national championship for the high jump at the age of sixteen, she never surrendered it; a new champion came only after her retirement at the conclusion of the Olympics. While the high jump was her signature event—"a spectacular leap" that led to her 1941 victory just one of ten consecutive national titles—she also possessed speed.[1] For her prowess as a sprinter, the press dubbed Coachman, "the Tuskegee flash." For five consecutive years in the mid-1940s,

1 The African American *Pittsburgh Courier* provided the description of Coachman's 1941 high jump victory. "Tuskegee Lassie Goes Up and Over to Retain Title," *Pittsburgh Courier*, 29 July 1941, 16.

her 50-meter sprint titles qualified her as the fastest woman in the United States. In 1943, she was named a member of the first All-American Women's Track and Field Team, continuing that yearly distinction until her retirement in 1948. When she returned from the Olympics to her hometown of Albany, Georgia, blacks and whites came together to celebrate her victory. And in the early 1950s, she became the first African American woman athlete to acquire a corporate endorsement when she appeared with fellow Olympic track star Jesse Owens in print advertisements for Coca-Cola.

But the glory of being an Olympic champion faded with the passing years and, in time, few people knew of her athletic feats, even in her hometown. Roughly twenty years after winning the gold medal, the extent to which history had been rewritten became shockingly clear. While teaching physical education in her hometown during the 1960s, she gave her students an assignment as they began their unit on the sport—read and report on the history of track and field. One of the students brought in a book that stated Wilma Rudolph was the first African American woman to win an Olympic gold medal. "But Mrs. Davis," her students remarked, "we thought you said you were the first." Coachman had spoken with them in the past about her Olympic experience. She informed them that the book was incorrect, but they remained skeptical. Reminiscing about the incident years later, she recalled that the only way to convince them was to bring her gold medal into class the following day.[2]

This is the story of African American women's relationship with competitive sport during the twentieth century. It is a relationship that allowed athletically talented black women, many of them from poor backgrounds, to attend college, travel, and experience life in ways that otherwise would have been unknown to them. It is a relationship that fostered widespread support and acclaim from members of the black community. And it is a relationship in which the athletes confronted and challenged contemporary perceptions of what it meant to be a woman and black in American society, and what it meant—both in white society and the black community—to be at the forefront of the struggle for civil rights.

When African American women began playing competitive sport in the 1920s, they did so through the support of their own, segregated communities. These communities often saw sport as a vehicle for both teamwork and competition, as well as individual and collective achievement in the face of a dominant white society. Coaches and mentors, neighbors, friends, entrepreneurs, and patrons collectively discovered young women who were athletically gifted and then developed a path for them to train and compete. Sometimes there was conflict about what was best for the athletes versus the community; nevertheless, high school girls received strong support from black communities whose goal was to help them succeed. And succeed they did, in track and field, tennis, and basketball. Black businesses sponsored industrial teams, establishing leagues for women to compete. Programs in high schools and historically black colleges and universities allowed for training and competition, enabling black women to explore their athletic talent. Black coaches scoured surrounding states for talented high school girls, and suddenly poor rural and working-class women found their route to college through competitive sport and work-study programs. College meant both advanced education and national and international travel as competition opportunities opened up at home and abroad. And as black women athletes competed against whites, they brought home national championships and Olympic medals. This pattern of community support and athletic success played out repeatedly over the decades of the twentieth century.

Black women's experience with sport was far from idyllic, however, often mirroring those of their white counterparts. Throughout the twentieth century, women athletes had to navigate stereotypes about

2 Coachman's married name is Davis. Alice Coachman Davis, Interview by author, tape recording, Tuskegee, Alabama, 10 February 2003.

their femininity, sexuality, and economic standing.[3] Sport was the playground for men, really always had been. As far back as the ancient Greek Olympics, women had been excluded from participating in, even watching, sporting events, and the modern world was not terribly different. When U.S. women did begin to play sports in the late nineteenth century, Americans questioned which sports they should participate in, how they should participate, what clothing they should wear, and whether competition, in a fashion similar to men, was appropriate for the "fair sex." Class identity combined with gender and prevailing notions of femininity to further label and constrain women's relationship with sport. When track and field and basketball became labeled as working-class sports, women who participated were characterized by disparaging gender stereotypes that questioned their femininity. As a sport of the elite, men and women who played tennis had to conform to its rigid social expectations. But for women, gender expectations were bound to class identity as well. Hitting the ball with too much power could result in masculine, working-class labels. In short, black and white women alike who participated in sport were often scrutinized, questioned, challenged, qualified, and even ridiculed by white society.

What African American women athletes had to contend with that white women did not were race and racism.[4] This may seem like an obvious statement, but it changed the dynamic of their relationship with sport in dramatic ways. These athletes had to deal both with how African Americans perceived them in terms of gender and class and how whites perceived them in terms of race, gender, and class. Race, then, became a defining element for these women among both African Americans and whites. In white society, they sometimes joined with white women athletes to combat common gender stereotypes that suggested that women who played sport were too masculine. In truth, however, race always made a difference. Black women had to contend with racial stereotypes that white women did not, such as the hypersexualized black female or the natural black athlete. Since race was a rallying cry within their own community, gender and class stereotypes persisted on a different level. The question for some within the black community became how to help black women athletes "overcome" their working-class backgrounds and combat gender stereotypes in white society. Excelling in athletic competition was, for many within the black community, significant for the race as a whole. As such, an important, though sometimes conflicted, relationship developed between black women athletes and their mentors, and those within the community who were connected to the broader civil rights campaign. Indeed, the way these women and their mentors navigated racism and racial relationships was one of the most compelling aspects of their careers.

---

3 Many scholars have already explored women athletes' navigation of such stereotypes. Susan K. Cahn, *Coming on Strong: Gender and Sexuality in Twentieth-Century Women's Sport* (New York: Free Press, 1994), is the seminal book-length study into femininity/sexuality, class, and women in sport, and its insights remain extremely relevant. Other important works include Gwendolyn Captain, "Enter Ladies and Gentlemen of Color: Gender, Sport, and the Ideal of the African American Manhood and Womanhood During the Late Nineteenth Centuries," *Journal of Sport History* 18 (Spring 1991): 81–102; Mary Jo Festle, *Playing Nice: Politics and Apologies in Women's Sports* (New York: Columbia University Press, 1996); Cindy Himes Gissendanner, "African-American Women in Competitive Sport, 1920–1960," in *Women, Sport, and Culture*, ed. Susan Birrell and Cheryl L. Cole (Champaign, IL: Human Kinetics, 1994); Gissendanner, "African American Women Olympians: The Impact of Race, Gender, and Class Ideologies, 1932–1968," *Research Quarterly for Exercise and Sport* 67 (June 1996): 172–82; Patricia Vertinsky and Gwendolyn Captain, "More Myth Than History: American Culture and Representations of the Black Female's Athletic Ability," *Journal of Sport History* 25 (Fall 1998): 532–61; Rita Liberti, "'We Were Ladies, We Just Played Basketball Like Boys': African American Womanhood and Competitive Basketball at Bennett College, 1928–1942," *Journal of Sport History* 26 (Fall 1999): 567–84; Pamela Grundy and Susan Shackelford, "Black Women Embrace the Game," in *Shattering the Glass: The Remarkable History of Women's Basketball* (Chapel Hill: University of North Carolina Press, 2005); Martha Verbrugge, *Active Bodies: A History of Women's Physical Education in Twentieth-Century America* (Oxford: Oxford University Press, 2012).

4 While the work of many theoretical scholars has been transformed by what Kimberlé Crenshaw called the intersectionality of race, class, and gender, my own approach is grounded less in theory and more in historical analysis and narrative. Kimberlé Crenshaw, "Mapping the Margins: Intersectionality, Identity Politics, and Violence against Women of Color," *Stanford Law Review* 14 (1991): 1241–99. For a recent overview of the theory, see Michele Tracy Berger and Kathleen Guidroz, ed., *The Intersectional Approach: Transforming the Academy through Race, Class, and Gender* (Chapel Hill: University of North Carolina Press, 2009).

While black women athletes competed, African Americans spent much of the twentieth century writing, marching, boycotting, and struggling to acquire equality under American law. While progress was slow, life in the United States looked very different for a woman of color competing in the 1920s, when black women first came on the African American sporting scene, than for one competing in the 1980s, when black women had been ruling the sport of national track and field for fifty years. Besides changes in the broader society, the world of sport had experienced its own transformation. In 1946, Kenny Washington and Woody Strode broke the thirteen-year exclusion of blacks in the NFL; four years later, Earl Lloyd broke the color barrier in the NBA. But no breakthrough during mid-century had the same impact on sport and society as the one Jackie Robinson made in the national pastime. When Robinson broke the color barrier in major league baseball in 1947, he became the standard against which other sports stories involving African Americans were compared. His athletic performance, racial pride, and willingness to let racial slurs roll off his back affirmed African American athletic ability, challenged prevailing concepts of racial inferiority, and made at least some whites consider race relations in a new light. White ballplayers refused to play with him. Eventually they became his friends. Managers who had been raised in the South worried that they could not overcome their own prejudice. They did. Teammates, coaches, and managers came to defend him—both his abilities as a ballplayer and his value as an individual. Moreover, he stood as a symbol for African Americans against racial discrimination and prejudice throughout his life. He was a proud black man in a largely segregated, white America, whom whites and blacks alike came to admire and respect. His career and his position in America following his retirement provided a racial context for many within the black community to interpret other advances in sport, including those of African American women.

Throughout their athletic careers, then, black women athletes found themselves at the forefront of the racism that characterized much of the American twentieth century. When they were not pushing back against color barriers, stereotypes, and perceptions of white America, they were often being scrutinized and groomed by black communities that wanted to ensure they were acceptable race representatives. They did not always accept their place as race heroes. Some athletes fell into the role more willingly and naturally than others. Some vocally rejected it, wishing instead that their careers could be acknowledged on nonracial terms. Such rejection could lead the adulation, celebration, and support of black civil rights sport leaders to turn on a dime. Even so, the desire and sheer force of will of black women athletes to compete in a society that marginalized them made a difference over time. The advances were sometimes small. In the 1940s, it was a matter of whether they got noticed in the sports pages of the white newspapers. In another twenty years, however, black women track and field athletes were on their way to becoming "our girls" in the American press. And by the 1980s, they had become a dominant force in the world of U.S. sport, even as they continued to confront gender and racial stereotypes. Their story is one of hard work, resilience, and perseverance in the face of an American society that initially scorned and ignored them, and finally came to accept them, albeit sometimes still in racial terms.

The focus of each chapter in the narrative that follows is an individual athlete, a woman whose combination of dedication, training, athletic skills, and timing resulted in an exceptional career.[5] Ora Washington was a champion tennis player and basketball star in the black community beginning in the

5 This narrative approach addresses the problem of limited sources, especially for the athletes who competed during the first half of the century. The black press began following women athletes within the black community as early as the 1920s, and, by mid-century, the white press was writing about them as well. However, the details that can be gleaned from the sports pages—scores, descriptions of games, matches, and track meets, and the names of players—often generate more questions than they answer. Where possible, interviews, personal papers, and autobiographies supplement the press accounts, yet oral and archival information are not abundant for "famous" athletes and virtually nonexistent for many women who competed against and alongside them.

late 1920s. When white organizations erected color lines to bar black players, athletes like Washington found athletic opportunities within sporting teams and organizations that African Americans created for themselves. The 1940s and 1950s produced two important black women athletic champions in two very different sports. Track and field was one of the few sports in the country that permitted competition among and between African Americans and whites at the national level. Alice Coachman, the Olympic champion track and field athlete of the 1940s, and women like her, reveled in the opportunity to compete nationally. Althea Gibson was an amateur tennis player of the 1950s who became the first African American Wimbledon and U.S. national champion. She was a natural with a tennis racquet, but she was also a tough, tomboyish black woman from Harlem, a stark contradiction to white tennis society. Sprinter Wilma Rudolph, a track star of the late 1950s and early 1960s, overcame crippling childhood illnesses to become a triple Olympic gold-medal winner. During her time as America's sprint queen, black women track athletes became the United States' best hope to defeat the Russian women in track in a world locked in a bitter Cold War. The racial turbulence of the late 1960s and the rebirth of the women's movement in the 1970s is the backdrop for the story of Wyomia Tyus. A champion sprinter and Olympic gold medalist, her career occurred during a time of profound changes for women and blacks in America. By the 1980s, African Americans were the standard bearers of women's track and field. Raised in the wake of the Title IX legislation that opened up more sporting opportunities for women, Jackie Joyner-Kersee earned the title of "world's greatest female athlete" when she won six Olympic medals and set eight world records. She emerged from the ghetto into a world of international track and field that, with its million-dollar endorsement contracts, looked very different from the sport Alice Coachman, Wilma Rudolph, or Wyomia Tyus competed in.

These are not mini-biographies, nor are they meant to be. But most of the athletes are not well known today, and, therefore, some biographical context is necessary in each chapter. Their individual stories reveal interesting and complex individuals—their struggles and triumphs; what they accomplished and what they had to give up in the process; the important people and communities that helped them achieve athletic success; and the ways in which they were likable, and sometimes, not so likable. Their stories unveil striking similarities. All of the athletes came from poor beginnings. Many of their childhoods were mixed with pleasant memories and hard times. While their families were intact, the home lives for many of them were not always idyllic. All six were natural athletes and played multiple sports well, with basketball being a common denominator among them all. Strong male mentors often made their educations and athletic careers possible, and many of them received invitations to leave home as teenagers to train elsewhere. For all but one, sport was their vehicle to a college education that probably would have eluded them otherwise. After they retired from sports, most of them struggled with life to varying degrees; they often had a hard time finding steady work despite their athletic fame and college education. And those who had broken racial, gender, or sporting barriers questioned their place or, more accurately, lack of place in American popular culture.

Two of the similarities are particularly striking. First, all of these women used sport as a way to broaden the typical life that lay ahead of rural or working-class African American women of the period. Most poor black women of the first two-thirds of the twentieth century found work in agriculture, service, or industrial sectors.[6] While growing numbers of historically black colleges throughout the country were available to teach trades and provide higher education, many African American families could not afford tuition. Beginning in the 1930s, sport and work-study programs that black colleges like Tuskegee Institute and Tennessee State University extended to gifted athletes became their path

6 Jacqueline Jones's monograph remains a valued overview of the work lives of black women. See Jacqueline Jones, *Labor of Love, Labor of Sorrow: Black Women, Work and the Family, From Slavery to the Present* (New York: Vintage Books, 1986).

to a skilled trade and/or higher education. By the late 1970s, white universities like UCLA were actively recruiting black women athletes and offering full athletic scholarships. Moreover, athletic competition provided travel experiences that many of these women would otherwise have been unable to afford. All the athletes traveled widely, first nationally, and by mid-century, internationally. Second, strong, influential, African American men made possible the athletic and college careers of these athletes. Most often the mentors were coaches, and they guided a number of other young African American women who excelled at sport through the same path. Most of them viewed sport as a way for their young athletic charges to better themselves, and they not only helped train the athletes but also encouraged them educationally and socially. The relationships between black women athletes and male coaches, mentors, and promoters, then, point to the community nature of betterment efforts within African American society, efforts that could easily cross gender barriers established by the dominant society. At a time when many in white America discouraged women from entering competitive sport, African American men were finding ways and developing programs to give young black women athletes a way to succeed in the sporting world and an opportunity at a better life.

Of course, using the stories of six athletes as a narrative for this history brings up the question of representation. Is it appropriate to think that these women could represent the many other black women athletes who competed throughout the decades of the twentieth century? There were other exceptional athletes over the years and many others who were very good. There were African American women who competed on white teams in the North that do not appear in depth in these pages. But the relationship that the athletes in this book had with sport clearly represents a path that many other African American women of their generations used to escape poor, rural, or working-class backgrounds; travel extensively; secure a college education; and reject the cultural stereotypes of African American women. Some additional names of athletes appear throughout the text as they intersect with the athlete in each chapter. Even so, many others are absent. I hope they, in some way, still see their story in these pages. In the end, it is a story of athletic women who faced and overcame a number of challenges as they strove for excellence, whose black communities gave them strong support, and who pushed back against stereotypes that attempted to define who they were as athletes and African American women. It is a story of champions whose talent, hard work, and determination to push back against racial and gender stereotypes resulted in a spectacular leap for black women athletes of the twentieth century.

11

WHAT KAEPERNICK STARTED

A FORMER NBA PLAYER REFLECTS

Etan Thomas

Seeing All of the Venom Spewed at NFL Player Colin Kaepernick Takes Me Back to the 2003 Invasion of Iraq.

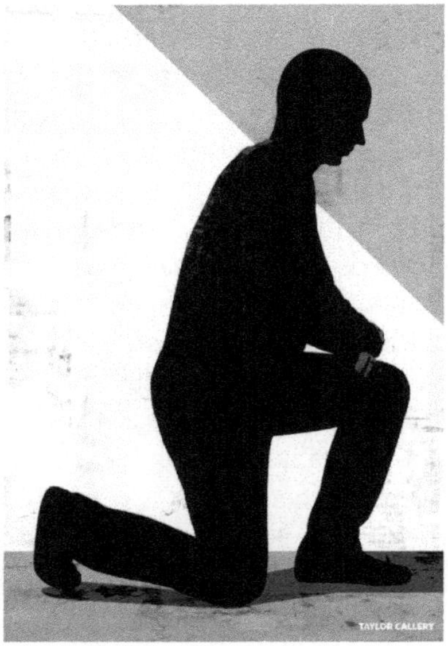

Today, even Republicans admit that there were no weapons of mass destruction, no direct connection to 9/11, and no reason to invade Iraq, but back in 2003 it was thought to be anti-American, even treasonous, to speak out against the Iraq invasion. I was playing for the Washington Wizards in the nation's capital and simply couldn't keep quiet about what I saw as blatant disrespect to our troops—sending them to die because of deliberate lies perpetuated by then-President George W. Bush. I began reciting my poems at rallies and marches around Washington, D.C. Sometimes thirty or forty people came. At other times, hundreds or even thousands showed up. I delivered each poem with the same tenacity no matter the size of the crowd. Here is an excerpt from one of my poems, titled "Bring Our Heroes Home":

> Out of the ashes of Iraq come soldiers dressed in fatigues of fire wearing helmets secured in smoke
> They've choked off the lies spewed out of the mouth of a burning bush
> The true warrior's existing wake
> Whose flames burned them at the stake
> Cremated their bodies
> And stuffed them in an urn wrapped in red, white, and blue ...

Rummaging through a forest set ablaze by one lethal match
With witty catch phrases forever attached to the side of their kingdom
Operation Iraqi Freedom Links to Al Qaeda Eminent Threats
And weapons of mass destruction ...

They've been skillfully thrown into the lion's den
Out of the frying pan and into the furnace
Their courage exceeds any measuring stick
But they can hear the footsteps of death creeping around the corner
For they've been led into the eye of the storm
Transformed into peacekeepers
Lending a helping hand for the poorly planned post-war strategy ...

I attempted to get my message out to the papers, but nobody wanted to cover it. I tried *The Washington Post* and *The Washington Times,* since those papers covered our team. But I was met with a resounding no.

Then, at one particular anti-war rally, I performed a poem called "The Field Trip." I named about ten different Republicans I wanted to take on a field trip to see the results of their policies. That rally went viral before going viral was a thing. There was no social media or Twitter back then, but soon the story of the rally was everywhere.

All the criticism leveled at Kaepernick takes me back to those days and the hate mail delivered to me at the then-MCI Center (now Verizon Center). I played with Michael Jordan and Gilbert Arenas, so I saw guys get stacks and stacks of fan mail delivered to them every day. I would get a few letters here and there, but after that rally, I started getting boxes delivered to me. Some of the letters were supportive, but a lot of them were filled with anger and hate.

I didn't have any other players speak against me the way Kaepernick has, but I did have a lot of players make it a point to come up to me during games and offer me words of support. Some of them were superstars.

I also caught a backlash from media types who disagreed with what I believed.

Today, I take my hat off to Colin Kaepernick for everything he is enduring, especially now in the age of social media. Every Tom, Dick, and Harry can develop what I call "Twitter courage" and type a hateful, evil condemnation of Colin Kaepernick. Sports writer Dave Zirin, who is my co-host on the radio show "The Collision" on WPFW 89.3 FM in Washington, D.C., once said:

"Twitter is the white hood of the twenty-first century. It's where bigots revel in their anonymity and rage against the current, where people can be both hateful and cowardly."

He is absolutely right.

Kaepernick reported that he actually received death threats as a result of his stand. That shouldn't really surprise anyone. Muhammad Ali, Mahmoud Abdul-Rauf, John Carlos, Tommie Smith, and countless other athletes who have taken a stand that was viewed as "unpatriotic" have received similar threats from cowards who hide behind anonymous letters—or, in this day and age, social media.

The criticism that has been hurled at Colin Kaepernick has been both disgusting and hypocritical.

Isn't it interesting that many of the same people, who are currently calling Kaepernick and others who have joined in the protests "unpatriotic" have been disrespecting our President and First Lady for the past eight years? Isn't it also interesting that those same people who describe Kaepernick's stance as disrespectful to veterans (although he specifically explained that he has the utmost respect for veterans) aren't as angry at George W. Bush who sent those veterans to die for a lie? Isn't it interesting that these same conservatives have voted against better health care and aid to vets after they come home?

A lot of people have a confused interpretation of patriotism. They are terribly concerned about Kaepernick but are unfazed and unconcerned with the countless veterans and current soldiers who actually need help. If you're not offended by the fact that one out of two veterans who have returned from Iraq or Afghanistan knows a fellow soldier who has attempted suicide, or by the two million vets who don't have insurance, or the 50,000 who are homeless, but you are offended by Colin Kaepernick taking a knee during the national anthem, you have greatly misplaced your patriotism.

What's beautiful to see is how Colin Kaepernick's message is spreading and how it is resonating with so many athletes, from high school football teams to Howard University cheerleaders.

At first, only 49ers teammate Eric Reid joined Kaepernick. But then more teammates, including Antoine Bethea, Eli Harold, Jaquiski Tartt, and Rashard Robinson joined in, raising their fists during the national anthem at San Francisco's September 18 game against the Carolina Panthers.

NFL player Jeremy Lane of the Seattle Seahawks sat during the national anthem. Kansas Chiefs cornerback Marcus Peters raised his fist, and told reporters he supports Kaepernick's efforts to raise awareness about our broken justice system. On *Sunday Night Football,* Patriots tight end Martellus Bennett and safety Devin McCourty also raised their fists for the national anthem.

Although he lost two endorsement deals, Denver Broncos linebacker Brandon Marshall also took a knee during the national anthem at the NFL regular season opener, and says he will continue to kneel.

Although a Miami-area police union asked deputies not to escort Dolphins unless players stand for the anthem, four Dolphins players—running back Arian Foster, safety Michael Thomas, wide receiver Kenny Stills, and linebacker Jelani Jenkins—on the fifteenth anniversary of the September 11 terrorist attacks in 2001, took a knee during the anthem after standing up for a 9/11 acknowledgment.

Rams defensive end Robert Quinn and wide receiver Kenny Britt also raised their fists. Not only are they taking the stand in solidarity with Kaepernick, but they are verbalizing and articulating exactly why they are taking that stand. Arian Foster tweeted, "Don't let the love for a symbol overrule the love for your fellow human."

Brandon Marshall was quoted as saying, "I'm not against the military. I'm not against the police or America. I'm against social injustice."

But what's even more impressive is how this message is resonating with high school athletes who, as we know, are greatly influenced by professional athletes. They are watching, learning, and taking stances of their own. Not because it's a new fad as some sports commentators remarked, in a feeble attempt to discredit and demean this movement, but because they have their own experiences with injustice and their own deeply felt reasons. Some have stood in the face of adversity, hatred, and threats of physical harm.

A Brunswick, Ohio, high school football player named Rodney Axson Jr. was threatened with lynching and called the N-word by his white teammates after he knelt to protest racism on Friday, September 2.

Garfield High School's football team and coaching staff, along with more than a half-dozen West Seattle High School players, took a knee while the national anthem played before their Friday night game.

They were not intimidated by critics including Trent Dilfer, Dabo Swinney, Kid Rock, Tony La Russa, or Kate Upton.

Mike Ditka, Jim Harbaugh, Vikings offensive lineman and Kaepernick's former teammate Alex Boone, Jason Whitlock, Boomer Esiason, Victor Cruz, Tiki Barber, U.S. Representative Lee Zeldin, and Shaquille O'Neal all use their platforms to discredit, condemn, and ridicule Colin Kaepernick and all of these other athletes for having the moral courage to stand up for what they believe in. One would think they would be just as vocal in condemning social injustice and the countless murders at the hands of the police that have gone unpunished. More than two dozen black people were killed during encounters with police in just the first six weeks after Kaepernick began protesting.

Where is their condemnation of that?

They were silent when, on September 16, police murdered unarmed Terence Crutcher in Tulsa, Oklahoma, who was guilty of having car trouble and expecting the police to help him out.

They had nothing to say when, on September 20, the Charlotte police killed a disabled black man whose name was Keith Lamont Scott, allegedly guilty of reading a book in his car.

In both of these recent cases, officers went out on paid administrative leave. As Colin Kaepernick said in his postgame interview after taking a knee during the national anthem, "There are bodies in the street and people getting paid leave and getting away with murder."

They should be outraged at that and not at whether Colin Kaepernick and other athletes are sitting or standing during the national anthem.

As a wise saying goes, "Justice will not be served until those who are unaffected are just as outraged as those who are."

Thank you, Russell Westbrook, for expressing your outrage about this case. And thank you Rajon Rondo, Iman Shumpert, Dwyane Wade, Matt Barnes, Anthony Morrow, Nick Young, Nate Robinson, and Kenny Vaccaro for speaking out about the Terence Crutcher murder in my hometown of Tulsa, Oklahoma.

Thank you, coach Steve Kerr, who when asked about Colin Kaepernick's decision to kneel during the national anthem in protest said, "No matter what side of the spectrum you're on, I would hope that every American is disgusted with what is going on around the country."

Thank you to coach Stephanie White of the Indiana Fever and the entire Indiana Fever team, who all took a knee before their playoff game.

I applaud all of the athletes for having the moral courage to withstand the backlash, the criticism, the outrage, the venom, and all of the hate, and use their position as a platform to speak out and bring awareness to an issue that has plagued our country for far too long. Much respect to them.

12

FUTURE DIRECTIONS IN RACE AND SPORT PARTICIPATION

Krystal Beamon and Chris M. Messer

Participation in athletic programs enables children and young adults to develop a wide range of skills. Moreover, it provides opportunities to develop trans-racial friendships, for entertainment, to cultivate belonging, and learn how to negotiate relationships while achieving shared goals. A staple in the U.S. economy, the sports industry generates millions of dollars in revenue in cities and states. For example, Super Bowl XLV alone was estimated to bring in between $200 and $300 million revenue to the North Dallas area (McCarthy 2011).

In terms of racism and racial hierarchies, although the U.S. athletics industry has moved beyond state-sanctioned segregation, racialized barriers to full participation remain. There are, for example, Blacks in areas of government and business at levels unmatched at any time in our nation's history. Of that we should be proud. To a degree, sports have been central to the development of anti-racist projects in the United States and have helped integrate some sports while others such as professional hockey remain predominantly White.

However, just like American society in general, work remains to be done in terms of race relations and sports. There have been great efforts to break down institutional discrimination in American society and in the sporting world. All major professional sports leagues and the NCAA are aware of the lack of minorities and women in decision-making positions and have policies in place to remedy this issue. Some progress has been made, but there remains an underrepresentation and a lack of opportunity for minority and female athletes to have professions related to sports after they are no longer on the field.

As we've highlighted throughout this book, it's not enough to simply discuss minorities as a single group that experiences the same obstacles in sport and society. Indeed, each minority group experiences unique challenges that have roots in their position in America's economic and cultural landscape. For instance, despite their cultural heritage of games, competitions, and physical activity, Native American players are rare on most current North American sports fields. Native Americans not only experience a lack of presence in sports, but also encounter negative imagery used for sports teams. This negative imagery can be seen in team names, mascots, and chants used by teams and fans. The fight to remove the stereotypical images of Native American mascots and nicknames in sports has been active for around four decades, and today involves many of the major Native American civil rights groups. Since the initiation of the debate some 40 years ago, more than 1,000 schools and colleges have abandoned their Native American mascots; however, many teams at all levels have yet to do so (Staurowsky and Baca 2004). Although slow change is not no change, significant strides remain to be made.

Similarly, Hispanics and Blacks experience their own unique challenges as well. While Hispanics disproportionately represent Major League Baseball players, Blacks disproportionately make up teams in football and basketball. There's nothing at all wrong with this fact alone. The potential problems lie in how much these groups have invested their resources and efforts to achieve what is statistically an unlikely outcome: professional status. This investment often comes with the cost of abandoning much more realistically attainable goals. And both of these groups experience unique challenges associated with identity. Hispanic players struggle to be accepted as "truly American." While the United States continues to grapple with immigration, baseball serves as a microcosmic view about attitudes and values related to what "American" means. On the other hand, Blacks are sometimes equated with an exclusively athletic identity by both themselves and society at large.

Representative Disparities

Despite the overrepresentation of certain racial and ethnic groups in certain sports, discussion should continue over a noticeable pattern of segregation. Black players are most visible in basketball and football. Hispanic players continue to show up most heavily in boxing and baseball. Hockey, golf, and tennis attract primarily White players—although the color barrier has been broken by star players such as Tiger Woods in golf and Venus Williams in tennis. Still, those athletes remain exceptions and one can't ignore a very visible absence of minorities in those sports. Segregation in sports is certainly dependent on the cultural factors we have discussed throughout this book as opposed to the stereotype of race-related physical characteristics. However, we can't ignore the equally important impact of socioeconomic status and access to sport. Golf, for instance, has less minority participation in large part because of the costs associated with playing on a regular basis. Minority groups such as Hispanics, Blacks, and Native Americans are the most economically disadvantaged in American society and therefore have much less access to golf and fewer opportunities for talent development.

Directions for Future Research

There are a number of directions that future research on race relations and athletics should take. First, it's imperative that researchers look more closely at the relationship between race and sport participation. As we've discussed at different points throughout this book, certain racial and ethnic groups disproportionately represent the majority of athletes in some sports, and in others they are severely underrepresented. Research should continue to identify the structural and socialization patterns that produce this phenomenon and critically analyze the consequences. Second, research should expand on racial and ethnic groups that are underrepresented in academic scholarship. We noted that some groups, such as Hispanics, Asians, and Native Americans, frequently go unstudied, particularly at the community level. Their experiences on any playing field need to be better understood in the larger context of sport participation and race/ethnicity. As researchers and students, we shouldn't assume that just because these groups may have very small levels of athletic participation, at least in certain sports, their experiences are unworthy of scholarly critique. In fact, we should also find out *why* these groups participate at the levels they do and the types of sport they play.

Third, scholars and students alike could glean more insight into sport and race with more research on the intersection of athletics and opportunity. We have argued, like Hartmann (2000), that sport is a contested terrain; that is, in some ways athletics can provide golden opportunities, but in other ways it can produce unrealistic expectations and a perpetuation of myths and stereotypes about racial and ethnic groups.

Bringing it All Together

As the first author sat at Rangers stadium and cheered for the home team, her kids cheered on their favorite player and they wildly chanted "CRUUUUUUZZZZZZ" along with thousands of other fans. In those moments no one is thinking "Is baseball too Hispanic?" None of the fans is concerned with immigration policies and whether Cruz shut out some "American" player for a slot on the Rangers roster. They were simply cheering on their favorite player who was getting the job done well for the home team. The home team: that is what sport creates for our society. A sense of "we-ness" that goes beyond race/ethnicity. We hope that America continues to follow the lead of athletics in this respect.

But sports are a microcosm of American society and, just as race still matters in American culture, it still matters in sports. The intersection of race and sports creates avenues for research and social commentary that go beyond the scope of the topics discussed in this book. Sports participation patterns and the segregation that we see in sports and sports administration will likely continue into the foreseeable future unless definitive steps are taken to eliminate such patterns. As we strive toward a truly color-blind society in America, sports can continue to lead the way as it has historically. Title IX opened up doors for women to participate on a much larger scale in a number of different sports. This increased access doesn't solely benefit women, but society at large. It debunks myths about women and athleticism and creates a broader appreciation for sport and its functions in society. Perhaps similar programs could be implemented with an emphasis on broadening racial and ethnic diversity across different sports, particularly at the high school level. Black women, for instance, should have just as much opportunity to participate in soccer as they do in basketball and track. Similarly, Black males should have greater access to high school sports such as baseball, which according to Keown (2011) is currently operating like a "country club" for higher-income Whites who can afford better equipment and training. Increased access to sport would ideally lead to greater diversity and further progress toward American race relations.

However, as we have illustrated throughout the course of this book, society must also work toward the development of realistic expectations. Athletes will continue to become overnight millionaires in some sports, but by far the vast majority of student-athletes won't. In fact, the vast majority won't even earn college scholarships to play sport. Therefore, it's imperative that sport be viewed only as one path to success, and arguably as one rare path to success. Athletics offers so many positive experiences and lessons to our youth and undoubtedly will continue to do so. But we must not ignore the problems that emerge as a result of sport becoming a multi-billion-dollar industry and the unique consequences for racial and ethnic groups.

Discussion Questions

1. In what ways do you think professional athletics restricts the opportunities available to men and women—particularly those from working-class backgrounds?
2. What role can professional athletics play in countering the racism that continues in the post-civil rights United States?

References

Hartmann, Douglas. 2000. "Rethinking the relationship between sport and race in American culture: Golden ghettos and contested terrain." *Sociology of Sport Journal, 17*, 229–53.

Keown, Tim. 2011. "Is Major League Baseball too Hispanic?" *ESPN*. Retrieved October 4, 2011 (http://espn.go.com/espn/commentary/story/_/id/7058357/are-there-too-many-hispanics-major-league-baseball)

McCarthy, Michael. 2011. "Super Bowl XLV set to bring record revenue to Texas." *USA Today*, (February 3). Accessed online at http://usatoday30.usatoday.com/sports/football/nfl/2011-02-03-super-bowl-revenue_N.htm

Staurowsky, Ellen, and Lawrence Baca. 2004. "Mascot controversy." Pp. 201–204 in *Native Americans in sports*, ed. C. Richard King. Armonk, NY: Sharpe Reference.

FURTHER READING

Privileged

Kyle Korver

If you have a digital edition of this book, please click on the link below to access the article:

https://www.theplayerstribune.com/en-us/articles/kyle-korver-utah-jazz-nba

If you have a print edition of this book, please use your cell phone to scan the QR code below to access the article:

Rio 2016: Gabby Douglas's Olympics Experience Fits the Pattern of How We Treat Black Female Athletes

Alex Abad-Santos

If you have a digital edition of this book, please click on the link below to access the article:

https://www.vox.com/2016/8/15/12476322/gabby-douglas-rio-olympics-racism

If you have a print edition of this book, please use your cell phone to scan the QR code below to access the article:

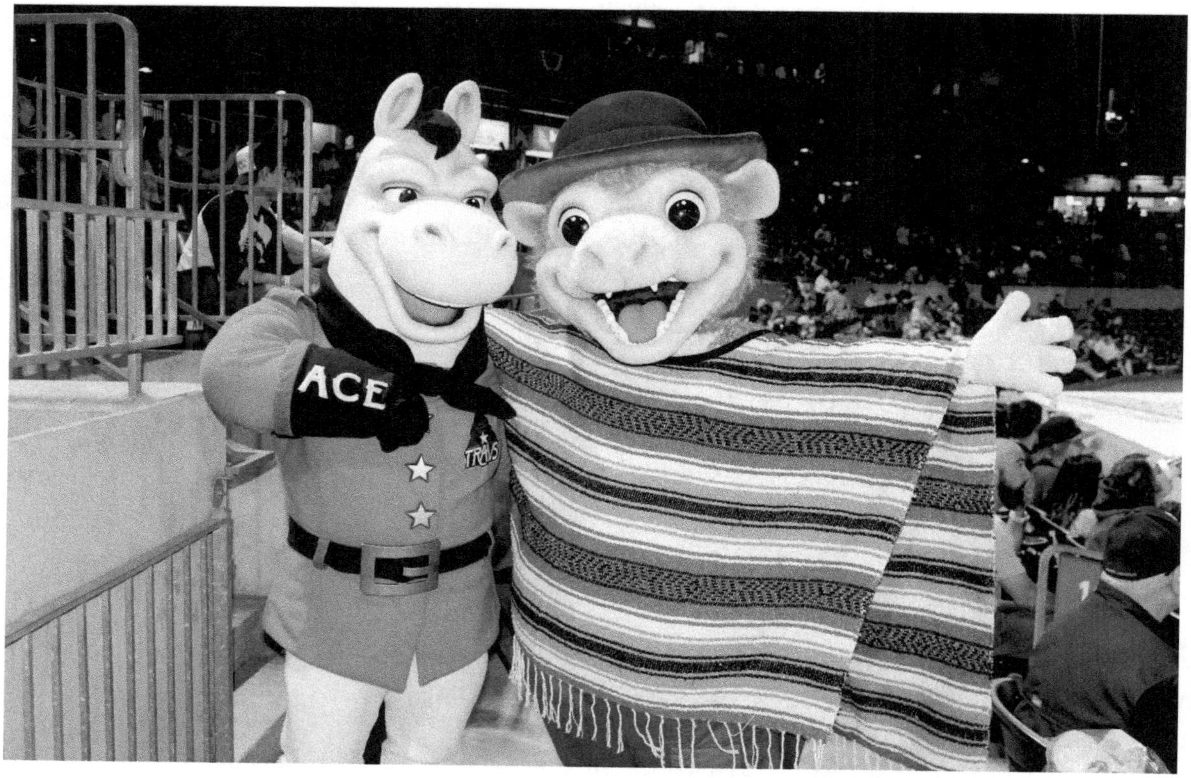
ACE
TRAVS

CHAPTER 6

SPORT AND CULTURAL APPROPRIATION

In the past 40 years, US society has changed, notably by becoming increasingly diversified. However, a celebration of acceptance of diversity does not always follow. Quite the opposite can occur when **nativists**, the dominant and native-born members of a society, see diversity as an attack or a threat to their cultural capital. This capital, acquired during hundreds of years of **colonialism** and domination, includes cultural characteristics such as English being the dominant spoken language, Christianity as the dominant practiced religion, and heterosexual lifestyles being the most authentic coupling accepted in society. The changes that occurred during the previous four decades have disrupted these supposed ideas, as a growing number of people living in the United States identify with the LGBTQ community, as well as gender nonconformance. During this time, same-sex marriages disrupted the social order that evangelical Christians attempted to impose through a rise in conservatism in politics. At the same time, the remarkable increase in the number of Spanish-speaking Latinx people in the United States has resulted in the rise of white nationalism and nativism in this country. This chapter examines **cultural appropriation** and sport. Cultural appropriation can be seen on holidays such as Cinco de Mayo, when non-Mexican people dress in sombreros and stereotypical Latinx attire, consuming tequila and tacos, unaware of what they are actually celebrating. When asked what the holiday recognizes, very few participants can answer that it was the Mexican army's successful defeat of an invading French army in Puebla, Mexico, in 1862. Their answers might include ignorant responses such as "Mexican Independence Day" or more honestly answering that they do not know. In 2017, Minor League baseball teams began a program to encourage Latinx fans to attend their local games by creating a Latin night. However, at most of these events, "Latin" really means "Mexican descent," ignoring that heterogeneous **ethnic category** of Latin. In the image at the beginning of the chapter, the Little Rock, Arkansas, Travelers' mascot is featured on the left, with the Latin mascot, an opossum dressed in Mexican colors, on the right. In sport, cultural appropriation is highly prevalent with the use of Native American images as mascots. However, there is not another living person whose image is used in these disparaging ways.

13

HOSTILE ENVIRONMENTS

ANTI-INDIAN IMAGERY, RACIAL PEDAGOGIES, AND YOUTH SPORT CULTURES

C. Richard King

A History Lesson

Today, nearly 1,500 schools, including more than 75 colleges and universities, employ pseudo-Indian imagery (Rodriguez, 1998; Staurowsky, 1999). They have a long history, dating back to the late 19th and early 20th century. They developed in conjunction with the rise of intercollegiate and professional athletics, a crisis in White masculinity, the closing of the frontier, urbanization, industrialization, and the subjugation of Native America (Churchill, 1994; Deloria, 1998; Drinnon, 1980). Over the course of the 20th century, Native American mascots have become a taken for granted element of American culture, reflecting the pleasures, possibilities, and powers they have granted their Euro-American performers. In this context, pseudo-Indian imagery in athletics and education congealed for myriad reasons, including comments by fans or sportswriters, historic relationships between an institution and indigenous peoples, and regional associations. Over the past century, they have become institutionalized icons, encrusted with memories, tradition, boosterism, administrative investment, financial rewards, and collective identity (See Connolly, 2000; Coombe, 1999; Davis, 1993; King & Springwood, 2001b; Nussell, 1994; Vanderford, 1994).

Native American mascots rely on stereotypes and cliches. They reduce indigenous peoples to a limited set of cultural features: the feathered headdress, face paint, buckskin paints, warfare, dance, and the tomahawk (chop). They recycle these key symbols to fashion moving, meaningful, and entertaining personas and performances that many take to be authentic, appropriate, and even reverent. The condensed versions of Indianness rendered through such signs and spectacles confine Native Americans within the past and typically within the popular image of the Plains warrior. Pseudo-Indian imagery, then, confines indigenous peoples within overlapping tropes of primitive difference: on the one hand, romantic renditions of noble savagery conjure bellicose warriors like Chief Illiniwek and the Fighting Illini of the University of Illinois or the Seminoles with their Chief Osceola at Florida State University; on the other hand, perverse burlesque

C. Richard King, "Hostile Environments: Anti-Indian Imagery, Racial Pedagogies, and Youth Sport Cultures," *Youth Culture and Sport: Identity, Power, and Politics*, ed. Michael D. Giardina and Michele K. Donnelly, pp. 148-152, 157-159.

parodies of the physical or cultural features of Indians invigorate the basest visions of ignobility, such as Chief Wahoo of the Cleveland Indians or Willie Wampum at Marquette University (King, 2001).

Increasingly, Native American mascots have become subject to debate (King & Springwood, 2001b; Spindel, 2000). Activists protest at sporting events featuring teams with such team spirits, while students and citizens openly express concern about school symbols; in turn, political organizations, from the American Indian Movement to the National Congress of American Indians, have denounced pseudo-Indian imagery in athletics. Together, these public challenges have fostered heated discussions and policy reassessments. Some schools like the University of Utah have altered their mascots, while many others, such as Marquette University and the University of Miami, have ended their use of pseudo-Indian imagery. Likewise, many school boards—from the Minnesota Board of Education to the Los Angeles School District—have passed resolutions requiring that schools change the Native American mascots. In addition, religious organizations and professional societies—including the Unitarian Universalist Association of Congregations, the National Education Association, the United Church of Christ, the Modern Language Association, the United Methodist Church, and the American Anthropological Association—have condemned the continued use of pseudo-Indian icons in education and athletics. And at the national level, the United States Commission on Civil Rights and the Trademark Trial and Appeal Board have taken stands against Native American mascots. Over the past quarter century, the total number of symbols has dropped noticeably. By one estimate nearly 1,500 Native American mascots have been changed, retired, or reworked since 1970 (Suzan Shown Harjo, personal communication, December 2, 2001).

Miseducation

Although it may be easy to forget when witnessing thousands of fans do the tomahawk chop or when reading the highlights of a sensational game, Native American mascots actually perform a pedagogical function concerning race, culture, and history. Native American mascots are quite literally teaching machines. Playing Indian at half-time and the associated commercial products and cultural practices associated with it address citizen-subjects within a number of interlocking "sites of pedagogy" (Dileo, 2002), including sports stadia, pep rallies, parades, and half-time shows, the hallways and classrooms of countless schools, media coverage, commercial ventures between schools or teams and corporations, public appearances by embodied mascots, as well as, pennants, tee-shirts, and baseball caps worn by fans. Importantly, the use of anti-Indian imagery, names, and logos in association with athletics does not impart racial lessons in isolation. Instead, it teaches through complex intertextual, symbolic, and performative dialogues with other formulations of Indianness, such as movies, commodities and advertising, the news media, boy scouts and similar youth groups, biased historical accounts, and fiction (see Berkhofer, 1978; Bird, 1996; Whitt, 1995), and with constructions of other forms of racialized difference, especially whiteness and blackness (see King & Springwood, 2001a). Native American mascots educate, or, as Pewewardy (1991, 1998, 2001) and Staurowsky (1999) would prefer, *miseducate*, the public about cultural difference, history, race relations, and what it means to be a citizen-subject.

Obviously, as detailed above, the use of Indian imagery in athletics reiterates false renderings of indigenous peoples. It reduces them to cartoon characters and well worn cultural clichés of the Chief, the brave, the warrior, the clown. It traps Native Americans with the past, in perpetual, unwinnable conflict with the superior White man. It confines them most often to the horse cultures of the plain, adorned in flowing headdresses and beautiful buckskin. It misappropriates and reinvents indigenous spirituality, dance, and material culture for the pleasure of largely White audiences. In 1999, the Society of Indian Psychologists of the Americas outlined the consequences of such stereotyping:

> We believe that it establishes an unwelcome academic environment for Indian students, staff, and faculty and contributes to the miseducation of all members of the campus community ... Stereotypical and historically inaccurate images of Indians in general interfere with learning about them by creating, supporting, and maintaining oversimplified and inaccurate views of indigenous peoples and cultures.

Perhaps most importantly, Native American mascots always have opened as occasions for the fashioning of the self as well as the Other: they construct White citizen-subjects as proud heirs of once great people sadly gone, reverent individuals who belong to community and nation, powerful conquerors and rightful owners of place and history, and men (and to a lesser extent women) privileged to honor and imitate imagined and invented alters, while rendering Indigenous others as inhuman objects and deaden masks, demonized threats to civilization and civility, romanticized containers of desire, liminal figures of (transgressive) possibility, and prized, profitable trophies testifying to the triumphant fatalism of EuroAmerican conquest. Playing Indian at half-time not only communicates deeply held values about what it means to be a (White) man in a broader social community, but also rewrites the history of the social as well. In fact, such symbols and spectacles of Indianness alternately underscore EuroAmerican triumph and superiority (the metaphoric taking from the vanquished enemy, the Indian head as trophy, the Indian name as talisman) and actually narrates the past through ritual claims to culture and place, ranging from mimicking dance and dress to mockingly encoding historical peace offerings. In a very real way, Native American mascots foster the rote memorization of how to live as racialized citizen-subjects: who won the war, who is superior, who is a citizen (Strong 2004), who can take from whom, who can take pleasure in mimicking and mocking whom, what happened in the past, what is fun, and so on. Indeed, the continued use of Indian imagery in athletics offers lessons in White supremacy (Staurowsky, 2007).

Oddly, many Americans suggest that Indian imagery in athletics honors indigenous peoples. In effect, Native American mascots contribute to a dominant (mis)reading of race and racism that tends to suggest racism is negative, located in the past, discernible in the malicious and ill intentioned actions a few individuals, and not related to their beliefs and behaviors. In other words, such symbols and spectacles which evoke (White) tradition, often recycle gendered notions of valor, bravery, and strength, appear authentic, seemingly dignified, and above all else, look "positive" do not register as racial symbols for most EuroAmericans desperate to live in a color-blind society, but rather reaffirm for them a sense of belonging, pleasure, respect, and naturalness of difference. As a consequence, Native American mascots perpetuate what Joyce King (1991, 5) has dubbed dysconscious racism,

> an uncritical habit of mind (that is, perceptions, attitudes, assumptions and beliefs) that justifies inequity and exploitation by accepting the existing order of things as given. It involves identification with an ideological viewpoint which admits no fundamentally alternative vision of society.

Cornell Pewewardy (2001, 258) suggests that the ubiquity of mascots, their resonance with common sense, and the constant repetition of sanctioned and spontaneous antics associated with them numbs citizen-subjects, encouraging them to take for granted the existing social arrangements, while failing to equip them with the critical capacity or will to read them differently.

Ultimately, the lessons taught by Native American mascots are deeply anti-Indian. Anti-Indianism, according to Elizabeth Cook-Lynn (2001, xx), has four key elements:

> [I]t is the sentiment that results in the unnatural death of Indians. Anti Indianism is that which treats Indians and their tribes as if they do not exist .... Second, Anti-Indianism is that which denigrates, demonizes, and insults being Indian in America. The third trait of Anti-Indianism is the use of historical event and experience to place the blame on Indians for an unfortunate and dissatisfying history. And, finally, Anti-Indianism is that which exploits and distorts Indian beliefs and cultures. All of these traits have conspired to isolate, to expunge or expel, to menace, to defame.

The continued use of American Indian imagery, nicknames, and logos clearly embody all of these elements. Of equal importance, so too do the practices and arguments employed by educational institutions to defend such symbols and spectacles of Indianness.

References

Berkhofer, R. F. (1978). *The white man's Indian: Images of the American Indian from Columbus to present.* New York: Vintage/Random House.

Bird, S. E. (Ed.) (1996). *Dressing in feathers: The construction of the Indian in American popular culture.* Boulder, CO: Westview.

Churchill, W. (1994). Let's spread the fun around. In *Indians are us? Culture and genocide in native north America* (pp. 65–72). Monroe, ME: Common Courage Press.

Connolly, M. R. (2000). What in a name? A historical look at Native American related nicknames and symbols at three U.S. universities. *Journal of Higher Education 71*(5), 515–547.

Cook-Lynn, E. (2001). *Anti-Indianism in North America: A voice from Tatekeya's earth.* Urbana: University of Illinois Press.

Coombe, R. J. (1999). Sports trademarks and somatic politics: Locating the law in critical cultural studies. In R. Martin & T. Miller (Eds.), *SportCult* (pp. 262–288). Minneapolis: University of Minnesota Press.

Davis, L. (1993). Protest against the use of native American mascots: A challenge to traditional, American identity. *Journal of Sport and Social Issues, 17* (1): 9–22.

Deloria, P. (1998). *Playing Indian.* New Haven, CT: Yale University Press.

Dileo, J. (2002). The sites of pedagogy. *Symploke 10* (1): 7–12.

Drinnon, R. (1980). *Facing west: The metaphysics of Indian-hating and empire building.* Minneapolis, MN: University of Minnesota Press.

King, C. R. (2001). Uneasy indians: Creating and contesting Native American mascots at Marquette university. In C.R. King and C. F. Springwood (Eds.), *Team spirits: Essays on the history and significance of Native American mascots,* (pp. 281–303). Lincoln: University of Nebraska Press.

King, C. R., & Springwood, C. F. (2001a). *Beyond the cheers: Race as spectacle in college sports.* Albany: State University of New York Press.

King, C. R., & Springwood, C.F. (Eds.). (2001b). *Team spirits: Essays on the history and significance of native American mascots.* Lincoln: University of Nebraska.

King, J. E. (1991). Dysconscious racism: Ideology, identity, and miseducation of teachers. *Journal of Negro Education, 60*(2), 133–146.

Nuessel, F. (1994). Objectionable sports team designations. *Names: A Journal of Onomastics 42*, 101–119.

Pewewardy, C. D. (2001). Educators and mascots: Challenging contradictions. In C. R. King and C. F. Springwood (Eds.), *Team spirits: Essays on the history and significance of Native American mascots* (pp. 257–279). Lincoln: University of Nebraska Press.

Pewewardy, C. D. (1998). Fluff and feathers: Treatment of American Indians in the literature and the classroom. *Equity and Excellence in Education, 3*, 69–76.

Pewewardy, C. D. (1991). Native American mascots and imagery: The struggle of unlearning Indian stereotypes. *Journal of Navaho Education, 9*(1), 19–23.

Rodriquez, R. (1998). Plotting the assassination of Little Red Sambo: Psychologists join war against racist campus mascots. *Black Issues in Higher Education, 15*(8), 20–24.

Society of Indian Psychologists of the Americas. (1999). Statement against the continued use of Indian symbols. Retrieved July 19, 2004, from http://aistm.org/society_of_indian_psychologists_.htm

Spindel, C. (2000). *Dancing at halftime: Sports and the controversy over American Indian mascots.* New York: New York University Press.

Staurowsky, E.J. (2007). "`You Know, We Are All Indian': Exploring White Power and Privilege in Reactions to the NCAA Native American Mascot Policy." *Journal of Sport & Social Issues, 31*(1): 61-76.

Staurowsky, E. J. (1999). American Indian imagery and the miseducation of America. *Quest*, 51(4), 382–392.

Strong, P.T. (2004). "The Mascot Slot: Cultural Citizenship, Political Correctness, and Pseudo-Indian Sports Symbols." *Journal of Sport & Social Issues, 28*(1): 79-87.

Vanderford, H. (1996). What's in a name? Heritage or hatred: The school mascot controversy. *Journal of Law and Education, 25*, 381–388.

Whitt, L. A. (1995). Cultural imperialism and the marketing of native America. *American Indian Culture and Research Journal, 19*(3), 1–31.

14

THE NATIVE AMERICAN EXPERIENCE

RACISM AND MASCOTS IN PROFESSIONAL SPORTS

Krystal Beamon and Chris M. Messer

Early European contact with Native American tribes resulted in cultural and physical **genocide.** According to the 2010 census, Native Americans make up less than 1 percent of the total population of the United States of America. This once thriving group that numbered over 10 million persons and spoke over 700 languages prior to colonization is projected to make up less than 0.5 percent of the American population by 2050 (Schaefer 2011). Today, the culture and language of many tribes are extinct, with tribal elders, anthropologists, and other scholars fighting to preserve and pass on remnants of both for future generations. Compared to other racial and ethnic groups, Native Americans have the highest rates of poverty, alcoholism, and suicide, and the lowest rate of educational attainment (Center for Native American Youth 2012).

The term Native American refers to an extremely diverse group of people. Although similarities exist, each tribe has a distinct culture with varying customs, religious and spiritual beliefs, kinship and political systems, and history. Due to the wide use of stereotypes in the media, isolation of Native Americans on reservations, and the invisible nature of mixed-raced Native Americans in urban areas, most Americans conceive of "Indians" in a very narrow manner. **Pan-Indianism,** or the growing solidarity among Native Americans, has created a tendency to focus less on tribal heritage and more on common injustices that Native Americans face as a whole. A key source of frustration relates to a set of cultural stereotypes that narrowly depict Native Americans as a remnant of history filled with savagery. More specifically, according to many pan-Indian civil rights groups, the commercialization of Native American images and the use of Native American mascots perpetuate a minimalistic understanding of their diverse experiences and cultures (Nuessel 1994; Williams 2007). It's important first to discuss the historical presence of Native Americans in sport, and later, the surfacing of mascots that depict Native American images.

Native Americans in Sports

Historically, Native American tribes have been physically active in games and athletics. Traditional Native American sports such as stickball, lacrosse, archery, running, and canoeing were often connected to spiritual, political, or economic worldviews (King 2004). They were important in training children, and the outcomes often held ritual significance. In the late 19th century, Native American boarding schools were developed with aims to "kill the Indian and save the man," taking Indian children out of their homes away from their families and indoctrinating them with European language, culture, religion, and sports (Churchill 2004: 14). While many Native Americans continued to participate in traditional games and sports, this forced **assimilation**, a form of ethnic genocide in boarding schools, produced a decline in traditional games.

Organized interscholastic sports were institutionalized by European Americans as a form of cultural control. Sports were used as a tool of domination in which Native American boys learned to see their traditional games as "inferior" and were taught that there were more "civilized" ways to compete. For example, according to Gems, football "taught Indians rules, discipline, and civilization" (1998: 146), which were considered European American virtues. The White headmasters perceived sports as an effective tool in channeling males into more acceptable European roles and behavior. As an unintended consequence, many boarding schools fielded successful athletic teams in football and baseball, taking on and winning against collegiate powerhouses such as Harvard and Syracuse between 1900 and 1932 (Haggard 2004).

The Carlisle Indian School and Haskell Institute produced exceptional athletes, such as Jim Thorpe, who is considered one of the most versatile athletes in American history. A Sac and Fox tribal member, Thorpe played professional baseball, football, and basketball and also won gold medals in the 1912 Olympics for the pentathlon and decathlon. He attended the Haskell Institute in Lawrence, Kansas as a youth (Wheeler 1979). As Gems (1998) notes, athletic participation at such schools allowed Native Americans in the early 1900s to assert their racial identity,

> by providing a collective memory of self-validation and the creation of kindred heroes as they successfully tested themselves against the beliefs of Social Darwinism and dispelled notions of white dominance ... In that sense football proved to be not only an assimilative experience, but a resistive and liberating one as well.
>
> (Gems 1998: 148)

No netheless, there was an obvious absence of Native American athletes reaching national success between World War II and the 1964 victory of Billy Mills at the Olympic Games (King 2004). Mills began running at the Haskell Institute in Kansas as a youth and became the second Native American to win a gold medal at the Olympics (Jim Thorpe was the first). His win in the 10,000-meter run was unexpected as he competed against a world record holder from Australia, Ron Clarke (Mills 2009). Mills often discussed why many traditional Native Americans did not participate fully in organized sports. Mills believed that engaging in a sporting program that does not acknowledge cultural heritage creates a fear among Native American athletes, a fear of going too far into White society and losing one's "Indianness" while participating in mainstream sports (Simpson 2009: 291).

In 1968, the American Indian Movement (AIM) was launched in Minneapolis, Minnesota and soon thereafter spread across the country. The movement sought to address problems affecting the Native American community such as poverty, police harassment, and treaty violations. During its initial stages, the movement was known for its pan-Indian philosophy and protests. Perhaps the most famous protest occurred in 1973 at Wounded Knee, South Dakota at the Pine Ridge Indian Reservation. Armed members of the movement occupied the area in protest at Native American poverty and U.S. government treaty violations. The event culminated in a 71-day standoff with federal law enforcement and ended only after two Native Americans were killed (Banks and Erdoes 2004). Today, AIM continues to fight against the same problems of poverty and treaty violations and also actively protests the use of Native American mascots (American Indian Movement n.d.).

Other organizations such as the National Indian Athletic Association (NIAA), founded in 1973, and the Native American Sports Council (NASC), founded in1993, were created to promote athletic participation and excellence among Native American athletes throughout North America. Today, the NASC sponsors sports leagues and provides training and other forms of support to potential Olympians. These organizations support the development of Native Americans through fitness, community involvement, and boosting self-esteem (Kalambakal 2004). Formerly a colonial tool used to force Native American children of both sexes to reject their heritage and adopt European-American cultural norms, these athletic organizations employ sports to steer youngsters in a positive direction and reduce the high rates of suicide, drug and alcohol use, and gang activity on the reservations (Kalambakal 2004). Through both the NIAA and NASC, sports education, sports camps, and clinics have led to an increase in Native American participation in mainstream sports in the Olympics, college, and professional sports; however, this "trend has yet to produce the numbers experienced during the early twentieth century" (Haggard 2004: 226).

Native American athletes are hardly visible in contemporary sports. Aside from a few teams and individual athletes in segregated Indian schools, Native American sport participation has been limited by many factors. Poverty, poor health, lack of equipment and facilities, and a lack of cultural understanding by those who control sports, as well as academic unpreparedness and negative academic stereotypes of Native American student-athletes, has limited the non-reservation sports opportunities of these athletes (Simpson 2009). This cultural group remains underrepresented as athletes at all levels despite the obvious talent and the popularity of basketball on Native American reservations. However, this talent garnered recent attention with the story of two sisters on the University of Louisville's women's basketball team, which finished as the national championship runner-up in 2013. Shone and Jude Schimmel were raised on the Umatilla Reservation in Oregon and were considered exceptional local talent. Playing a style they call "rez ball," the sisters captivated local audiences growing up. Their national success has led to an explosion of interest in basketball among the local reservation youth and a sense of pride among Native Americans in general (Block 2013).

Youth sports are associated with forms of capital including social capital that can advantage Native youth. For example, children and youth who participate in organized sports perform better academically, are less likely to drink or do drugs, have higher self-esteem, and lower rates of obesity and diabetes (Bailey 2006; Broh 2002; Eitle and Eitle 2002; Ewing et al. 2002; Pate et al. 2000). Native Americans are underrepresented in youth sport leagues and have higher rates of alcoholism, high school dropout, suicide, obesity, and diabetes than any other minority group (Bachman et al. 1991; Center for Native American Youth 2012; Gray and Smith 2003). Greater participation may be a valuable resource for Native American youth.

Native Americans also remain underrepresented at the elite levels. In NCAA Division I, II, and III sports, Native American men and women make up 0.4 percent of student-athletes (NCAA 2012b). As illustrated in Figure 14.1, White men and women make up the largest majority of NCAA Division I, II, and III student-athletes in most sports, while Native Americans are widely underrepresented in all sports. In fact, even in lacrosse, a sport thought to have roots in the Cherokee traditional game "stickball," Native American men and women make up less than 0.5 percent of collegiate players. The highest representation of Native American NCAA student-athletes is seen in softball, where Native American women make up 0.7 percent of all players.

	All sports (Division I)	Football	Basketball	Track and field	Soccer	Baseball	Softball	Lacrosse
White Men	62.5	55.1	43.5	64.9	68.5	84.7		88.2
White Women	70.6		55.7	66.2	80.7		81.1	88.2
Black Men	29.4	35.4	45.5	21.6	7.2	3.9		2.7
Black Women	16		32.7	20.4	3.7		5.8	2.8
Hispanic Men	4.2	3	2.8	4.6	9.9	5.6		1.5
Hispanic Women	4.2		3	4.1	5.6		6	2.1
Native American Men	0.4	0.5	0.2	0.4	0.2	0.4		0.3
Native American Women	0.4		0.4	0.4	0.3		0.7	0.2
Asian Men	2	0.7	0.5	1.4	1.6	0.9		0.9
Asian Women	2.4		0.8	1.4	1.5		1.2	1.2

FIGURE 14.1 NCAA Student-Athlete Racial Composition by Selected Sport 2010–2011

Source: Lapchick 2011

While they are underrepresented as students on college campuses along with most minority groups, Native Americans are far less represented as collegiate athletes compared to Blacks and Hispanics. In fact, the most visible representation of Native American culture in popular commercialized sports is found among mascots. In addition to the many professional sports teams, hundreds of high schools and close to 100 universities have Native American images for mascots and nicknames—not to mention the countless little league and peewee teams that follow suit using these images to represent their teams. Along with class and access issues in youth sports, these disparaging mascots may be linked to the lack of participation of Natives in youth sports and the benefits that go along with participation.

Contemporary Racism in Sports: Native American Symbols as Mascots

Native American mascots have remained a common fixture in the world of athletics at all levels from peewee leagues to professional teams. The Washington Redskin has been the mascot of one of the most popular NFL teams, located in our nation's capital, since 1932. The term is considered a disparaging reference to many Native American people. According to Stapleton (2001), "redskin" is a term with a 400-year history and first emerged in sport during a time when the American government actively sought to assimilate Native Americans. In his book *Skull Wars*, Thomas (2000) writes,

> There is today no single word more offensive to Indian people then the term "redskins," a racial epithet that conjures up the American legacy of bounty hunters bringing in wagon loads of Indian skulls and corpses—literally the bloody dead bodies were known as "redskins"—to collect their payments.
>
> (p. 204)

Although many Native Americans are offended by the term, 88 percent of Americans surveyed oppose a name change for the team (Sigelman 2001).

In a survey of the top 10 most common team mascots, most were birds or beasts of prey, with the exception of two: "Warriors" and "Indians" (Franks 1982). The only two nickname categories that are not predatory animals refer to Native Americans. Many would ask, what's the problem? Are we not honoring indigenous people for being such fierce warriors?

To perceive Native Americans through the eyes of mascots and sports nicknames creates a myopic and inaccurate version of the rich traditions, culture, history, and contemporary existence of the population. Native American mascots are based on the stereotypical "Cowboy and Indian" Wild West images of America's indigenous peoples, with no regard for the diverse cultures and religious beliefs of tribal groups. This manner of stereotyping Native Americans began very early upon European contact. Colonizers portrayed "Indians" as "barbaric," "wild," "bestial," and most of all "savage" (Berkhofer 1978). In fact, Americans' view of "Indians" as predatory beasts has been ingrained from the inception of our nation. George Washington wrote that "Indians" were "wolves and beasts who deserve nothing from whites but total ruin," and President Andrew Jackson stated that troops should seek out "Indians" to "root them out of their dens and kill Indian women and their whelps" (Stannard 1992: 240–41). Racist and dehumanizing descriptions produced mass fear of Native Americans as an entire race or category of people. This fear negates the concept of "honoring" tribes as the basis for naming teams as fierce warriors or other Native American-derived images.

As America grew, these stereotypes were used to justify the systematic genocide of Native Americans, as they were seen as a threat to the safety of colonizers. These images remain a part of American culture, as many Americans continue to visualize the image of a "savage warrior" with feathers and war paint when thinking of Native Americans. One can go into any costume shop and find a Native American costume complete with tomahawk and a feathered headdress. These images have become embraced by **popular culture** and controlled by the **dominant group** instead of Native Americans themselves.

Activism Around Native American Imagery

Native American mascots and the use of Native American imagery in advertising and branding (i.e., Land O'Lakes butter, Sue Bee honey, Jeep Cherokee, Crazy Horse Malt Liquor, Winnebagos) grew during the era of racial segregation and legalized discrimination in America (Meerskin 2012). The use of Native American peoples as mascots ranges from generic titles such as Indians, Braves, Warriors, or Savages to specific tribal designations such as Seminoles, Apaches, or Illini. These have been prevalent since the turn of the century, at a time when Little Black Sambo, Frito Bandito, and other racially insensitive branding was commonplace in "less enlightened times" (Graham 1993: 35). While Little Black Sambo and Uncle Rastus have long since been abandoned, the equally insensitive **Chief Wahoo** remains. These images exaggerate physical and cultural aspects of Native Americans and reduce them to one stereotypical representation: savage warrior.

The fight to remove the stereotypical images of Native American mascots and nicknames in sport has been active for nearly four decades. It occurred alongside the **civil rights movement** of the 1960s as the **National Congress of American Indians** (**NCAI**) began to challenge the use of stereotypical imagery in print and other forms of media (Staurowsky and Baca 2004). The use of Native American mascots also fell under attack when this campaign was launched in 1968. NCAI contended that the use of Native American imagery was not only racist but further reproduced the perception of Native American peoples as sub-human. By 1969 universities began to respond, as Dartmouth College changed its nickname from "the Indians" to "Big Green." Many followed suit, including the universities of Oklahoma, Marquette, and Syracuse, which all dropped Indian nicknames in the 1970s. Currently, an estimated 1,000 academic institutions have relinquished use of Native American mascots or nicknames.

Other institutions have resisted and remain invested in retaining their racist mascots. Close to 1,400 high schools and 70 colleges and universities have refused to cede to calls for change (Staurowsky and Baca 2004). Although Native Americans protest at every home opener with signs that read "We are human beings, not Mascots," MLB's Cleveland Indians maintain the use of the caricatured Chief Wahoo. The Washington Redskins have lost trademark protection, but continue to fight through litigation to maintain the use of the team's mascot. The University of Illinois Fighting Illini fought to maintain their mascot, **Chief Illiniwek**, amid major controversy for over a decade before finally retiring the chief in 2007. The Florida State Seminoles also maintain the use of their Native American imagery, citing an endorsement from the Seminole tribe as justification. All argue that they are honoring the history of Native Americans by using them as mascots. For example, the Cleveland Indians proclaim that the team's designation was chosen to honor the first Native American to play professional baseball, Louis Francis Sockalexis. The University of Illinois argued that their mascot was an honor to the extinct tribe that once inhabited the state. Although Florida State University has been given "permission" to maintain the use of its mascot and nickname by the Seminole tribe and its chief, "there are American Indians protesting outside every Florida State game, including some Seminole people. They say the mascot looks like a Lakota who got lost in an Apache dressing room riding a Nez Perce horse" (Spindel 2002: 16).

Many organizations using Native American designations argue that some Native American individuals and tribal groups have no issue with the use of the mascots and indeed feel a sense of pride. And many fans of these teams agree. In his study of local public opinion, Callais (2010) found that supporters of retaining Native American mascots base their position on maintaining tradition and promoting a color-blind society through a tribute to Native Americans.

While some individual tribes and persons may approve of this practice, all major Native American organizations have denounced it and called for a cessation of the use of their images as mascots, nicknames, and in the branding of products. Mascots are "manufactured images" of Native Americans, and their continued promotion results in a loss of power to control use of those images.

> Indigenous mascots exhibit either idealized or comical facial features and "native" dress, ranging from body-length feathered (usually turkey) headdresses to more subtle fake buckskin attire or skimpy loincloths. Some teams and supporters display counterfeit Indigenous paraphernalia, including tomahawks, feathers, face paints, and symbolic drums and pipes. They also use mock Indigenous behaviors such as the tomahawk chop, dances, chants, drumbeats, war-whooping, and symbolic scalping.
>
> (Pewewardy 1999: 2)

These images were manufactured by their respective schools, universities, and teams. They were created in the minds of those who established them during a time of racial hatred, stereotyping, and when Native Americans were seen as a threat (Callais 2010). The "costumes" of the mascots are derived from stereotypical and widely oversimplified views of a diverse group of people. In reality, each feather and bead, the facial paint, and especially the dances have a distinct, significant, deeply spiritual, and religious meaning to each tribal group. Particular dances mark "the passage of time, the changing of the seasons, a new status in a person's life" and "dancing expresses and consolidates a sense of belonging" (Spindel 2002: 189). In the eyes of many Native Americans, to put on the "costume" and perform a "war dance" at halftime is to mock their religion. How would it go over to have a team designated the "Black Warriors" with a mascot named Chief Watutsi dressed in a loincloth dancing around with a spear? While this mascot would not probably last a single day, Native Americans have been unable to have the use of their images stopped, despite a 40-year struggle to do so.

All in Fun?

Charlene Teters, the Native American activist who called national attention to the University of Illinois fighting Illini, describes how her children reacted when they first witnessed Chief Illiniwek in the documentary *In Whose Honor* (Rosenstein 1997). She describes her son sinking into his chair as he tried to become "invisible." One of the primary arguments against the use of Native American mascots is how it affects children of all races, but especially Native American children. The flippant and inaccurate depiction of Native American culture and identity "causes many young indigenous people to feel shame about who they are as human beings" (Pewewardy 1999: 342). These feelings become a part of the identity and self-image of Native American children, working together with the objective experiences of poverty and deprivation to create low self-esteem and high rates of depression (Pewewardy 1999). One in five Native American youth attempts suicide before the age of 20. In fact, suicide is the second leading cause of death for Native American youth between the ages of 15 and 24 (Center for Native American Youth 2012). This is two and a half times higher than the national average. While there are many factors that contribute to this statistic, such as poverty and drug and alcohol abuse, the use of Native American mascots further damages the self-image of Native American youth. Mascots dehumanize Native Americans and present images, sacred rituals, and other symbols in a way that negates the reverence instilled in Native children, thus negatively impacting their self-esteem. In fact, the American Psychological Association (2001) states emphatically that the use of Native American mascots perpetuates stigmatization of the group and has negative implications for perceptions of self among Native American children and adolescents.

For non-indigenous children, the use of Native American stereotypes as mascots perpetuates the mythical "Cowboys and Indians" view of the group. In a study conducted by Children Now, most of the children studied were found to perceive Native Americans as disconnected from their own way of life (Children Now 1999). Debbie Reese, a Nambe' Pueblo who travels across the country educating children and teachers concerning Native American stereotypes, recounts the many times that children described native people as "exotic," "mythical," or "extinct" and asked if she drove cars or rode horses (Spindel 2002: 224). Most Americans do not come into meaningful contact with traditional Native Americans very often, if at all. Thus, these stereotypical images of mascots and mythical beings are how we learn about Native American culture. Unfortunately, they disallow Americans from visualizing "Indians" as real people, but encourage viewing them as fierce warriors or even clowns dancing around with tomahawks, war paint, and feathered headdresses.

Children and adults alike are profoundly influenced by stereotypical images. The **stereotype threat** is a popular social psychological theory that has been researched empirically since introduced to the literature in 1995 (Steele and Aronson 1995). Claude Steele, a Stanford University professor of social psychology, defines a stereotype threat as "the pressure that a person can feel when she is at risk of confirming, or being seen to confirm a negative stereotype about her group" (Steele and Davies 2003: 311). For instance, when women are reminded that they are women, they perform poorly on math tests due to the stereotype that women are not good at math (Spencer, Steele, and Quinn 1999). Applied to the stereotypical images of Native Americans perpetuated through mascots, these violent and trivialized images may be associated with the lowered self-images of Native youth or the current statistic in which violence accounts for 75 percent of deaths among Native Americans between the ages of 12 and 20 (Center for Native American Youth 2012).

The use of Native American mascots is an example of institutional discrimination. Chief Wahoo and other such images have become as American as baseball itself. They are ingrained into the inter-working of our society and its institutions. Major societal institutions such as the economy, sports, and education discriminate against Native Americans by continuing to denigrate living human beings through mascots and team designations. Perhaps if the elite levels of sport (professional and inter-collegiate) terminated their use of Native American mascots and raised awareness on the issue, K–12 schools would follow suit. This could serve as an instructional piece for schools as they confront the issue of stereotyping, a process that begins early in one's childhood.

The U.S. Civil Rights Commission released a statement in 2001 condemning the use of Native American mascots. In fact, the National Congress of American Indians, American Indian Movement, National Education Association, National Association for the Advancement of Colored People (NAACP), countless state and local school boards, and the American Psychological Association have all issued similar resolutions. Such images and symbols have been found to perpetuate stereotypes and stigma-tization, and negatively affect the mental health and behaviors of Native American people (American Psychological Association 2001). As stated by Native American activist Dennis Banks, "what part of ouch do they not understand?" (Rosenstein 1997).

Conclusion

The issues that Native Americans currently experience in sport—underrepresentation and stereo-typing—bring us back to the image of sport as contested terrain. While many believe that the use of Native American mascots is a way of paying tribute, many Native Americans themselves battle to gain more control over the portrayal of their own identity. Athletes are often portrayed as "savages" and "animals," images that Native Americans have fought hard to be disassociated from. And while universities and professional teams generate millions of dollars from the sale of merchandise using Native American imagery, "real" Native Americans remain one of the most impoverished racial groups in society. With a group that experiences disproportionately high rates of dropout, obesity, and suicide, perhaps more effort should be spent on encouraging Native American youth athletics participation, which may help reduce these very problems. Furthermore, their heightened level of participation in sport could also result in society adopting a more positive outlook and understanding of Native Americans, an identification that goes beyond equating Native Americans and sports with mascots.

Discussion Questions

1. How do you feel about the use of Native American mascots? Do they dishonor Native Americans?
2. Under what circumstances, if any, would it be acceptable to use Caucasian Americans such as the Puritans as sports mascots?
3. What stereotypes exist of a group to which you belong? How would you respond if those stereo-types were used for marketing brands of food, automobiles, or professional sports teams?

4. How can this issue be resolved? Should all teams that have Native American designations be forced to find alternative nicknames or mascots? Why or why not?

References

American Indian Movement. n.d. "National coalition on racism in sports and media." Accessed online at http://www.aimovement.org/ncrsm/index.html

American Psychological Association. 2001. "An emergency action of the board of directors: Resolution against racism and in support of the goals of the 2001 United Nations world conference against racism, racial discrimination, xenophobia, and related intolerance." Accessed online at http://www.apa.org/pi/racismresolution.html

Bachman, Jerald, John Wallace, Patrick O'Malley, Lloyd Johnston, Candace Kurth, and Harold Neighbors. 1991. "Racial/Ethnic differences in smoking, drinking, and illicit drug use among American high school seniors, 1976–89." *American Journal of Public Health*, 81, 372–77.

Bailey, Richard. 2006. "Physical education and sport in schools: A review of benefits and outcomes." *Journal of School Health*, *76*, 397–401.

Banks, Dennis, and Richard Erdoes. 2004. *Ojibwa warrior: Dennis Banks and the rise of the American Indian Movement*. Norman, OK: University of Oklahoma Press.

Berkhofer, Robert. 1978. *White man's Indian: Images of American Indians from Columbus to the present*. New York: Random House.

Block, Melissa. 2013. "Two sisters bring Native American pride to women's NCAA." *NPR*. Retrieved April 8, 2013 (http://www.npr.org/2013/04/08/176597459/two-sisters-bring-native-america-bride-to-womens-ncaa)

Broh, Beckett. 2002. "Linking extracurricular programming to academic achievement: Who benefits and why?" *Sociology of Education*, *75*, 69–95.

Callais, Todd. 2010. "Controversial mascots: Authority and racial hegemony in the maintenance of deviant symbols." *Sociological Focus*, *43*, 61–81.

Center for Native American Youth. 2012. "Fast facts on Native American youth and Indian Country." Accessed online at http://www.aspeninstitute.org/sites/default/files/content/upload/1302012%20Fast%20Facts.pdf

Children Now. 1999. "A different world: Native American children's perceptions of race and class in the media." Accessed online at http://www.childrennow.org/uploads/documents/different_world_native_americans_1999.pdf

Churchill, Ward. 2004. *Kill the Indian, save the man: The genocidal impact of American Indian residential schools*. San Francisco, CA: City Lights Books.

Eitle, Tamela, and David Eitle. 2002. "Race, cultural capital, and the educational effects of participation in sports." *Sociology of Education*, *75*, 123–46.

Ewing, Martha, Lori Gano-Overway, Crystal Branta, and Vern Seefeldt. 2002. "The role of sports in youth development." Pp. 31–47 in *Paradoxes of Youth and Sport*, ed. Michael Margaret Gatz, Michael Messner, and Sandra Ball-Rokeach. Albany, NY: State University of New York Press.

Franks, Ray. 1982. *What's in a nickname? Exploring the jungle of college athletic mascots*. Amarillo, TX: Ray Franks Publishing.

Gems, Gerald. 1998. "The construction, negotiation, and transformation of racial identity in American football: A study of Native and African Americans." *American Indian Culture and Research Journal*, *22*, 131–50.

Graham, Renee. 1993. "Symbol or stereotype: One consumer's tradition is another's racial slur." *The Boston Globe* (January 6): 35.

Gray, Amy, and Chery Smith. 2003. "Fitness, dietary intake, and body mass index in urban Native American youth." *Journal of American Dietetic Association, 103*, 1187–91.

Haggard, Dixie. 2004. "Nationalism." Pp. 224–26 in *Native Americans in sports*, ed. Richard King. Armonk, NY: Sharpe Reference.

Kalambakal, Vickey. 2004. "National Indian Athletic Association." P. 223 in *Native Americans in sports*, ed. C. Richard King. Armonk, NY: Sharpe Reference.

King, C. Richard. 2004. *Native Americans in sports*. Armonk, NY: Sharpe Reference.

Meerskin, Debra. 2012. "Crazy Horse malt liquor and athletes: The tenacity of stereotypes." Pp. 304–10 in *Rethinking the color line*, ed. C. Gallagher. New York: McGraw Hill.

Mills, Billy. 2009. *Wokini: A Lakota journey to happiness and self-understanding*, New York: Hay House.

National Collegiate Athletic Association. 2012b. "Race and gender demographics." Accessed online at http://web1.ncaa.org/rgdSearch

Nuessel, Frank. 1994. "Objectionable sport team designations." *Names, 42*, 101–19.

Pate, Russell, Stewart Trost, Sarah Levin, and Marsha Dowda. 2000. "Sports participation and health-related behaviors among U.S. youth." *Archives of Pediatrics and Adolescent Medicine, 154*, 904–11.

Pewewardy, Cornel. 1999. "The deculturalization of indigenous mascots in U.S. sports culture." *The Educational Forum, 63*, 342–47.

Rosenstein, Jay (dir.). 1997. *In whose honor?* [Film]. New Day Films.

Schaefer, Richard. 2011. *Racial and ethnic groups* (10th edn.). Upper Saddle River, NJ: Pearson.

Sigelman, Lee. 2001. "Hail to the Redskins? Public reactions to a racially insensitive team name?" Pp. 203–209 in *Contemporary issues in the sociology of sport*, ed. A. Yinnakis and M. Melnic. Champaign, IL: Human Kinetics.

Simpson, Kevin. 2009. "Sporting dreams die on the 'Rez.'" Pp. 285–91 in *Sport in Contemporary Society*, ed. D. Eitzen. Boulder, CO: Paradigm.

Spencer, Stephen, Claude Steele, and Diane Quinn. 1999. "Stereotype threat and women's math performance." *Journal of Experimental Social Psychology, 35*, 4–28.

Spindel, Carol. 2002. *Dancing at halftime: Sports and the controversy over American Indian mascots*. New York: New York University Press.

Stannard, David. 1992. *American holocaust: Columbus and the conquest of the New World*. New York: Oxford University Press.

Stapleton, Bruce. 2001. *Redskins: Racial slur or symbol of success?* San Jose, CA: Writers Club Press.

Staurowsky, Ellen, and Lawrence Baca. 2004. "Mascot controversy." Pp. 201–204 in *Native Americans in sports*, ed. C. Richard King. Armonk, NY: Sharpe Reference.

Steele, Claude, and Joshua Aronson. 1995. "Stereotype threat and the intellectual test performance of African Americans." *Journal of Personality and Social Psychology, 69*, 797–811.

Steele, Claude, and Paul Davies. 2003. "Stereotype threat and employment testing." *Human Performance, 16*, 311–26.

Thomas, David. 2000. *Skull wars: Kennewick man, archaeology, and the battle for Native American identity*. New York: Basic Books.

Wheeler, Robert. 1979. *Jim Thorpe, world's greatest athlete*. Norman, OK: University of Oklahoma Press.

Williams, Dana. 2007. "Where's the honor: Attitudes toward the 'Fighting Sioux' nickname and logo." *Sociology of Sport Journal, 24*, 437–56.

FURTHER READING

Cultural Appropriation on Full Display in Wisconsin and Beyond in the Form of Mascots

Kelly Ward

If you have a digital edition of this book, please click on the link below to access the article:

https://www.dailycardinal.com/article/2018/02/cultural-appropriation-on-full-display-in-wisconsin-and-beyond-in-form-of-mascot-names

If you have a print edition of this book, please use your cell phone to scan the QR code below to access the article:

"Fighting Irish" Notre Dame Symbol Not Racist Like American Indian Ones

Eugene O'Driscoll

If you have a digital edition of this book, please click on the link below to access the article:

https://www.irishcentral.com/opinion/others/fighting-irish-notre-dame-symbol-racist-american-indian

If you have a print edition of this book, please use your cell phone to scan the QR code below to access the article:

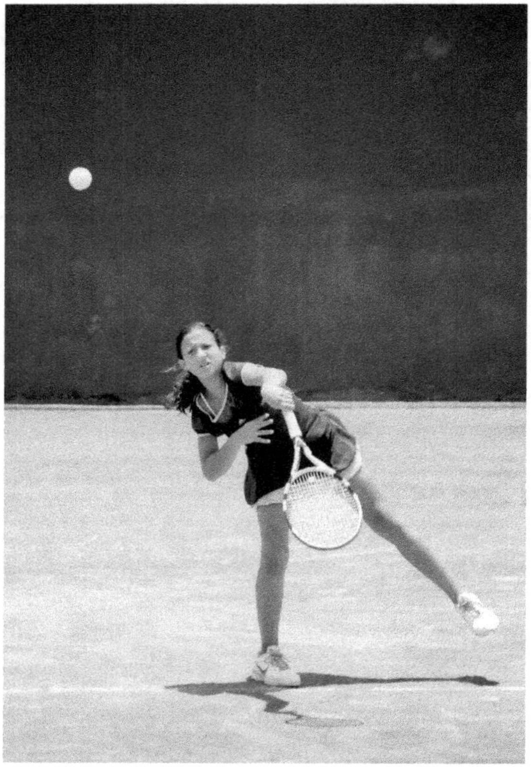

CHAPTER 7

GENDER AND SPORT

During the summer of 1999, I attended a World Cup match at Soldier Field in Chicago, Illinois. The United States hosted the World Cup that year, and Team USA went on to a historical win. It was my first international soccer experience, and I remember asking a friend of mine if our country had a men's team. For me, "the" national team was our women's team. Little did this teenager know that there was an incredible disparity in pay and media coverage between Team USA's men's and women's programs. The World Cup win in 1999 was their second championship title. Today, Team USA women have four World Cup victories and four Olympic gold medals. Moreover, the team earned a medal in all eight of the World Cup tournaments. The greatest success of their counterparts, Team USA men's soccer program, was making it to the round of sixteen in 1994 when the United States hosted the World Cup. Most recently, the men failed to qualify for the 2018 FIFA World Cup. When discussing USA soccer, there is "the" national team and "the women's national team," a phenomenon known as **gender marking**. This is when a men's program is the most authentic team, and the women's program is marked with their gender first. For example, we have the NBA and the WNBA. Additionally, women in sport have an expectation to be strong and athletic while maintaining **appropriate femininity**. The institution of sport governs this with uniform requirements as well. In the image here, the young woman is wearing the required tennis uniform that includes skirt-like attire rather than shorts like the men. Chapter 7 examines the marginalization of gender in the world of sport and the disparity in economic opportunities.

Figure Credit

Fig. 7.1: Copyright © 2011 by Myousry6666, (CC BY-SA 4.0) at https://commons.wikimedia.org/wiki/File:Women_in_sport_(7).jpg.

15

THE INFLUENCE OF GENDER-ROLE SOCIALIZATION, MEDIA USE AND SPORTS PARTICIPATION ON PERCEPTIONS OF GENDER-APPROPRIATE SPORTS

Marie Hardin and Jennifer D. Greer

Perceptions of Sports as Gender-Appropriate

As children are introduced to sports, their experiences are based on gender roles and expectations (Hargreaves, 1994; Nilges, 1998). The construction of sports as appropriate replicates gender-typed toys: rough-and-tumble symbols for boys, domestically oriented symbols for girls. Messner (2002) writes that day-to-day interactions of children with each other and with adults still privilege boys and men in the athletic status system and marginalize girls and women.

Early work on how sports are typed in regard to gender was done by Metheny (1965), who proposed a set of attributes used to categorize a sport as feminine or masculine; sports recognized as masculine involve contact and the use of force or heavy objects (Koivula, 2001). Later, Postow (1980) argued that sports-related attitudes such as devotion to a team, stamina, and competitive spirit also are perceived as masculine. Thus, team sports are considered more masculine than individual sports. Sports in which aggressiveness is considered an essential part of the game, including ice hockey and football, have been regarded as masculine (Koivula, 2001). Sports that have historically been perceived as feminine, such as figure skating or gymnastics, are those that allow women to exhibit gender-role attributes such as grace and beauty while participating (Koivula, 2001). These typologies reinforce ideas of difference; they showcase constructions of men as stronger and faster, thus deserving a higher rank in the overall social order, than women. Generally, men and women type sports similarly; exceptions sometimes occur with basketball, which may be categorized as a more masculine sport by boys than by girls (Riemer & Feltz, 1995).

Although Cashmore (2005) argues that the typologies developed by Metheny (1965) and others are "about as fresh as disco music and mullets" (p. 157), research indicates that even in recent

Marie Hardin and Jennifer D. Greer, "The Influence of Gender-Role Socialization, Media Use and Sports Participation on Perceptions of Gender-Appropriate Sports," *Journal of Sport Behavior*, vol. 32, no. 2, pp. 209-211, 224-226.

years, sports have been gender-typed in traditional ways (Koivula, 2001; Matteo, 1986; Riemer & Feltz, 1995; Solmon, Lee, Belcher, Harrison, & Wells, 2003). More recent studies, however, have identified that some sports are perceived as more neutral—indicating a slight shift in perception that sports must be either masculine or feminine. A recent study (Koivula, 2001) involving 400 university students found that participants categorized sports as feminine, masculine, or gender-neutral based on their perceptions of the sports' aesthetics, speed, and risk. Sports such as tennis, volleyball, and swimming were ranked as neutral, gymnastics and aerobics were ranked as feminine, and baseball, soccer, and football were typed as masculine. Respondents incorporated the perceived purpose of a sport and its risk when assigning labels. Koivula (2001) points out that definitions of a gender-appropriate sport can change because gender is constructed based on historically and culturally specific conditions. Action sports, which have attracted more participants and more attention from media in recent years, have not been examined in past studies related to gender-typing.

The Influence of Sports Participation

Since passage of Title IX, sports participation by girls and women has grown exponentially. In 1972, 1 in 27 girls played high school sports; in 1998, one in three did (*Sports Illustrated for Women*, 2002). Sports participation by boys also has increased, although not at the same rate (Carpenter & Acosta, 2005). Most growth in participation by girls and women has been in sports that have been typed neutral or masculine, such as soccer. The most frequent college varsity sports for women are basketball, volleyball, cross country, soccer, softball, tennis, track and field, golf, swimming, and lacrosse—none of which is aesthetically oriented (Acosta & Carpenter, 2004).

The expanding role of sports in the lives of girls (and boys) in the United States could lead to more progressive ideas about what constitutes a gender-appropriate sport, but research has not supported that possibility. Several studies have revealed that male athletes have more conservative, traditional attitudes toward gender roles than do male non-athletes (Andre & Holland, 1995; Boyle, 1997; Houseworth, Peplow, & Thirer, 1989). Studies in the 1980s and 1990s demonstrated that high school and college students judged participation in gender-appropriate sports as socially more desirable than participation in sports deemed gender-inappropriate; for instance, girls who participated in gymnastics were deemed more desirable as a date (for boys) and as a friend (for girls) than were girls who played golf or softball (Holland & Thomas, 1994).

Matteo (1986) found that the more strongly a male college student adhered to traditional gender roles, the less likely he was to participate in sports not considered masculine. Young women, even if they strongly adhered to gender roles, were more likely to try masculine sports, perhaps because masculine sports are considered more valuable in U.S. culture (Matteo, 1986). Perceptions of a sport as masculine, feminine, or neutral also may impact perceptions of ability. Solmon et al. (2003) found that college-aged women who perceive a sport as gender-neutral are more confident about participating than are women who identify a sport as masculine.

Impact of Media Messages

Research indicates that the U.S. sports/media complex has positioned sports as male terrain; its "masculinist cultural center" has been a site for boys and men to learn hegemonic masculinity (Messner, 2002, p. 92). Messner has outlined lessons of the "televised sports manhood formula:" sports belong to men; aggression is integral to sports and to masculinity; and violence is natural and oftentimes necessary. Lessons from the televised sports manhood formula "are evident, in varying degrees, in the football, basketball, extreme sports, and SportsCenter programs and their accompanying commercials" (p. 124).

Media emphasize the "sports manhood formula" and overwhelmingly feature core men's sports (Bernstein, 2002; Bishop, 2003; Messner, 2002; Pedersen, 2002). Sports media generally dedicate only 5% to 8% of coverage to women's sports even though 40% of sports participation is by women (Adams & Tuggle, 2004; Kane, Griffin, & Messner, 2002). Further, network coverage emphasizes women's sports considered traditionally gender-appropriate. For instance, NBC's Olympic coverage showcases women's figure skating (winter) or gymnastics (summer) while Olympic sports such as women's shot put or discus are virtually invisible, and women's team sports receive less prime-time coverage than individual sports (Tuggle, Huffman, & Rosengard, 2002). Adams & Tuggle (2004) found that women's team sports such as basketball, soccer, and softball received less coverage in more recent years than in the early-to-mid 1990s.

U.S. sports media outlets enjoy great popularity. In the late 1990s, 94% of children surveyed said they consumed sports media, and many said they did so daily (Messner, 2002). "Sports media are thus likely to be one of the major influences on children's views of gender, race, commercialism, and other key issues" (2002, p. xix). Messner argues that children are socialized into traditional views of gender and sport even by the new genre of "action" sports (also called alternative or extreme sports) such as skateboarding and snowboarding. Such sports are so popular that teenage sports fans in 2002 voted skateboarder Tony Hawk "coolest big-time athlete" (Wheaton, 2004). Action sports have moved into the mainstream through heavily commercialized coverage of the "X Games" on television and the integration of snowboarding into the Winter Olympics in 2006. These sports are mostly individual activities that emphasize both risk (masculine) and aesthetics (feminine); they are also non-contact. Wheaton argues that action sports offer possibilities for more progressive ideas about gender.

References

Acosta, R. V. & Carpenter, L. J. (2004). Women in intercollegiate sport: A longitudinal, national study. National Association for Girls and Women in Sport. Retrieved January 1, 2005 from http://www.aahperd.org/nagws/template.cfm?template=acostacarpenter.html

Adams, T., & Tuggle, C. A. (2004). ESPN's SportsCenter and women's athletics: 'It's a boys' club.' *Mass Communication & Society, 7*, 237–248.

Andre, T., & Holland, A. (1995). Relationship of sport participation to sex role orientation and attitudes toward women among high school males and females. *Journal of Sport Behavior, 75*, 241–254.

Bernstein, A. (2002). Is it time for a victory lap? *International Review for the Sociology of Sport 3* 7(fall-winter), 415–428.

Bishop, R. (2003). Missing in action: Feature coverage of women's sports in Sports Illustrated. *Journal of Sport and Social Issues, 27*, 184–194.

Boyle, J. E. (1997). *Organized sports participation, masculinity, and attitudes toward women*. Unpublished thesis. Virginia Polytechnic Institute and State University, Blacksburg.

Carpenter, L. J., & Acosta, R. V. (2005). *Title IX*. Champaign, Ill.: Human Kinetics.

Cashmore, E. (2005). *Making sense of sports* (4th ed.). London: New York.

Hargreaves, J. (1994). *Sporting females: Critical issues in the history and sociology of women's sports*. London: Routledge.

Holland, A., & Thomas, A. (1994). Athletic participation and the social status of adolescent males and females. *Youth & Society* 25, 388–407.

Houseworth, S., Peplow, K., & Thirer, J. (1989). Influence of sport participation upon sex role orientation of Caucasian males and their attitudes toward women. *Sex Roles, 20*, 317–325.

Kane, M. J., Griffin, P., & Messner, M. (2002). *Playing unfair: The media image of the female athlete.* [Motion picture]. (Available from Media Education Foundation, 60 Masonic Street, Northampton, MA 01060)

Koivula, N. (2001). Perceived characteristics of sports categorized as gender-neutral, feminine and masculine. *Journal of Sport Behavior, 24*, 377–393.

Matteo, S. (1986). The effect of sex and gender-schematic processing on sport participation. *Sex Roles, 75*, 417–431.

Messner, M. (2002). *Taking the field: Women, men, and sports.* Minneapolis: University of Minnesota Press.

Metheny, E. (1965). Symbolic forms of movement: The feminine image in sports. In E. Metheny (Ed.), *Connotations of movement in sport and dance* (pp. 43–56). Dubuque, IA: Brown.

Nilges, L. M. (1998). I thought only fairy tales had supernatural power: A radical feminist analysis of Title IX in physical education. *Journal of Teaching in Physical Education*, 17, 172–194.

Pedersen, P. M. (2002). Investigating interscholastic equity on the sports page: A content analysis of high school athletics newspaper articles. *Sociology of Sport Journal, 19*, 419–432.

Postow, B. C. (1980). Women and masculine sports. *Journal of the Philosophy of Sport, VII*, 51–58.

Riemer, B. A., & Feltz, D, L. (1995). The influence of sport appropriateness and image on the status of female athletes. *Women in Sport & Physical Activity Journal, 4*, 1.

Solmon, M. A., Lee, A. M., Belcher, D., Harrison, L., & Wells, L. (2003). Beliefs about gender appropriateness, ability, and competence in physical activity. *Journal of Teaching in Physical Education, 22*, 261–279.

Sports Illustrated for Women (2002). Media Kit. New York: Time, Inc.

Tuggle, C., Huffman, S., & Rosengard, D. (2002). A descriptive analysis of NBC's coverage of the 2000 Summer Olympics. *Mass Communication & Society, 5*, 361–375.

16

EFFECTS OF TITLE IX ON INTERCOLLEGIATE ATHLETICS, 1972–2012

Nancy Lough

Key Terms

- gender equity
- grant-in-aid
- proportionality
- sex discrimination
- Equity in Athletics
- Disclosure Act (EADA)

When Title IX was passed as a section of the Education Amendments that President Richard M. Nixon signed in 1972, it was intended as an education law to remedy sex discrimination within American educational institutions. Bernice Sandler has been credited with drafting portions of the legislation, spurred by her personal experience of being denied a tenure-track position in the late 1960s because she "came on too strong for a woman" (Edwards, 2010, p. 303). Sandler began studying the issue, resulting in the accumulation of 250 complaints of sex discrimination against colleges receiving federal contracts. This list of complaints served as the impetus for the initial introduction of a bill requiring gender equity in education. The bill changed over time, with language used replicating Title VI of the Civil Rights Act of 1964, in which "sex" was substituted for "race, color, or national origin," resulting in the following: "No person in the United States shall, on the basis of sex, be excluded from participation in, be denied the benefits of, or be subjected to discrimination under any educational program or activity receiving Federal financial assistance" (20 U.S.C. 1681).

Originators of the law purposely worked to draw as little attention as possible during the process, concerned attention would weaken the chances of the law passing. As Sandler indicated, "We had no idea how bad the situation was—we didn't even use the word sex discrimination back then—and we certainly had no idea the revolution it would start" (Wulf, 2012, para. 4). The resulting significance of Title IX has been the profound increase in opportunities for women, both in sports and in higher education. While gains for women in college sports have been impressive, with a 622% increase in participation numbers from 1971–1972 to 2009–2010, gains in education have been equally impressive. In 1972 women earned less than 10% of both law and medical degrees and only 13% of doctoral degrees. By 2012, nearly half of all law and medical degrees and more than half of all doctoral degrees were earned by women.

As a result, some have pointed to Title IX as the most important step toward gender equality, beyond the Nineteenth Amendment giving women the right to vote. Yet the original intent to provide equal educational opportunity for women quickly became lost within a high-profile debate centered on football. Sports became the lightning rod for those opposed to Title IX. Both the National Collegiate Athletic Association (NCAA) and the College Football Association expressed alarm, as they contended Title IX would harm college football.

Two divergent points of view prevailed throughout the decades following Title IX's passage. On one side, Title IX was credited with creating improved gender equity within U.S. colleges and universities, by empowering generations of women to successfully pursue higher education. Contrastingly, those who opposed the law blamed Title IX for the elimination of men's sports programs. Opposition to Title IX never declined, requiring continued vigilance on the part of those who support the law.

Why was Title IX Needed?

In the decades leading up to Title IX, discrimination against women who sought degrees and careers in higher education was common. For example, during a three-year period in the state of Virginia prior to Title IX, 21,000 female applicants were denied admission to college, while all male applicants were accepted. Several barriers existed throughout the United States for women interested in higher education. Admissions criteria were often 30 to 40 points higher for women applicants than men. Quotas admitting one or two women were an accepted standard within law schools, medical schools, and even doctoral-degree-granting programs, where classes of men could be upwards of 100 or more. This culture of discrimination was also evidenced by requirements for women to live on campus, while men were free to select where they would live. The on-campus housing requirement often was an additional expense, thus acting to impede the opportunity for those women without financial means for the added cost.

While these barriers restricted access to higher education for women, the situation in college sports was no different. Before Title IX, athletic opportunities at the collegiate level were often in the form of "play days" organized by women physical educators. Perhaps most telling, the legendary Billie Jean King, who won multiple Grand Slam titles, was not provided an athletic scholarship, labeled grant-in-aid by the NCAA, to compete in tennis at UCLA. This example points out how the first steps toward a remedy for sex discrimination were awareness and acknowledgment a problem existed.

The congressional passage of Title IX demonstrated the highest level of support toward seeking gender equality in federally funded educational programs. Yet initial interpretations of the law questioned whether it applied to intercollegiate athletics. While the Department of Health & Human Services delayed the initial deadline for institutional compliance until 1978, the Office of Civil Rights (OCR), charged with enforcement of Title IX, did not issue a policy interpretation statement until 1979. The most critical aspect of the 1979 interpretation was labeled the three-prong or three-part test (Johnson, 1994).

Compliance with Title IX requires an institution demonstrates *one* of the following:

> Part One: Substantial Proportionality. Satisfaction of this part occurs when participation opportunities are "substantially proportionate" to the respective undergraduate enrollment for men and women.
>
> Part Two: History and Continuing Practice. Satisfaction of this part occurs when an institution can show a history and continuing practice of expanding programs in response to developing interests and abilities of the underrepresented sex.
>
> Part Three: Effectively Accommodating Interests and Abilities. Satisfaction of this part occurs when the interests and abilities of female students have been met by the institution, even where there are disproportionately fewer females than males participating in sport. (U.S. Department of Education, 1997)

Despite this clarification, many institutions were unclear to what degree they were expected to comply with Title IX. The first true legal test required resolution by the Supreme Court in 1984, which for a time meant Title IX did not apply directly to intercollegiate athletics. There have been four distinct stages in the evolution of Title IX, including resistance, marginalization, advocacy, and backlash (Lough, 2012). In each of these stages, major milestones contributed to development of the law as it is understood today.

Stage 1: Resistance

In the initial period following the passage of Title IX, the rhetoric was often divisive. The conflict was centered primarily on the NCAA's contention that a choice needed to be made between football and women's sports. The NCAA petitioned Congress to be considered "exempt" from Title IX on multiple occasions. The perception was that allocating funding to support women's sports would compromise the established men's programs. During the initial grace period given for implementation and clarification, several amendments were drafted by the NCAA to make men's revenue-producing college sports exempt from Title IX. All were rejected. Then in 1975, final regulations were issued, establishing a three-year time frame for institutions to become compliant with the law. This regulation was reviewed by Congress and signed into law with additional provisions banning sex discrimination. Similarly, the 1979 Policy Interpretation provided the three-prong test for determining compliance, which provided guidance on the requirements for sport participation opportunities. With this, the Office for Civil Rights was assigned oversight authority for Title IX.

The time period from the passage of Title IX through the end of the 1970s, was one marked by limited understanding resulting in a lack of enforcement. One estimate suggested NCAA women's Division IA sports accounted for 14% of the overall athletics budgets in 1977, which meant 86% of all expenditures were on men's sports. For decades the men's programs had benefited from receiving mandatory student fees with this revenue allocated exclusively to men's athletics operating budgets. This was one of many practices demonstrating gender discrimination, yet among college sports leaders it was perceived as fair. Widely accepted practices such as this point to the crux of the struggle for acceptance that women's sports faced in this initial stage of resistance. Change is most often met with resistance, which is one partial explanation for reluctance to share resources. Finally in 1981, after numerous failed attempts to avert Title IX, the NCAA officially adopted women's sports.

Stage 2: Marginalization

The marginalization stage is noted for the milestone litigation resulting in suspended operation of women's sports programs among athletic departments from 1984 through 1988. The landmark case of *Grove City College v. Bell* questioned whether programs had to be in *direct* receipt of federal funds to be held to Title IX compliance. The resulting U.S. Supreme Court decision provided two instructive points. First, indirect federal funding did result in Title IX jurisdiction, but in this ruling "the jurisdiction of Title IX applied only to the subunit within the institution that was the *direct* recipient of the federal funding" (Carpenter & Acosta, 2005, p. 195). The second part of this decision resulted in athletic departments no longer falling within the scope of Title IX. In essence, federal funding was linked mostly to grants and financial aid for students; however, in the case of athletics, if an athlete received this type of funding, it was not via the athletic department. Since athletic departments did not directly receive federal funding, there was no need for compliance with Title IX. This case is particularly instructive even today, as the ruling demonstrated that many athletic and institutional leaders were willing to stop the progress that had been made and, in some cases, take steps backward.

During this same period the rapid decline in women's athletic programs and departments led by women, and concomitantly the dissolution of the Association for Intercollegiate Athletics for Women (AIAW), was unfolding. The AIAW had served in the leadership role for women's college sports for decades, offering 41 national championships in 19 sports for more than 6,000 teams representing 960 member institutions (Carpenter & Acosta, 2005). The AIAW had been successful in obtaining television contracts for its women's basketball national championship, which unfortunately led to the NCAA perceiving the AIAW as a competitor. Given the influence the NCAA had with the media, it effectively blocked the AIAW from acquiring new television contracts, which compromised a key revenue source. The AIAW then sued, but lost its antitrust case against the NCAA. The AIAW then dissolved, due largely to an inability to compete with the money the NCAA offered to member schools who qualified for national championships.

The advocacy stage came about largely as a result of the Civil Rights Restoration Act, which in effect restored the original intent of Title IX. Throughout the next decade, the lack of investment in women's sports and failures to focus on Title IX compliance by universities resulted in several lawsuits. The need for litigation to begin the progress toward Title IX compliance marks the beginning of the advocacy stage.

Stage 3: Advocacy

After the first 20 years of Title IX, more opportunities for women's sport participation existed, but sex discrimination continued. The Office of Civil Rights was admittedly reluctant to punish institutions, largely because removal or elimination of federal funding from an institution of higher education was simply too harsh a consequence to levy. The ramifications would be far reaching and clearly beyond the scope of problems existing in the athletic program. As a result, those advocating for change turned to litigation.

One of the most crucial court decisions came from the *Franklin v. Gwinnett County Public Schools* in 1992. While this case was not centered on sports, it was illuminating because it demonstrated that monetary awards, in the form of punitive and compensatory damages, could be awarded to successful Title IX plaintiffs. In this case, the actual issue involved sexual harassment. Initially, Franklin filed a complaint with the OCR, but the result did not meet her expectations. By exercising her private right of action, the case reached the Supreme Court, where a unanimous decision affirmed monetary damages may result from a Title IX lawsuit. This was an important point, since it served as a wake-up call to higher education institutions. In essence, noncompliance with Title IX now posed the threat of substantial financial loss. Some institutions realized the most fiscally appropriate action would be to adhere to compliance standards. However, the male model of college sports was a deeply gendered subculture, which meant advocacy would be met with resistance.

With little help from the OCR, female athletes increasingly pursued litigation to remedy the discrimination in college sports. As higher education began to feel the challenge of an economic downturn in the early 1990s, athletics budgets were reduced and a common response was to eliminate sports, often focusing on women's programs. Multiple lawsuits challenged universities that chose to eliminate women's sports. Perhaps one of the most notable was the case in which the National Organization for Women (NOW) sued the entire California State University system (19 schools at the time). In this case the Cal State system lost, resulting in a settlement that forced it to develop a plan to provide women sport participation opportunities more closely reflecting the student body ratio of females to males. To achieve the new targets, some institutions chose to eliminate men's sports, instead of adding women's sports. This practice led to media accounts repeatedly blaming Title IX and women's sports for elimination of men's nonrevenue sport programs. Rhetoric around gender equity was typically framed as "battle of the sexes," a "dispute," "fight," or "tug of war" (Staurowsky, 1998, p. 7).

Still the most definitive case to date was *Cohen v. Brown University*. Initiation of the lawsuit was in response to Brown's decision to cut sports for both men and women. Cohen represented the female athletes suing to reinstate their sports. Brown believed the cuts were fair. However, at the time of the cuts, the ratio of male to female athletes was 63.3% to 36.7%. This case is particularly illustrative of a practice many institutions pursued, which was to eliminate an equivalent number of female and male sports. Brown University spent millions of dollars defending its position, which led to more clarity on a number of issues tied to gender equity. First, terminating the same number of sports for men and women is not a "safe passage" to compliance. Second, the "relative interests" theory was pursued as a key argument by Brown. The idea was that by surveying students regarding their interest in sports, the ratio of responses could then be used as a gauge to measure proportionality and thereby demonstrate compliance with Title IX. The courts rejected this approach.

In addition to striking down the "relative interests" argument, the court also rebuked the use of "quota" and "affirmative action" language when pursuing Title IX compliance. Additionally the ruling clarified that actual participants, not participation opportunities, need to be reported. Similarly, using ratios acquired from a survey would freeze opportunity levels and thereby sustain past discriminatory practices. Because a new group of students can potentially represent a new level of interest, a survey of interests typically captures only one moment in time, as opposed to developing interests and abilities.

Cutting men's sport was suggested by the Supreme Court as one potential remedy to discrimination, noting the OCR had deemed proportionality as a "safe harbor." With mounting pressure following the *Brown* ruling, The NCAA Gender Equity Task Force created the most comprehensive definition to guide institutions toward Title IX compliance: "An athletics program can be considered gender equitable when the participants in both the men's and women's sports programs would accept as fair and equitable the overall program of the other gender. No individual should be discriminated against on the basis of gender, institutionally or nationally, in intercollegiate athletics" (NCAA Gender Equity Task Force). Put in clearer terms, if the men's basketball team would trade all aspects of its program, including coaches, travel, uniforms, practice, and competitive facilities with the women's basketball program, then gender equity has truly been achieved. Also, around this time, the task force recommended the creation of emerging sports, to address growing interest and continue the development of sport opportunities for women.

Perhaps one of the most impactful steps was creation of the Equity in Athletics Disclosure Act (EADA) in 1996, which was a federal mandate for disclosure of data by every NCAA athletic department and included categories such as operating expenses for all sports, per capita expenses for all sports, recruiting and scholarship allocations, salaries for head and assistant coaches, and revenues and expenses for basketball and football. The EADA was proposed to provide an avenue for parents and athletes to assess the level of commitment each school provides for its athletic programs. The notion was that a more informed decision could be made when selecting a college or university. Also, the belief was athletic programs would be held more accountable through this annual disclosure of data. Yet, in a study examining EADA data, Hattery, Smith, and Staurowsky (2007) found gender inequities have clearly continued, even as the fourth decade of the law was unfolding.

Stage 4: Backlash

While each prior stage involved aspects of backlash against Title IX, the thirtieth anniversary of the law marked the beginning of a period of significant challenges. In 2002 the Bush administration formed a commission to study Title IX. Spurred on by critics such as the National Wrestling Coaches Association (NWCA), the Commission on Opportunity in Athletics held hearings across the country over a period of eight months. Ultimately, Title IX was not reformed in any significant way, although proponents were reassured that the progress made over the past 30 years could easily be reversed if the law was weakened or eliminated. Following the commission hearings, in 2003 the OCR issued further clarification indicating Title IX does not encourage or expect reduction of men's sport programs, as many had suggested the proportionality test advocated.

Similarly, criticism of prong three continued, with the primary concern being that universities fail to meet either the spirit or intent of Title IX when using manipulative strategies to demonstrate "interest" among women has been met. Following a 2005 clarification debacle, the OCR issued new guidelines in 2010 regarding the use of interest surveys. Notably, the OCR indicated a survey cannot stand alone, and its evaluation will focus on both the content and target population of the survey. In essence, prong three can be used to determine compliance but only if the demonstration of interest employs sound survey methods and seeks information from the underrepresented population.

In total there are 13 areas for compliance including equipment and supplies, scheduling, travel and per diem, tutors, coaches, facilities, medical care and training, housing, publicity, support services, and recruiting. To demonstrate a disparity in any of these areas the differences must be based on sex with a negative impact on athletes of one sex, and the disparity must be so substantial as to deny equal opportunity to athletes of the one sex. This is not to say that all areas must be exactly equal or equivalent. Permissible differences are recognized by the OCR based on the unique aspects of each sport. For example, event management costs are far higher for football than any other sport, as are equipment costs for all sports requiring protective equipment. While there is not room here to discuss each of the 13 areas, scholars have shown disparities in a number of these areas. Yet Staurowsky and Weight (2011) found Title IX knowledge is lacking among both athletes and coaches. Without a full understanding of gender equity, all 13 areas covered by Title IX, discriminatory practices are likely to go unchallenged.

Unintended Consequence

Paradoxically, growth in sport participation opportunities for women occurred as the numbers of women coaches and administrators diminished. For more than 30 years, Acosta and Carpenter (2012) kept track of these trends. Despite a record number of sports offered, the representation of female coaches has remained below 50% for decades. Women athletic directors, also few in number, have seen little growth even though the pipeline for leadership should be filled with an unprecedented number of former college athletes. For a better understanding of this issue, readers are encouraged to access Acosta and Carpenter's (2012) full report.

STAKEHOLDER PERSPECTIVE

NCAA Emerging Sports for Women

In 1994 the NCAA's Gender-Equity Task Force recommended a list of emerging sports as a way to continue to grow opportunities for women. During the past 17 years, rowing, ice hockey, water polo, and bowling have become championship sports. To remain on the list, emerging sports are required to attain a minimum of 40 varsity programs within 10 years or show steady progress toward the goal. Marilyn Moniz-Kaho'ohanohano, chair of the NCAA's Committee on Women's Athletics (CWA), indicated the CWA was supportive of forwarding triathlon for consideration as an emerging sport. Triathlon is believed to be a natural fit for colleges and universities, with more than 150 campuses currently supporting triathlon clubs. At the 2013 national collegiate championship, triathletes from 46 states participated, including more than 400 women. USA Triathlon's data further support interest, with women representing more than 40% of all collegiate participants. Moniz-Kaho'ohanohano said the CWA was impressed with the level of support offered by USA Triathlon, including a coach's certification program and events in 50 locations utilized to introduce triathlon to new communities while developing future participants.

Marymount University is one of a list of institutions adding the sport, which will increase to 15 the sports offered in the 2012–2013 seasons. Dr. Chris Domes, Marymount's vice president for student development and enrollment management, said "We're very excited because these will be the first sports added at Marymount since 2003, when we launched men's and women's cross country. More sports mean more opportunity for athletes; in our experience, these are students who tend to do well academically and who serve as leaders and role models on campus. As an NCAA Division III school, Marymount values athletics as part of a well-rounded educational experience; we also recognize the important role that sports can play in building community and promoting school spirit."

Relatedly, some believe the decline in women coaches is reflective of a climate that does not value women. For decades, women's sports coaches were fired for speaking out regarding gender inequities. Yet the scope of Title IX regarding retaliation for whistle blowers did not reach the Supreme Court until 2005 in *Jackson v. Birmingham Board of Education*. This case, pursued by a male girls' basketball coach, resulted in the court expanding the range of permissible plaintiffs. In essence, the ruling indicated that Title IX protects victims of retaliation, even when the plaintiff was not a direct victim of the discrimination. This watershed ruling opened the door for coaches who had lost their jobs as a result of advocating for gender equity in their programs. The numbers of coaches and administrators who

CASE STUDY

Sport Media Guides

Messner (2002) argued sport media is the primary vehicle that legitimizes "unequal power relations between the sexes" and makes female athletes and their bodies "contested ideological terrain." Following Title IX, media portrayals of female athletes replicated social norms, even though sports was believed to empower women and serve as a means to foster change. Guided by the notion "media coverage of sport offers fertile ground for any investigation that explores images, symbols, and myths related to power," Kane and Buysse (2005) analyzed Division I media guide covers from the 1990s to the early 2000s seeking differences in gender portrayals. Media guides from 12 sports at 68 colleges in six major Division I athletic conferences, resulted in 528 guides for analysis. Media guides were chosen because they are considered a marketing tool used to advertise teams to sponsors, donors, alumni, and key stakeholders, while also used as a recruitment tool for future college athletes. Three aspects were examined: Were the athletes in or out of their uniforms, on or off the court, and in active or passive poses? In earlier studies, women's teams were often depicted as "ladylike" being portrayed in dresses, in passive poses, and in a nonsports environment.

The authors found males and females were portrayed in uniforms on most media guide covers. Approximately 80% of the women and 86% of the men were portrayed in their competitive venue. Females were portrayed in active poses in 71% of the media guides compared to 78% for men. The results "clearly indicate strong and consistent trends regarding the seriousness with which male and female athletes were portrayed" (Kane & Buysse, 2005, p. 223). A visual analysis also revealed women in hockey, softball, basketball, and tennis were most likely to be in active poses, compared to sports of golf and gymnastics. Not surprisingly, traditionally feminine sports were sometimes portrayed in a passive pose, adhering to gender stereotypes. This analysis demonstrated "significant shifts in the representations of sportswomen from the early 1990s to 2004, shifts that led to the construction of females as serious, competent athletes" (p. 231). Notably, Kane and Buysse found these recent portrayals of college sportswomen represented a stark contrast to the images found in mainstream media. They concluded:

> The impact of Title IX, and its relationship to higher education, is behind our second suggestion for why stereotypic narratives did not rule the day ... In large measure because of Title IX, more and more girls are exposed to formalized, competitive sports at an early age. This not only creates a greater interest in sports among females but also produces a sense of entitlement that is often expressed in the expectation of an athletic scholarship ... consequently, colleges and universities are now required to make meaningful athletic opportunities and experiences available to women. One way to do this is to structure women's athletics around the highly competitive and commercialized "male model" of sports. Women's intercollegiate athletics have thus become more commercialized and, as a result, institutions of higher education now have a stake in making them more appealing to a broader audience. (pp. 234–235)

Questions to Consider

1. Given the 13 areas for Title IX Compliance, in which area(s) would this issue reside? Why?
2. Given the need for college sports programs to generate revenue and garner media attention, discuss the need for women's athletic programs to emulate the commercialized "male model."

fell victim to this form of discrimination is unknown, but clearly the backlash would have continued had this critical ruling not come about in 2005.

Most recently the scope of Title IX has been broadened within higher education, as this educational law has also been utilized to address inequities in access to higher education, career education, employment, the learning environment, math, science and technology, sexual harassment, and standardized testing, as well as treatment of pregnant and parenting students. As further evidence of how college sports continues to be predominantly a male model, the NCAA failed to recognize the need to protect athletes during pregnancy until 2005. For many women, the protection provided by Title IX also presented various forms of backlash.

The Fortieth Anniversary and Emerging Fifth Stage

Forty years of Title IX has not resulted in the elimination of sex discrimination, even within college sports, where it has received the most attention. Instead, Title IX as applied to intercollegiate athletics has been deemed "the most visible gender controversy" (Suggs, 2005). Even recent accounts continue to illustrate the divergent views initiated in the 1970s. Title IX has been credited with increasing sport participation opportunities for women, while also being blamed for cuts to men's collegiate sport teams. Upon examining narratives regarding Title IX's impact, Hardin and Whiteside (2009) confirmed the notion that many believe women do not deserve the equality Title IX affords them.

Conclusion

Twenty years after the initial passage, a shift toward gender equity began due largely to litigation pursued by women athletes interested in restoring or improving athletic opportunities. To date, the OCR has never used its authority to penalize a school for noncompliance, and at the same time, every institution of higher education sued for noncompliance with Title IX in intercollegiate athletics has lost in court. From the beginning, college football proponents pointed to Title IX as the cause for financial challenges, which has been refuted consistently in scholarly work. Examples over the past 40 years lead many to believe that the eradication of Title IX would result in the elimination of women's programs and thereby educational opportunities. At the heart of this legislation created to eliminate sex discrimination is the fact that each opportunity to participate in athletics is in fact an educational opportunity. Few would argue that men deserve more opportunities to pursue a degree in higher education than women. Yet this is the essence of the arguments used to privilege men's sports over women's. Continued advocacy and education are needed as accurate knowledge of Title IX remains limited, even among coaches of women's sports, athletes, and athletic administrators.

Questions for Discussion

1. Do you think the spirit and intent of the federal law written in 1972 is a reality today? Why or why not?
2. Why has a law written to improve educational opportunities become known primarily as a "sport law"?
3. Of the three methods to demonstrate compliance, which appears to be most effective? Why?

References

Acosta, R. V., & Carpenter, L. J. (2012). *Women in intercollegiate sport: A longitudinal, national study thirty-five year update 1977–2012*. Retrieved from http://www.acostacarpenter.org

Brown, G. (2013). CWA asks to add triathlon as an emerging sport. NCAA.org. Retrieved from http://www.ncaa.org/wps/wcm/connect/public/NCAA/Resources/Latest+News/2013/May/CWA+asks+to+add+triathlon+as+an+emerging+sport

Carpenter, L., & Acosta, V. (2005). *Title IX*. Champaign, IL: Human Kinetics.

Civil Rights Restoration Act of 1987, 20 U.S.C. section 1687 (1988).

Cohen v. Brown University, 991 F. 2d 888 (1st Cir. 1993); 101 F. 3d 155 (1st Cir. 1996), cert. denied 520 U.S. 1186 (1997).

Edwards, A. R. (2010). Why Sport? The development of sport as a policy issue in Title IX of the Education Amendments of 1972. *Journal of Policy History, 22*, 300–336.

Franklin v. Gwinnett County Public Schools. Retrieved from http://caselaw.lp.findlaw.com/scripts/getcase.pl?court=us&vol=503=60

Grove City College v. Bell. Retrieved from http://caselaw.lp.findlaw.com/scripts/getcase.pl?court=us&vol=465&invol=555

Hardin, M., & Whiteside, E. E. (2009). The power of "small stories": Narratives and notions of gender equality in conversations about sport. *Sociology of Sport Journal, 26*, 255–276.

Hattery, A., Smith, E., & Staurowsky, E. (2007). They play like girls: Gender equity in NCAA sports. *Journal for the Study of Sports and Athletes in Education, 1*(3), 249–272.

Johnson, J. K. (1994). Title IX and intercollegiate athletics: Current judicial interpretation of the standards for compliance. *Boston University Law Review, 74*, 553–589.

Kane, M. J., & Buysse, J. A. (2005). Intercollegiate media guides as contested terrain: A longitudinal analysis. *Sociology of Sport Journal, 22*, 214–238.

Lough, N. (2012, April). *Equity in education: 40 Years of Title IX; A panel discussion*. Sponsored event held in the Hendrix Auditorium, UNLV College of Education, Las Vegas. http://wrinunlv.org/2211/equity-in-education-celebrating-40-years-of-title-ix/.

Messner, M. (2002). *Taking the field: Women, men and sports*. Minnesota: University of Minnesota Press.

NCAA Gender Equity Task Force. *Gender equity*. Retrieved from http://www.ncaa.org/about/resources/inclusion/gender-equity

Staurowsky, E. (1998). Critiquing the language of the gender gap equity debate. *Journal of Sport & Social Issues, 98*(22), 7–26.

Staurowsky, E., & Weight, E. (2011). Title IX literacy: What coaches don't know and need to find out. *Journal of Intercollegiate Sport, 4*, 190–209.

Suggs, W. (2005). *A place on the team: The triumph and tragedy of Title IX*. Princeton, NJ: Prince ton University Press.

U.S. Department of Civil Rights Office. Retrieved from www.ed.gov/about/offices/list/ocr/index.html

U. S. Department of Education. (1997). Title IX: 25 years of progress. Retrieved from www.ed.gov/pubs/TitleIX/

U.S. Department of Justice. Retrieved from www.usdoj.gov/crt/cor/coord/titleix.htm

Wulf, S. (2012, March 26). Title IX: 37 words that changed everything. *ESPNW.com*. Retrieved from http://w.espn.go.com/espnw/title-ix/7722632/print

FURTHER READING

Caster Semenya Ruling: Sports Federation Is Flouting Ethics Rules

Roger Pielke

If you have a digital edition of this book, please click on the link below to access the article:

https://www.nature.com/articles/d41586-019-01606-8

If you have a print edition of this book, please use your cell phone to scan the QR code below to access the article:

U.S. Women's Soccer Team Sues U.S. Soccer for Gender Discrimination

Andrew Das

If you have a digital edition of this book, please click on the link below to access the article:

https://www.nytimes.com/2019/03/08/sports/womens-soccer-team-lawsuit-gender-discrimination.html

If you have a print edition of this book, please use your cell phone to scan the QR code below to access the article:

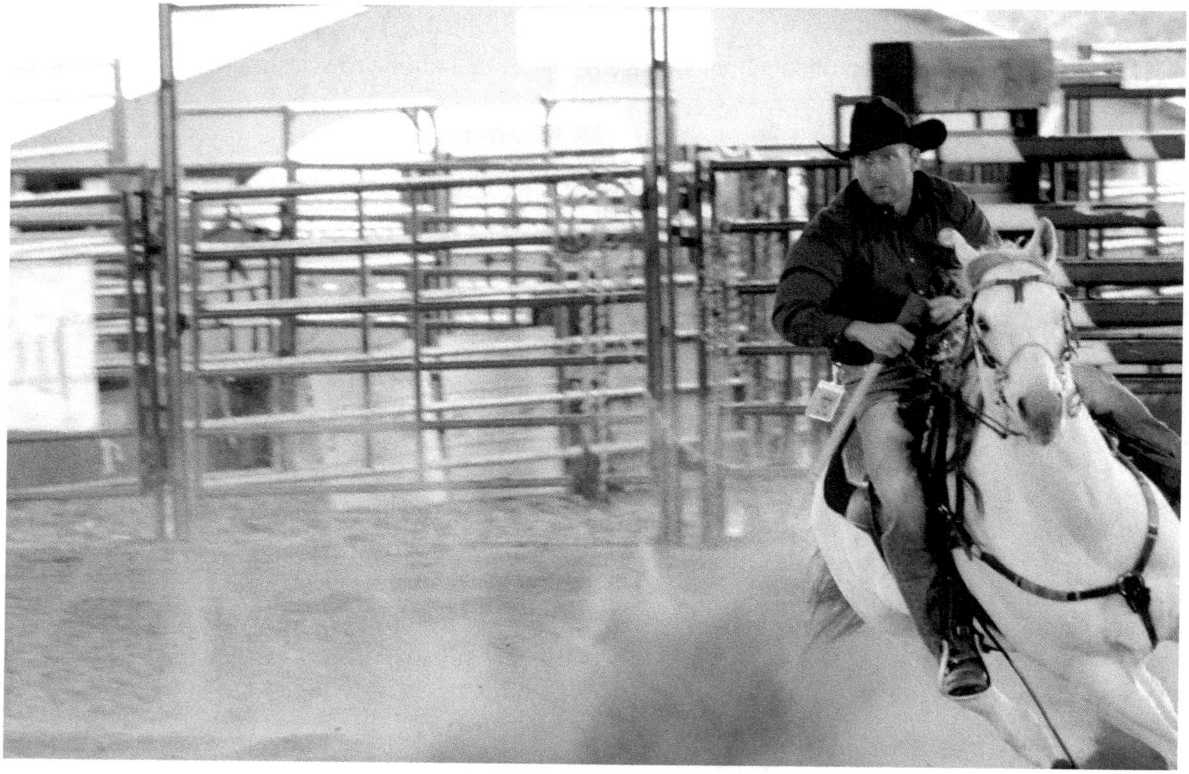

CHAPTER 8

LGBTQ ATHLETES IN SPORT

On Valentine's Day in 2006, Country Music Hall of Fame artist Willie Nelson released the song "Cowboys Are Frequently, Secretly Fond of Each Other." Nelson timed this release to express his support for the LGBTQ community, as well as his support of gay marriage. The song debuted on Howard Stern's radio broadcast and was available on iTunes shortly after that. Ned Sublette originally wrote the song in 1981. The song remained "in the closet" for twenty-five years. When Ned Sublette wrote the song, the gay liberation movement had already made great strides in bringing LGBT people out of the closet and into the public spotlight since the pivotal **1969 Stonewall riots** in New York City.

Gay liberation was not exclusive to the major metropolitan cities of New York, Chicago, and San Francisco. In 1976, rodeo cowboy Phil Ragsdale founded the Reno Gay Rodeo. Today, the International Gay Rodeo Association hosts rodeo competitions around the world that are open to any gender identity or sexual orientation. When he founded the Reno Gay Rodeo, Ragsdale believed that the phrase "gay cowboy" seemed to be a contradiction to many people in mainstream society because of **homophobic** stereotypes. This contradiction is similar to sociologist Eric Anderson's study of gay athletes and **hegemonic masculinity**—the gay athlete is a paradox because "gay [male] athletes comply with the gendered script of being male," yet they "violate another masculine script through the existence of their same-sex desires."[1] The gay male perspective on masculinity is challenged by the notion of hegemonic masculinity because it argues that femininity replaces masculinity, and gay cowboys challenge this notion. The sporting arena of the Gay Rodeo reinforces a "hegemonic model as the heroic ideal" for LGBT athletes (See Chapter 8 image of Kevin Springer at the Diamond State Rodeo in Little Rock, Arkansas).[2]

The gay rodeo challenged societal stereotypes of gay men by targeting one of the dominant narratives of the 1970s—gay identity as feminine. A QR code in the Further Reading section examines the gay rodeo and an event that took place in Golden, Colorado, in 2019. Today, the International Gay Rodeo circuit continues to challenge stereotypes about LGBT athletes, as these competitors continue to fight for their rightful place in sport.

1 Eric Anderson, *In the Game: Gay Athletes and the Cult of Masculinity* (Albany: State University of New York Press, 2005), 45; Anderson is drawing from the work of sociologist Brian Pronger, *The Arena of Masculinity: Sports, Homosexuality, and the Meaning of Sex* (New York: St. Martin's Press, 1990); the gay male perspective on masculinity is challenged by the notion of hegemonic masculinity because it argues that femininity replaces masculinity, and gay cowboys challenge this notion.

2 Rebecca Feasey, *Masculinity and Popular Television* (Edinburgh: Edinburgh University Press, 2008), 98.

17

MY (ATHLETIC) LIFE

Nancy Goldberger

I don't think it's too much of a stretch to say that being a member of the athletic community saved my life. Of course, this is certainly something I could not have foreseen as a young girl, growing up in the pre-Title IX[1] Midwest. In my years as a child and pre-teen, I played every sport possible, usually in an informal manner such as playground pick-up games or on a vacant lot after school or on weekends. There were no sports groups for girls in school. Even after Title IX came into effect, it took years before the small-town schools I attended in southern and central Illinois even tried to offer organized teams or the opportunity of equal access for participation.

During that time of my life, the sheer joy of sport and camaraderie of playing sports fueled my existence. Rare were the times I declined an invitation to play a game, whether it was baseball, football, basketball, or even tetherball. The sport didn't matter. I found participation in athletics life-giving and extremely satisfying. Even though there were not formally organized leagues and clubs to serve as an outlet for my athletic endeavors at the time, I found plenty of opportunities to play until about the age of 14. During the mid-1970s, gendered expectations were alive and well. Upon entering the teen years, girls often stopped being invited to play pick-up games or to join in sports. Social norms at that time did not look kindly upon a teenage girl wielding a baseball bat or throwing a football spiraling into the waiting arms of a receiver. Instead we were persuaded to cheer on the team and act more "ladylike." Realizing that I was being encouraged by friends and family to leave participation in sports behind, I tried my hand at other things. I competed in speech contests, science fairs, and so forth, activities decidedly more socially acceptable. I discovered that I could participate in these things and not be on the receiving end of a derisive look or comment from those around me who seemed to care about my fitting in. While I enjoyed those activities, nothing could stave off my unquenchable thirst for sport.

1 "Title IX of the Education Amendments Act of 1972 is a federal law that states: 'No person in the United States shall, on the basis of sex, be excluded from participation in, be denied the benefits of, or be subjected to discrimination under any education program or activity receiving Federal financial assistance'" (http://www.ncaa.org/about/resources/inclusion/title-ix-frequently-asked-questions). This amendment was a game changer in the area of athletics, positively impacting the opportunities for women to have equal opportunity to participation, athletic scholarships, and treatment (equipment, coaching, etc.).

Once I reached driving age, I discovered that there was a community summer softball league looking to add players to teams. Able to transport myself to and from practices and games, I joined a team and reveled in the opportunity for athletic participation. I played rec softball through high school, never once with my parents or family in the stands. While no one prevented me from participating, the message was loud and clear: We do not approve, and we will not support you in these activities.

While I was not fully aware, this message was a first warning from my family in regards to what they saw as the dangers that awaited a "girl like me," including my eventual discovery that I was a cisgender lesbian. Finding this out about myself in the first semester of my freshman year, I buried myself deep in the closet throughout college. I was keenly aware that should anyone else discover my secret, the religiously conservative educational institution I attended would expel me without hesitation if they had any whiff of perceived impropriety. This felt, to me, like the equivalent of a dishonorable discharge from the armed forces in a military family. Knowing this would bring instant and lasting humiliation upon me and my family (my father was a pastor of a large church in a small town), I tried my best to keep a low profile. I still, however, sought out ways to play sports.

I know now that leading a closeted life fosters feelings of shame, self-doubt, self-loathing, and constant concern about being discovered along with a host of other negative issues. But at 18 years old, I did not have the knowledge I have now, nor the support system. At that time, I began to feel overwhelmed in what seemed to be a suffocating environment. Any interest I had in classes faded. I no longer desired to go home for breaks or holidays as that felt even more oppressive. I started to feel as though there was no way out for me. If I lived a life my family would endorse, I would certainly die on the inside. If I lived a life that aligned with my identity, I would lose the only family I had ever known. There seemed to be no way out from this situation. I felt very alone and without hope. I was aware of a nagging little voice that told me in the quiet of the night that I was no good, that I was a disappointment to all who knew me, that I did not deserve to live. I never felt completely at ease wherever I was, save one place: on a team.

It was during this time of tremendous personal struggle that the value of participation in athletics became of utmost importance to me. I made the effort to go to classes only because it allowed me to play sports. At first I just joined the women's recreational leagues that were available to any interested female student. I found playing with these informally formed, yet fun and competitive teams, to be satisfying, and they brought me great joy. Feeling bolstered, I wanted more. You see, at this point, I gained more than just athletic satisfaction. When I picked up a bat or ball and stepped on a playing field, I belonged. My contribution to my team gave me purpose, satisfaction, and hope. Sports kept me going, gave me something to live for. I can honestly say that participation in athletics kept me alive when I felt at my lowest.

Once I began to experience a sense of belonging, I felt myself living more fully into the promise of who I was becoming as an individual. As my confidence grew, I joined the university track & field team as well as the field hockey team. Even though I had never played field hockey before, I was confident enough to take on roles that challenged me, such as becoming the goal keeper during my junior year. By senior year I was named captain of the team. This recognition from my teammates meant the world to me. It was such an honor to have their vote of affirmation and to serve as the team leader. Since maintaining a certain GPA was mandated to play for the university, my grades rebounded, and I ended up completing my Bachelor's degree in education with only one extra semester of course work. My ability to parlay my success on the field into academic success was no fluke. I know now that once I was able to experience a true sense of self and a real sense of belonging, the rest of the pieces began to fall into place for me. But this is not the end of my story.

After college, I taught in parochial school for the next few years. I was still in the closet as I would have been summarily dismissed from my teaching duties had my true identity been discovered. Even though I loved teaching, I longed to live a more authentic life. I knew I needed to completely extricate myself from this system in order to make my life my own. I left teaching after five years and became a book and magazine editor. This change not only removed the stigma of working within an intolerant religious system, it opened the world of work-sponsored athletic leagues. Making this move allowed me to find new opportunities to engage in athletics again. After a few years, I was team organizer for work volleyball and softball leagues. I reveled in the opportunity to work and play with people who accepted me for who I was—a hard-working dedicated employee who could also throw a mean strike to end the inning and win the game. My sexual identity did not matter, only that I was a positive contributor to the teams I worked and played with. I was, however, still living a fairly straight-looking life, passing as straight when I had to for family and at functions. It still felt like a part of me was playing it safe, unable or unwilling to take that last step out of the closet and into the fullness of the light of truth.

In 1992, softball proved to be more important than I could ever have imagined. That was the year that an invitation to join a softball team connected me to the person who would become my life partner. When she asked me to join her softball team, I did not know that she then had to quickly put one together. This effort, however, provided an arena where we could get to know each other. This was probably the single biggest compliment I have ever received in my life. We quickly discovered that we made a good team on and off the field.

A few years later, we delighted in finding and joining local LGBTQA-focused organizations that supported sports clubs. It was through these clubs that I met a wonderful array of individuals who not only enjoyed the satisfaction of playing sports, but knew the real value of belonging to a team on a very personal level. Being a part of a community of people who not only accept you for who you are but who are indeed like you in many ways is the next level of belonging. We often shared common experiences (e.g., facing discrimination in our families, being harassed on the street by those intolerant of non-heterosexuals, etc.), and we could help each other get through the toughest of times that most of the others in our lives did not know about or understand.

Over the several decades that I participated in teams through the Chicago Metropolitan Sports Association (CMSA) or the Women's Sports Association (WSA), I met some of the women who had forged a path to belonging. They were amazingly brilliant and brave individuals who believed in the value of sport together. They had also struggled through discrimination of those who would strip away avenues of expression based on gender identity and emerged victorious. I enjoyed their legacy for many years, playing volleyball, softball, and football. It was also through these organizations that I met newer members of the LGBTQA community. Realizing that they were also seeking to belong through athletics made it easy for me to become a team organizer, welcoming new members each season and including them in the fold. It is through my participation in these organizations that I have made some of the strongest, most enduring friendships in my life. Sports again gave me the opportunity to become not only an active participant, but also to serve as a leader to help build an inclusive and supportive community for others.

It was while we were playing in these leagues that my partner and I decided to pursue our dream of becoming parents. In the mid-1990s, it was not commonplace for non-heterosexual couples to have this option. I knew of only one other lesbian couple who travelled this path. However, we felt very passionate about this and our sport family supported us. They knew us, they believed in us, and they had our backs when others in our lives decided to turn away. We experienced discrimination from others along the way. The doctor we found who could help us realize our dream sat with us and announced that he did not want to take a lesbian couple as clients because "there are good Christian women" who worked in his practice. He refused to submit the clinic visits to the insurance, making us bear the full cost out-of-pocket and creating a negative environment for us during the process. If there had been other options, we would have pursued them. But at the time, this was the only path we could find, so we tolerated the doctor's arrogance and discrimination.

There were other instances along the way where heterosexual couples would have experienced warm, loving support, but we did not. The computerized baby registry only accommodated places for the names of the mother and father. When the extended family baby shower was held, I was not recognized as anything other than as a guest. It was truly awful to feel invisible and suffer the indignity of these events. Greatest among these was one deeply personal incident. You see, this pregnancy was the final straw for most of my conservative birth family. On the day our daughter was born, I picked up the phone and called my siblings to share the good news. I was not prepared for the debilitating shock I experienced when I heard my siblings respond that my father condemned this event, that they agreed with him, and until I "turned away from this way of life" that they did not want to have anything else to do with me. They rallied against me, and I was summarily disowned. The biggest fear of my youth had become reality. However, knowing that I did not have to go it alone, that I had a strong, loving partner and a community of support behind us, this new lowest point of my life was manageable. The other side of the coin, you see, was one of the highest points of my life. When I became a parent in 2001, my birth family tried to crush me and bring deep pain to this incredibly beautiful moment in my life. But after I endured their hurtful diatribe, I knew their self-righteous pontifications were just words intended to control me. I had become a strong enough person to survive without them. What mattered to me was the family I had created out of love, not the family that operated on hate. I don't know that I would have made it to this place without having athletics in my life.

It's no accident that I have earned Master's degrees in higher education and in women & gender studies. I feel very fortunate to have survived my undergraduate years and an unsupportive birth family. I know in my heart that participation in athletics has been tremendously critical in helping me discover who I am. Playing sports has allowed me to push past challenges and boundaries, to step up when I could contribute, and to reach back and pull others up with me. I now work in a large university in Chicago. I feel fortunate every day that I get to interact with undergraduate and graduate students who are often facing their own challenges. My goal is to not only help them successfully cross the finish line of their academic goals, but to help them live their own life more authentically. My education—in the classroom and on the field—has prepared me well to serve these students, and for that I am eternally grateful.

These days, after suffering a couple of broken bones (playing football and coaching youth soccer), I have stepped out of the role of participant and coach. I still play volleyball when I get the chance, and I can be occasionally coerced to throw pitching practice for softball when I go to watch my partner play. These days, however, most of my athletic involvement is watching our teenage daughter play club and high school sports. She knows that these opportunities haven't always been available, and she has a deep appreciation for what athletic participation brings to her life and ours. She has benefitted immensely from being an athlete, and I am a dedicated fan, cheering from the stands at every game. I've seen the sense of self that she has developed, and I have seen significant evidence of the positive benefits that athletics have had on her life so far.

This past summer, she and I attended one of my partner's games at the lakefront in Chicago. It was a beautiful day for a game. I sat on the sideline and chatted with the team until it was time for them to warm up. It was then that I became acutely aware of the group of people who had gathered behind me. As I turned to look, I did a double take, not really believing my eyes. There was a group of about 20 women and children, all milling about, and getting ready to watch the game. My eyes welled up a bit as I realized these were the partners and children of players on the field. What had been a rather radical concept 16 years earlier was now in full swing. Women having children with their female partners has become more commonplace today, and a fair number of those families are involved in athletic competition. They, too, were experiencing the sense of community and support that exists on these fields of play. Turning back around, I tapped my partner on the shoulder and said, "Look. Our legacy." She smiled and nodded. I call that a grand slam.

18

"AIN'T I A WOMAN?"

TRANSGENDER AND INTERSEX STUDENT ATHLETES IN WOMEN'S COLLEGIATE SPORTS

Pat Griffin

The title of this chapter is borrowed from Sojourner Truth's powerful demand that white feminist abolitionists in the nineteenth century expand their awareness to include the needs of black women in their fight for race and sex equality. Her question, "Ain't I a Woman," seems fitting for the twenty-first century also with regard to the inclusion in women's sports of transgender women and men and women who have intersex conditions. Increasing numbers of athletes who are transgender or have intersex conditions are challenging gender boundaries in sports as they insist on their right to participate according to their self-affirmed genders. Recent controversies surrounding the eligibility of South African runner Caster Semenya to compete in women's events and the participation of transgender athletes, such as George Washington University basketball player Kye Allums and professional golfer Lana Lawson, challenge the traditional boundaries of sex and gender in sport.

This chapter explores how the gender and sex binary assumptions upon which the organization of sports competition is based can create problems when people whose gender identities or variations in sexual development do not conform to these assumptions assert their right to participate. I discuss how transgender and intersex athletes challenge assumptions about the essential nature of the category "woman." At the same time, I show how sexist and heterosexist stereotypes converge to affect the gender performance of all women in sports, with a particularly limiting effect on people whose gender identity, gender expression, biological sex, and/or sexual orientation do not conform to cultural norms.

After a description of relevant language related to this topic, I review selected historical events describing concerns about women athletes' sex, femininity, and heterosexuality. I then explore how these concerns and the gender-binary assumptions undergirding them affect policies governing the eligibility of transgender and intersex athletes to participate in women's collegiate athletic events. I conclude the chapter with a discussion of current efforts to provide transgender and intersex athletes with opportunities to participate in school-based women's athletic competitions.

A Word About Words

The language of sex and gender can be confusing and complicated. Many of the concepts feminist scholars and gender activists use challenge conventional notions about gender and sex. Moreover, the language is evolving, and many feminist scholars and gender activists disagree about how the language should be used. For example, the terms "sex" and "gender" are used interchangeably by some writers, while others find it useful to provide specific and separate definitions for each of these terms. I find it helpful, at least on a conceptual level, to define these two key terms separately.

According to Gender Spectrum, an education and advocacy organization for gender-variant children and teens, "sex" is biological and includes physical attributes, such as sex chromosomes, gonads, sex hormones, internal reproductive structures, and external genitalia. At birth, individuals are typically categorized as male or female based on the appearance of their external genitalia. This binary categorization ignores the spectrum of biological sex characteristics that confound attempts to fit everyone neatly into either male or female categories. The term "gender" is similarly complicated. According to Genderspectrum.org, "Along with one's physical traits, it is the complex interrelationship between those traits and one's internal sense of self as male, female, both or neither as well as one's outward presentations and behaviors related to that perception." I find it helpful to make this differentiation, especially when discussing these terms in relationship to sports, where physical attributes are integral aspects of the discussion.

Gender is not inherently related to sex. A person who identifies as transgender has a gender identity (an internal sense of gender: being male or female, trans, or other gender sensibility) that does not match the sex (or gender) they were assigned at birth based on an inspection of their physical characteristics. A transgender woman or girl may be born with a body identified as male and, on the basis of that body, assigned to the gender category "boy," even though she identifies as a girl. The reverse is true for a transgender man or boy. Transgender people choose to express their genders in many ways: changing their names and self-referencing pronouns to better match their gender identities; choosing clothes, hairstyles, or other aspects of self-presentation that reflect their gender identities; and generally living and presenting themselves to others consistently with their gender identities. Some, but not all, transgender people take hormones or undergo surgical procedures to change their bodies to better reflect their gender identities. Transgender encompasses a vast range of identities and practices; however, for the purposes of this essay, I use the term "transgender" more specifically to refer to women who have transitioned from their assigned male gender at birth to their affirmed gender as women and to men who have transitioned from their assigned female gender at birth to their affirmed gender as men.

People with intersex conditions may be born with chromosomes, hormones, genitalia, or other sex characteristics that do not match the patterns that typify biological maleness or femaleness. Many intersex people are not aware of their intersex status unless it is revealed as part of a medical examination or treatment. People with intersex conditions are assigned a gender at birth; many live and identify with that assigned gender throughout their lives, although many do not. In this essay, I use "intersex women" to refer to women with intersex conditions who have always identified as women (for more information about intersex conditions, go to www.accordalliance.org).

The participation of transgender and intersex women poses related but different challenges to gendered divisions in sports. Transgender women and intersex women are viewed by many sports leaders, women competitors, and the general public as men or as "not normal" women whose participation in women's sports threatens the notion of a "level playing field." In the context of sex-segregated women's sports, these athletes' bodies are viewed as male, and they are often perceived to have an unfair competitive advantage over non-intersex or non-transgender women athletes. But trans and intersex visibility and participation belies the myth of the level playing field and the myth of binary gender on which it rests.

Sports and the Gender Binary

Although some school athletic teams, such as sailing, are composed of men and women who compete without regard to the sex or gender of participants, mixed-sex competition is the exception at all levels of sports. In most sports that women and men play, schools sponsor separate men's and women's teams—basketball, volleyball, swimming, track and field, lacrosse, or soccer, for example. This sex division is based on the assumption that sex-separate competitive opportunities are the best route to equal opportunity and fair competition for all. Title IX, the 1972 landmark federal legislation prohibiting sex discrimination in education, includes guidelines for providing comparable school-based athletic opportunities for girls and women and boys and men on sex-separate teams to provide equal participation opportunities (Brake 2010; Hogshead-Makar and Zimbalist 2007).

Dividing participants into sex-separate teams is based on two assumptions: (1) Sex and gender are binary and immutable characteristics, and (2) salient physical differences between males and females substantially affect athletic performance to the advantage of males in most sports.

Rather than a binary of athletic performance based on sex, it would be more accurate to describe sex differences as a spectrum, with females and males occupying overlapping positions. Although it is fair to say that most adult male athletes are bigger, taller, and stronger than most adult female athletes, some female athletes outperform their male counterparts in sport. So, even among athletes who are not transgender or intersex, sex-separated teams do not always adequately accommodate the diversity of skill, motivation, and physical characteristics among female and male athletes. Some boys or men might find a better competitive match competing on a girls' team, and some girls' athletic performances are more comparable to those on a boys' team.

Some girls and boys have been allowed to participate on teams designated for the other sex, particularly if a school only sponsors a team in that sport for one sex. For example, girls sometimes compete on boy's wrestling or football teams, and boys sometimes compete on girls' field hockey or volleyball teams. However, cross-sex participation on sports teams is always an exception and is often greeted with skepticism by other competitors, parents, and fans. Even among prepubescent girls and boys where size and strength are similar or where girls are often taller, stronger, and faster than boys, sports are typically divided by sex. Such is the entrenched nature of the belief in a static and immutable gender and sex binary in sports.

For most athletes whose gender identity is congruent with their gender assigned at birth or whose physical sex anatomy is congruent with their sex assigned at birth, the answer to the question of which team to play for is simple. However, for athletes whose gender identity does not match the gender they were assigned at birth or for athletes with differences of sexual development, the separation of sports into participation categories based on binary sex has often resulted in humiliation and discrimination. Transgender and intersex athletes challenge the gender binary in sports and force sports leaders to reflect on how and where to draw gender boundaries for the purposes of identifying on which teams an athlete is allowed to compete.

Because women athletes have always challenged the hegemonic notion of athleticism as a masculine trait and because sports participation has historically been a male privilege to which girls and women were not entitled, the fight for equal sports opportunities for women is ongoing. Gendered expectations for girls and women have not comfortably included such characteristics as "competitive," "athletic," or "muscular"; as a result, women athletes have always had to prove their "normalcy" based on socially constructed assumptions about femininity, heterosexuality, and an unquestioned acceptance of a gender binary. Women who excel in sports *and* whose appearance, behavior, and/or identity does not conform to traditional notions of who is a woman, how a woman should look and act, and who a woman should be sexually attracted to are viewed with suspicion and as illegitimate participants in women's sports competitions (Cahn 1994; Festle 1996; Griffin 1998).

History of Gender Anxiety in Women's Sport

During the early twentieth century, women participating in athletic competitions were subjected to white middle-class criticism from medical doctors, media commentators, psychologists, and others who warned of a range of catastrophic effects of athletic competition they believed would cause physiological and psychological damage. Based on the belief that white women were physically and psychically frail, sports participation was viewed as dangerous to their health and well-being. The prevailing medical and social perspective was that women who did compete in sports were subjected to a number of "masculinizing" effects on their appearance, behavior, and sexual interests that would prevent them from living as "normal" women whose proper roles were wives and mothers. Thus, the early seeds of gender suspicion about women athletes were planted. Advocates for women's sports participation and women athletes themselves often responded defensively to these criticisms by highlighting their femininity (according to racially white heteronormative standards) and heterosexual interests, and by portraying their sports interest as a complement to their focus on motherhood and marriage (Cahn 1994).

These fears are best illustrated in public reaction to Babe Didrikson, a multisport athlete who won Olympic medals in track and field and played baseball, basketball, and tennis before later focusing on professional golf. Didrikson was a well-known cultural icon whose brash manner, quick sense of humor, and competitive fire always made for a good story. Unfortunately, Didrikson was treated as a gender freak and ridiculed for her lack of femininity, her "masculine" appearance, and her athletic prowess. Called a "muscle moll" and worse, it is no wonder that by midcentury, Didrikson initiated an intentional public-relations campaign to reassure the American public that she was a "normal" woman after all, despite her athletic achievements (Cayleff 1995). She began wearing dresses and talking about her love of cooking, and, to seal the deal, she married wrestling champion George Zaharias. These efforts succeeded in quieting the concerns of male sports reporters and the general public about Didrikson's femininity and heterosexuality.

As women's competition in Olympic sports and professional golf and tennis became more visible in the 1940s through the 1970s, another wave of suspicion about the gender and sexuality of women athletes prompted some women's sports advocates and athletes themselves to take an apologetic stance by focusing on disproving sexist assumptions about the "masculine" lesbian women who lived in the sports world. These efforts included the institution of feminine dress codes, instructions about makeup application and hair styling, and direction of media attention to the "pretty ones," who served as goodwill ambassadors who contradicted the unsavory image of "masculine" women athletes (Gerber, Felshin, and Wyrick 1974).

These fears, coupled with the belief that women are inherently athletically inferior to their male counterparts, caused increased gender suspicions about outstanding athletic performances by female athletes. These questions were raised in the 1964 Olympics by Russian hammer-throwers and shot-putters Tamara and Irina Press, whose muscular appearances and medal-winning performances provoked suspicion that they were actually men posing as women.

In 1976, Renée Richards, a transgender woman, was denied entry in the Women's U.S. Open by the U.S. Tennis Association (USTA) on the basis that she was not a "born woman." The New York Supreme Court ruled against the USTA and enabled Richards to compete in the women's event. Despite this court ruling, the Ladies Professional Golf Association (LPGA) maintained a "born woman" requirement for membership until 2010; when faced with a lawsuit by transgender woman golfer Lana Lawson, the LPGA dropped its prohibition against transgender participants. Transgender women, such as Richards and Lawson, are viewed by some suspicious tennis players and golfers as illegitimate women who have male bodies that confer an unfair competitive advantage when competing against so-called "natural" women.

In 1966, in response to fears of male cheaters competing as women, the International Olympic Committee (IOC) instituted mandatory "gender" verification testing of all female competitors. (The tests were called "sex tests," and their purpose was to confirm that competitors were female-bodied and, later, that their chromosomal makeup was female.) The first such tests required all Olympic competitors entered in women's events to appear naked before a panel of "experts," who, by visual inspection, determined whether the prospective competitors were eligible to compete as female.

Not surprisingly, athletes and other sports observers criticized this humiliating process. Medical experts also criticized the process, because, in addition to the invasive and voyeuristic nature of the "gender test," it was also a crude and ineffective means of determining whether a competitor was female.

Eventually, more "scientific" procedures were developed in which women athletes were subjected to buccal smear tests in which mouth swabs yielded cellular samples from which the chromosomal makeup could be identified. Athletes whose chromosomal makeup was other than XX were determined to be ineligible to compete as women. Women who "passed" the test were given "certificates of femininity" and allowed to compete.

These supposedly more-scientific tests also failed to achieve their intended goal. Rather than identifying male imposters, the only competitors who were ever disqualified were women with atypical chromosomal makeup who had lived their entire lives as women and were not attempting to gain an unfair competitive advantage. The resulting traumatic and public shaming that followed their identifications as "not women" not only terminated their athletic careers but damaged their personal lives as well.

Current Policy Governing the Participation of Transgender and Intersex Athletes

These "gender" tests revealed the folly of identifying a simple and fair, not to mention respectful, means of determining who is a woman. Nonetheless, although mandatory "gender verification" testing was discontinued prior to the 2000 Olympic Games, individual women athletes who trigger suspicions about their sex are now tested on a case-by-case basis. Unfortunately, these sex challenges are typically triggered by such ambiguous and culturally biased gender criteria as short hair, small breasts, preferences for "masculine" clothes, deep voices, muscular physiques, and excellence of athletic performance. Thus, the challenge of identifying who is and is not a woman for the purpose of determining eligibility to compete in women's sports events continues to be controversial.

During the 2009 Track and Field World Championships, South African runner Caster Semenya astounded the international track establishment with her gold-medal performance in the women's eight-hundred-meter run, leaving her competition far back on the track. Semenya was identified as a female at birth, has always identified as a woman, and is accepted as a woman by her family and friends. However, unconfirmed speculations are that she has an intersex condition. Immediately following her victory, some of her competitors and race officials from other countries filed challenges to the International Association of Athletics Federation (IAAF) under the IAAF's case-by-case "gender-verification" policy. (Mirroring the IOC, the IAAF policy had replaced mandatory "gender" verification testing of women athletes in favor of a case-by-case process.)

After months of subjecting Semenya to medical examinations, public speculation about whether she is a woman, public humiliation, and egregious breaches of confidentiality by the IAAF, she was allowed to keep her gold medal. Eleven months later, after secretive IAAF deliberations, she was cleared for competition in women's events. The IAAF released this decision without an explanation of its process, criteria, or reasoning. When Semenya won her first two races after returning to competition and finished third in another, some of her competitors again began complaining that they were unfairly forced to compete against a man or, at the very least, a "woman on the fringe of normalcy," as one competitor described Semenya.

Whether being intersex confers any performance advantage is open to speculation. No scientific data are available to indicate that it does or does not. However, Semenya's competitors assume that she is a man or not a "normal" woman and that she has an unfair competitive advantage that should disqualify her from competing in women's events. These objections to Semenya's eligibility to compete as a woman are based on her margin of victory over the other women in the 2009 World Championships and on her "masculine" physical appearance, clothing, and deep voice. All these characteristics challenge the gender binary upon which sports competition is based as well as binary assumptions about who is a woman and therefore eligible to compete in women's events.

In 2004, in a surprisingly proactive decision by a typically conservative organization, the IOC adopted a policy outlining criteria enabling transgender athletes to compete in IOC-sponsored events:

- The athlete's gender must be legally recognized on official identity documents.
- The athlete must have completed genital reconstructive surgery and had his or her testes or ovaries removed.
- The athlete must complete a minimum two-year postoperative hormone treatment before she or he is allowed to compete.

The IOC policy is the first attempt by a mainstream sports organization to identify specific criteria governing the participation of transgender athletes. However, transgender-rights advocates criticize the policy, noting the class and sex bias built into the policy as well as problems related to privacy and medical confidentiality. Moreover, some transgender medical experts have provided some data indicating that a one-year waiting period is adequate for the athletes' hormonal levels to be within the range of non-transgender women and men. To date, no transgender athlete has competed in the Olympic Games under this policy.

Despite its considerable flaws, USA Track and Field, the U.S. Golf Association, and a few state high school athletic governing organizations have adopted the IOC policy (for example, those in Colorado, Connecticut, and Rhode Island). The participation criteria identified in the IOC policy would make it virtually impossible for transgender student athletes to compete in high school sports. The requirements of genital reconstructive surgery, mandatory sterilization, and changing the sex indicated on official identity documents impose financial and legal burdens that even many adult transgender athletes cannot or choose not to pursue. The two-year waiting period is not supported by medical data and is not practical in school sports, where a student athlete's eligibility is already limited to four or five years.

As of 2011, no national governing organization for high school sports has adopted a policy concerning the participation of intersex athletes in school-based sports events. However, in 2008, the Washington State Interscholastic Activity Association (WIAA) adopted the most progressive policy to date governing the participation of transgender student athletes on high school sports teams. This policy requires neither surgery nor change of identity documents. Transgender students can participate in their affirmed genders after appealing to the state interscholastic activities association and providing written documentation of the student's gender from the student and parent/guardian and/or a health-care provider. To date, the policy has been used successfully to enable transgender students to participate on sex-separate teams.

At the collegiate level, the National Collegiate Athletic Association (NCAA) released a statement in 2004 clarifying that the organization does not prohibit transgender student athletes from competing in NCAA-sanctioned events but that student athletes must compete in the sex identified on their official identity documents. NCAA legal advisers believed that this provision was a simple solution to addressing the question of transgender participation in NCAA athletic programs. Because of significant differences among state requirements for changing the sex indicated on official identity documents, however, this requirement is discriminatory and creates complications when athletes from different states compete against each other. More recently, the NCAA has recognized the need for a more nuanced and inclusive policy. In 2011, it adopted the first-ever national policy regarding transgender athletes in collegiate athletics; the policy allows transgender athletes to compete in sex-segregated sports if, and only if, their hormonal treatment is consistent with current medical standards—standards that themselves suggest different treatment requirements for trans men and trans women (Lawrence 2011).

As of 2010, only two collegiate openly transgender student athletes had competed in NCAA-sponsored events. Keelin Godsey competed on the women's track and field team at Bates College and in the Olympic trials in the women's hammer throw. Allums currently is a member of the George Washington University women's basketball team. Godsey and Allums are female-bodied transgender men who are not taking testosterone so they can continue to compete in women's events. Because they are not taking testosterone, an NCAA-banned substance, and are competing in the sex identified on their official identity documents as specified by the NCAA and IOC, Godsey and Allums are eligible to compete on women's teams.

Whether the perceived threats to women's sports are identified as male imposters, transgender women, transgender men not taking testosterone, intersex women, butch-looking straight women, or lesbians, protecting the boundaries of women's sports from these gender transgressors by upholding the gender binary has become increasing difficult as the myth of the gender binary and the myth of the level playing field have been exposed.

The Myth of the Level Playing Field

Just as some people view lesbians as threats to women's sports because they fear association with the stereotypes of lesbians as unsavory, so, too, do many athletes and the general public view transgender and intersex women athletes with particular suspicion. Although lesbians may be viewed as women who look or act like men, some people view transgender and intersex women as actually *being* men, in most places making them ineligible to compete in women's sports. The most-often-cited concern about the participation of transgender or intersex women in women's sports is that they threaten a "level playing field." Many competitors, coaches, and parents assume that transgender and intersex women, because of their male bodies, have an unfair competitive advantage over women who are not perceived to be trans or intersex.

Even without the participation of transgender or intersex women in women's sports, the playing field is hardly level. The entire focus of sports competition is to gain a competitive advantage, as long as that advantage is defined as being within the rules. Training hard to gain a competitive advantage is fair. Taking performance-enhancing drugs is not fair. Competitive advantages in women's sports come in many different forms: social, economic, environmental, psychological, and physiological, to name a few. Some women grow up in cultures where girls' sports participation is supported by social norms. These girls have a competitive advantage over other girls whose cultures restrict female athleticism. Girls whose families have the financial resources that enable them to train with the best coaches, to use the best equipment, to have access to good nutrition and health care, and to compete with the best athletes have a competitive advantage. Girls who live in places with clean air and water and safe streets have a competitive advantage. Girls who have inner resources of mental toughness and competitive drive have a competitive edge over physically talented but less mentally tough opponents. Some women have competitive advantages over opponents in their sports because of their genetics. Even some genetic conditions, such as Marfan syndrome, which results in unusual height, can be a competitive advantage in some sports where being tall is an advantage. All these competitive advantages are viewed in sports as fair and part of the game. All these advantages expose the myth of the level playing field even among women who are not transgender or intersex.

Why then is it that all these competitive advantages are accepted as fair variations among women athletes that can account for athletic-performance differences, but the competitive advantages that may or may not be enjoyed by some transgender or intersex women are viewed as unfair and threats to a level playing field warranting banishment from women's competition?

Competitive advantages assumed to be conferred by perceived maleness or masculinity are viewed as unfair competitive advantages. Transgender women, intersex women, or any women who do not conform to social expectations of femininity and heterosexuality are threats to the image of athletic women as gender conformists. As long as women athletes can be cast as feminine, heterosexual women, they do not pose a threat to the dominance of men in sports and male privilege in sports. This is the price of acceptance that women in sports have had to pay since the early twentieth century, when they began participating in sports in large numbers.

Gender Binary Meets Transgender and Intersex Athletes: What is the Way Forward?

Women who by their inability or refusal to conform to binary gender norms in sports also challenge the mythical gender binary altogether. Given that athletics as an institution has been built on sexist assumptions about the natural superiority of men's sports performance over that of women and that the gender binary forms the basis for how sports are structured into sex-separate participation categories, how should women's sports address the question of including transgender and intersex athletes?

Policy development designed to address this question can take several forms: (1) Protect the gender binary by using sex-verification testing to exclude "non-women," (2) address challenges to the gender binary on a case-by-case basis, (3) eliminate gender as a sport-participation category, and (4) expand gender categories to include participants whose bodies and/or gender identities do not conform to the gender binary.

Protect the gender binary with mandatory sex-verification testing of all female participants. This policy has been discredited as impractical, discriminatory, invasive, and ineffective. The IOC abandoned this policy in 1999, and nothing suggests that any improvement of testing procedures will bring it back as a mandatory process.

Use sex-verification testing on a case-by-case basis as challenges to individual female participants arise. This is the IOC/IAAF policy now in effect. The controversy surrounding the challenge to Semenya's eligibility to compete in women's events illustrates many of the problems with this policy. The criteria for challenging an individual athlete's gender are based on a combination of sexist assumptions about female athletic performance and bodies, socially constructed gendered expectations for appearance and behavior, and a selective belief in the level playing field in sports in which some competitive advantages, particularly those based on genetic differences, are viewed as fair while others are not. Testing on a case-by-case basis eliminates the impracticality of testing all competitors entered in women's events and avoids the mass anxiety inherent in the process. However, the sex testing of individual competitors on a case-by-case basis is based on myths about gender and a level playing field that subject the athletes who are targeted to an invasive and humiliating, and often public, process. The effects of these tests are questionable given the arbitrary nature of determining when a woman's physiological makeup crosses a socially constructed line to become "too" male to qualify to compete against other women.

The IOC policy for determining the eligibility of transgender women athletes on a case-by-case process includes criteria that require surgical intervention and legal documentation of transition that create insurmountable obstacles for most transgender people. The policy also requires an excessive waiting period once hormone treatment has begun that is not supported by current medical research.

Eliminate sex and gender as sports-participation categories. Some LGBT legal advocates believe that eliminating men's and women's sports in favor of other criteria for determining sports participation is the only way to address the complexities and challenges of including transgender and intersex athletes. These advocates argue that dividing sports participation on the basis of a sex and gender binary is inherently unfair. Some feminist legal critics of Title IX believe that the law, by assuming that sex-separate teams are the best route to equality for women in sport, has enshrined sex inequality and relegated women's sports to a permanent second-class status. Their assumption is that Title IX establishes a "separate but equal" goal even though this legal concept has been discredited in lawsuits challenging racial and disability discrimination (McDonagh and Pappano 2008).

The logic and goals of such legalistic arguments for the elimination of sex-separate sports as a way to address the myth of the gender and sex binary, inequality in women's sports, and the inclusion of transgender and intersex women athletes are appealing in some ways. Dividing sports by such performance-related physical criteria as height, jumping ability, or weight might be a reasonable strategy to eliminate discrimination based on sex and gender identity. Using actual performance in sports, such as running or swimming speed, agility, balance, points scored, or batting averages, also provides alternatives for dividing competitors into teams to level the playing field.

Although is it true that the gender binary creates a questionable division between the athletic interests, talent, and performance of men and women, it is also accurate to say that, for adults, most male athletes are bigger and stronger than most women athletes. As a result, dividing school teams by such "non-gendered" criteria as physical characteristics and athletic performance at this point in the history of women's sports would likely result in most athletic teams consisting of men and a few select women (including trans and intersex athletes). Second teams, if school chose to field them, would probably consist of men and women in more equal numbers (including trans and intersex women). Third teams, in the unlikely event that schools chose to expand their support for more than two teams per sport, would probably consist of mostly women (including men and some trans and intersex athletes) and some men.

It is also questionable whether these performance-based criteria are really non-gendered. Many of the physiological differences between male and female bodies do give men a competitive advantage over women, depending on the sport. However, gendered social and cultural expectations still encourage and reward male athletes more than they do female athletes. Sexism in sports still limits women athletes' access to sports and the resources that support athletic teams. Much like the rationale behind affirmative action as a way of correcting past race and sex discrimination, sex-separate sports enable women to overcome past sex discrimination in sports. Studies documenting the impressive increases in girls' and women's participation in sports and the increasing quality and quantity of women's sports experiences since the passage of Title IX demonstrate the law's undeniable positive effects (Carpenter and Acosta 2004). At the same time, despite these successes, resistance to Title IX compliance and persistent sexism are still obstacles to full women's equality in sports.

I worry that eliminating women's sports in favor of "non-gendered" sports opportunities will, at this point in the development of women's sports, relegate the majority of women athletes either to the junior varsity or to the sidelines. Sport is gendered by social and cultural expectations. Even criteria meant to be "gender-free" are still embedded in historical and contemporary societal structures of sex inequality that disadvantage female athletes while advantaging male athletes. I keep imagining an incredibly talented athlete, such as the University of Connecticut women's basketball player Maya Moore, sitting on the bench for a varsity college team made up of mostly taller, stronger men or starting on a junior varsity team that receives less attention and fewer resources than the varsity team. Moreover, Moore is an exceptional athlete. How does the elimination of women's teams benefit the majority of college women athletes (including trans women and intersex women) who are not as talented as she is?

Expand gender categories to include participants whose bodies and/or gender identities do not conform to the gender binary. I believe that, despite compelling criticisms of the problems posed by dividing sports participation into sex-separate participation categories, this structure is the best way, at this point in women's sports history, to achieve sex equality in sports. Sex-separate sports teams provide the most participation opportunities for the most girls and women. Title IX, although not perfect, has demonstrated that, when opportunities are available, girls and women come to play in increasingly larger numbers with every successive generation. I do not believe that this would be so if girls and women were competing not only against each other but also against boys and men for these opportunities.

If sex-separate sports are indeed the best route to sex equality, the question is how can we expand our criteria to include competitors in women's sports who challenge the rigidity of the gender binary? Can we respect the self-affirmed gender identities of transgender athletes and the differences of sex development in intersex women by including them in our definitions of "woman" so their right to participate on women's teams is also protected?

Current Efforts to Create Inclusive Collegiate Athletic Policy Governing the Participation of Transgender and Intersex Athletes

In October 2009, the National Center for Lesbian Rights and the Women's Sports Foundation co-sponsored a national think tank titled "Equal Opportunities for Transgender Student-Athletes." The attendees were legal, medical, athletic, and advocacy leaders with expertise in transgender issues. The think tank's goal was to develop recommended policies for high school and collegiate athletic programs. The report from this think tank, *On the Team: Equal Opportunities for Transgender Student-Athletes,* includes a comprehensive discussion of issues, policy recommendations for high school and college athletics, and a list of best practices for sport administrators, coaches, student athletes, and parents (Griffin and Carroll 2010).

The following guiding principles served as a foundation for the think tank's discussions and the policy recommendations included in the report:

1. Participation in interscholastic and intercollegiate athletics is a valuable part of the education experience for all students.
2. Transgender student athletes should have equal opportunity to participate in sports.
3. The integrity of women's sports should be preserved.
4. Policies governing sports should be based on sound medical knowledge and scientific validity.
5. Policies governing sports should be objective, workable, and practicable; they should also be written, available, and equitably enforced.
6. Policies governing the participation of transgender students in sports should be fair in light of the tremendous variation among individuals in strength, size, musculature, and ability.
7. The legitimate privacy interests of all student athletes should be protected.
8. The medical privacy of transgender students should be preserved.
9. Athletic administrators, staff, parents of athletes, and student athletes should have access to sound and effective educational resources and training related to the participation of transgender and gender-variant students in athletics.
10. Policies governing the participation of transgender students in athletics should comply with state and federal laws protecting students from discrimination based on sex, disability, and gender identity and expression.

To maintain the integrity of women's sports while including transgender and intersex women athletes on women's sports teams requires that sports-governing organizations at all levels develop policies enabling women who challenge the gender binary to play. These policies must be focused on providing equal opportunities to a broad spectrum of women and be based on current medical and legal information rather than on unchallenged acceptance of the gender binary, female athletic inferiority, and a selective view of what constitutes a level playing field. This endeavor will require confronting our anxieties about blurring gender and sexuality boundaries and recognizing the arbitrary manner in which we define who is a woman to maintain a comfortable but oppressive understanding of gender and sexuality. We must recognize that the enforcement of exclusionary definitions of who qualifies as a woman denies some students the opportunity to play on school sports teams. We must understand that enabling transgender and intersex students to participate on women's sports teams is an important step toward greater equality for all women and strengthens women's sports in the same way that addressing the needs of lesbians, women with disabilities, and women of color strengthens the broader social movement for women's equality.

Most colleges and universities include as part of their education missions commitments to equality and fairness. As reflected in nondiscrimination statements and educational programming focused on social justice and diversity, schools endeavor to invite students and staff to think more critically about privilege and disadvantage based on social and cultural identities. Policy development in collegiate athletics should reflect the broader goals and values of the schools they are part of and not allow competitive goals or financial gain to shape policies (Buzuvis 2011). Policies governing the inclusion of transgender and intersex student athletes must be based on a commitment to providing all students with equal opportunities to participate on school sports teams, while at the same time protecting the integrity of women's sports as the best strategy for achieving sex equality in sports.

Bibliography

Brake, Deborah. *Getting in the Game: Title IX and the Women's Sports Revolution.* New York: New York University Press, 2010.

Buzuvis, Erin E. "Transgender Student-Athletes and Sex-Segregated Sport: Developing Policies of Inclusion for Intercollegiate and Interscholastic Athletics." *Seton Hall Journal of Sports and Entertainment Law* 21 (2011): 1–59.

Cahn, Susan. *Coming on Strong: Gender and Sexuality in Twentieth-Century Women's Sport.* New York: Free Press, 1994.

Carpenter, Linda Jean, and R. Vivian Acosta. *Title IX.* Champaign, IL: Human Kinetics, 2004.

Cayleff, Susan E. *Babe: The Life and Legend of Babe Didrikson Zaharias.* Urbana: University of Illinois Press, 1995.

Festle, Mary Jo. *Playing Nice: Politics and Apologies in Women's Sports.* New York: Columbia University Press, 1996.

Gerber, Ellen W., Jan Felshin, and Waneen Wyrick. *The American Woman in Sport.* Reading, MA: Addison-Wesley, 1974.

Griffin, Pat. *Strong Women, Deep Closets: Lesbians and Homophobia in Sport.* Champaign, IL: Human Kinetics, 1998.

Griffin, Pat, and Helen J. Carroll. *On the Team: Equal Opportunities for Transgender Student-Athletes.* National Center for Lesbian Rights and the Women's Sports Foundation, 2010. Available at www.nclrights.org/site/DocServer/TransgenderStudentAthleteReport.pdf?docID=7901.

Hogshead-Makar, Nancy, and Andrew Zimbalist, eds. *Equal Play: Title IX and Social Change.* Philadelphia, PA: Temple University Press, 2007.

Lawrence, Marta. *Transgender Policy Approved.* September 13, 2011, NCAA.org. Available at www.ncaa.org/wps/wcm/connect/public/NCAA/Resources/Latest+News/2011/September/Transgender+policy+approved.

McDonagh, Eileen, and Laura Pappano. *Playing with the Boys.* New York: Oxford University Press, 2008.

19

JUST KEEP SWIMMING

INTERSECTION OF NON-BINARY AND ATHLETE

G Ryan

Being a swimmer will always be a part of who I am. It means I understand frozen hair in the winter, the smell of chlorine in class, and the lines on the bottom of the pool perpetually imprinted on my eyes. I didn't start swimming with the goal to swim in college, get a scholarship, or win trophies and medals. No, I started swimming because my older brother swam, and I had to prove I could do anything he could. I kept swimming after that because I loved the challenge and the discipline, and because I reveled in the fact that the clock doesn't lie or play favorites. And the people I've had the opportunity to meet, both competitors and teammates, are incredible. But as I entered college, I started to feel the constraints of my sport, rather than the ways in which it supported me. I began to recognize the limitations that might arise between my athletic identity and my gender identity. I was growing to better understand myself as a person, and I couldn't see how I would fit into swimming. I identify as genderqueer, and I didn't have a role model in the sports arena to base my actions off of. Was it even possible to continue to compete? And if so, what parts of myself would I have to sacrifice? I still don't have all the answers, but I do know more now than I did then.

I came out as queer in regards to my sexuality in high school. I was taking my classes online, so my only social connections existed within my team. I was nervous about it from that perspective, because I didn't want to alienate the only people I had meaningful interactions with throughout the day. And since I was spending four or more hours a day with my teammates, it would be better if those relationships were not unduly strained. I was wonderfully naïve to the whole idea of "coming out" at that time. I thought it would be this grand declaration with everyone present and the audience would erupt into fractured opinions and outcries. Well, it was far less dramatic than that, to no one's surprise but my own. First to my immediate family, then in small groups to my friends, I stammered out in variations on a script that I was queer and didn't really want to date guys. It turned out my sexuality wasn't a problem. It really wasn't even noteworthy. Most of the responses were along the lines of "Yeah, I figured" or "I pretty much guessed that." So, it became a non-event, despite my concerns. My family was supportive, and again, not particularly surprised. I thought that would be the end of everything, that I had

G. Ryan, "Just Keep Swimming: Intersection of Non-Binary and Athlete," *Queer Voices from the Locker Room*, ed. Cu-Hullan Tsuyoshi McGivern and Paul Chamness Miller, pp. 127-132.

come into my own and had also braved the reactions of others. But it was really only the beginning of my journey to discovering myself.

I've worn long shorts and baggy shirts most of my life. Having an older brother was a boon, because whatever he grew out of inevitably ended up in my closet. The age gap of seven years became an issue though, because he left for college when I was only eleven. I started having to actually navigate clothing stores, rather than raiding his drawers. By high school, when I started defining myself as queer, I had come to terms with the fact that I was more comfortable in short hair and boxers, in button downs and ties. I liked the anonymity of not having to conform to conventional gender rules, but it was draining to always have to defend myself in locker rooms and bathrooms. I had to give myself the permission to not only dress the way that I wanted, but to have a mix of emotions when it came to analyzing my appearance. I am allowed to feel upset or frustrated when getting dressed. There are things I can do to minimize those feelings, but then between my clothes and short hair, I tend to get excluded from any women's spaces. Once I am in my swimsuit, folks are fine, because suits don't really hide a lot. I picked the wrong sport really. I was and still am uncomfortable walking around in just my suit, because it emphasizes the parts of my body that trigger dysphoria. I can hide my chest with a binder and shirt, but in a suit, there is no way to disguise it. It is something I have to face each and every day.

As I entered my senior year of high school, I prepared to go on recruiting trips to various universities. I had to pause as I packed, wondering if my cargo shorts and baseball caps would be a problem with new groups of people from all around who didn't really know me. It was a jolt for me because I thought I had become comfortable enough with my identity that I didn't care about other people's reactions. I've learned since that I will never not care about them, but I have the power to choose to focus on the positive or the negative ones. I won't deny that there were times that I wished to look more traditionally feminine, but only to reduce the confrontations I experienced with other people. I tried some skirts, some frilly blouses, and I once let my teammates put makeup on me. And as much as I may have looked the part standing still, I couldn't begin to pull it off. I walked funny, I still sat with my legs splayed, and I felt so uncomfortable I was fidgeting and waiting to get home to throw on my comfortable clothes.

Despite my concerns, the recruiting visits went off without hitches, at least from the perspective of my interactions with the teams. Traveling to and from the institutions was a different story. Airports have always been a challenge, and continue to be one of the most stressful environments for me. At TSA, if I am scanned as a male, my binder or sports bra sets off the machine, or if scanned as a female, my boxer shorts usually do. A pat down means outing myself, one way or another. After I'm through security, the "fun" isn't over. If I use the women's restroom, I get weird looks, people see me and walk out and then back in, or I'm verbally accosted for being in the "wrong place." The men's room is usually a safer bet when traveling by myself, but when with my team, I don't even consider that an option, because I believe it would make everyone, swimmers and coaches, men's team and women's team both confused and uncomfortable. I would rather avoid that scene if I can. Thankfully, the bathrooms on planes are gender inclusive, so as long as I can wait until after takeoff, I can avoid the guessing game of "How am I being seen today?"

When I came out as queer sexually, I was uncertain how it would affect my relationships with my teammates. Thankfully I wasn't concerned that it would seriously alter my athletic opportunities, and I was confident that it would not have an impact on my eligibility for the team or associated activities. Since swimming is an objective sport, I didn't have to be concerned about any kind of bias during competition. The clock really doesn't care. But I did get nervous when I came to the realization of my genderqueer identity. I was unfamiliar with the concept until college. I learned that there was a whole spectrum of genders, with a wide range of interpretations and definitions. For me, to be genderqueer is to be somewhere in the middle of being a man and a woman. There is no set definition or a list of expectations, and so it left me free to express myself how I pleased. With that, I understood that it might be difficult to explain it to others, and I knew that there wasn't an established place for me in sports.

I started to explore on my own this new world I was discovering. I hadn't known of non-gendered restrooms, pronouns, or the support available to me on campus. I came across the resource center and became immersed in learning about myself and others like me. I had access to a map of the gender-neutral bathrooms on campus. I had someone ask me what my pronouns were for the first time. I formed connections with people who identified in similar ways, and found that those who identified very differently were still open and understanding. Rather than worrying about how others perceived me, I was able to explore who I was and who I wanted to be. As I was learning in my life outside the pool, I became comfortable with living authentically and not censoring myself, and it was increasingly more and more uncomfortable to return to my old persona in the athletic arena.

I knew that "coming out" again would be a long process. And by long, I mean that it would be a constant and ongoing practice for the rest of my life, a journey based on continuing to educate myself and others. I had been trying to avoid it for a while, attempting to maintain the precarious balance of my dual personality so that there were fewer explanations to my family and my team. While I wasn't really surprised when that failed to satisfy me, I still wasn't sure that I could launch into being out as non-binary in a space that bases so many fundamentals on the separation of the "two" genders. Deciding that I could no longer switch between being G and being Gillian, especially with the latter feeling more and more insincere each day, I started to figure out just exactly how I was going to broach the subject of my gender identity with the people I cared about.

Towards the end of my first year of college, I made several decisions. I decided to come out again to my family, this time as genderqueer. And, I decided to ask my team and coaches not to refer to me as "a woman." This was a compromise I struck with myself, treating this as a trial run for how this kind of change would be handled within the team. I was not excited about the conversations with my family, but in all honesty, I was extremely anxious and nervous about talking to my coaches and teammates. I thought that especially in an athletic space, what I was asking for was weird; it was different, and in a situation where working together and unity are highly valued, I was concerned about causing a rift that I would be unable to repair. I was no longer a daughter, a sister, or "one of the girls" on the team. As challenging as it was, it was a relief to not have to pretend that those labels were accurate or comfortable. It took time to find my own comfort zone, the labels that felt comfortable. And throughout the process, already some of those have shifted and changed. One of my ongoing challenges is communicating those changes to other people. My identity is not yet fixed, but I am secure enough in my own mind to start slowly sharing my story with others. I try to live as honestly and genuinely as I can, and I wish to continue that, as hard as it might be.

I am grateful that I was surrounded with people who value me for the person I am, and not for the labels I ascribe to. My coaches, my teammates, and everyone else I have interacted with in the athletic department were willing to listen and learn. It took time, and folks are still working on using "they" and "them" as my pronouns. But what surprised me was the hesitation in asking questions. So many people's first question to me was "Is it okay to ask these things?" On one hand, I believe that exhibits an awareness and respect for a person's private life, and it is important to first gain permission before attempting to dissect someone's identity. On the other hand, my question in return was, "How will you learn if you don't ask?" I think there is a fear of offending people, which is legitimate, but acts as a hindrance for things we don't understand. It's useful so that one doesn't blurt out something inappropriate, but the truth is that asking hard questions is a necessary step in gathering knowledge. I am usually willing and happy to answer questions. Being able to talk about my experiences and share resources I know about is something I consider a privilege. But everyone has off days. If for whatever reason, I am unable to have an effective and reasonable conversation at the time, I will ask that my space is respected. I want to share what I know so that people can alleviate misunderstandings and confusion. In my opinion, this is a vital step towards acceptance.

I think one of the hardest things to learn is that in order for anything to change, it is necessary to very specifically ask for that change to happen. My first year could have been more comfortable, but I didn't know how much liberty or support I had. I didn't know what I could ask for, and I failed to express what things or circumstances heightened my discomfort. I didn't know the people around me well enough to guess if the reaction to asking for inclusive language would be positive, negative, or mostly ignored. That changed significantly during my second year of college, when I had gained personal confidence and when I had made more connections within my team. I learned what I needed to know about my coaches to be confident in broaching tougher subjects. My teammates and coaches now call me G, and are starting to use the pronouns I align with. In group meetings, discussions, or emails, the address of "women" has been removed. My work out clothes and uniforms are now unisex sizing and cut. None of these were particularly hard to achieve, but the act of speaking up was crucial in accomplishing all of them.

I found that it was not a lack of willingness that was the barrier to change. The issue was a lack of education. The access to information can seem limited for those within athletics, as the precedent of LGBTQ athletes is slim, and even more so for trans and non-binary athletes. The vocabulary surrounding this community is daunting in and of itself, especially if there is little prior experience. It is a challenge sometimes to try and facilitate and encourage this access, this exchange of information. It can be exhausting, but at the same time, immensely worthwhile. My day to day interaction with my team is much better than when I first arrived, and the environment continues to improve. The hurdles that remain are more systematic within both my sport and the world of athletics. These are not in the control of my coaches, and so I don't know how best to attempt to alter them. I really don't feel comfortable competing for a women's team, but I would not be competitive on a men's team. It still feels like I'm impersonating someone else when I step up on the blocks, but I refuse to give up swimming. I wish there were gender neutral locker rooms, both at home and when I travel. The issue seems to come down to how sports are currently organized: men compete against men and women compete against women. There isn't a place for people who aren't either. I felt like I have to continually choose between being comfortable in my body and being a competitive athlete, and that shouldn't have to be a choice. I don't know what systematic design would be most inclusive, but I do know that it has to start somewhere. Anyone who is a woman should be able to compete on a women's team without their body being policed, regardless of whether they are trans or cis. And while there is no simple answer for non-binary folks, a good place to begin is by having a conversation. What things can we do to make the current athletic arena more comfortable and inclusive?

In a way, I want to love swimming, and tout all the amazing aspects of the sport and all of the opportunities it has provided me. At the same time, if I'm being honest I feel that the sport itself enforces restrictions on me that I can't combat without rendering myself ineligible to compete. Sports are supposed to be about inclusivity, bringing people together, and competing for the thrill and joy of it. Can't we just focus on that and stop telling people who they are or how they should be? I guess a simple way to put it is I would like a space in athletics where I can unapologetically be myself, and race to the best of my ability. In some of my discussions with administrators at my own school, the good news is that some of these changes are in the planning stages. While most things likely won't be implemented in my final two years of college, I am optimistic that they are changing nonetheless.

The arena of athletics has immense power to be at the forefront of social change, because so many different people can relate to it. Through shared experiences, athletes can connect and work together to improve the world we all live and compete in. In order to achieve this, it takes people to open up to change and actively practice inclusivity, rather than remain with the status quo and passively accept exclusion. I believe in this vision. I hope that by continuing to race and compete, and attempting to reach the highest level that I can, I can further this progress so that people like me can train and compete in a more inclusive and understanding place. I don't know what to expect going into my third year. I am halfway through my college eligibility, and already there has been positive change. I want to keep pushing the envelope, to see how far it goes for myself and everyone else that comes after. I don't know what I will find, but I am excited to move forward.

FURTHER READING

Former College Football Captain Was Openly Gay

Cyd Zeigler

If you have a digital edition of this book, please click on the link below to access the article:

https://www.outsports.com/out-gay-athletes/2013/2/21/4015526/brian-sims-football-gay

If you have a print edition of this book, please use your cell phone to scan the QR code below to access the article:

Penn State's Lesbian Hater

Jim Buzinski

If you have a digital edition of this book, please click on the link below to access the article:

https://www.outsports.com/2013/4/4/4185770/penn-states-lesbian-hater

If you have a print edition of this book, please use your cell phone to scan the QR code below to access the article:

This Trans Volleyball Player Is Headed to the NCAA

Chloe Psyche Anderson

If you have a digital edition of this book, please click on the link below to access the article:

https://www.outsports.com/2016/6/1/11814342/transgender-ncaa-volleyball-chloe-psyche-anderson

If you have a print edition of this book, please use your cell phone to scan the QR code below to access the article:

Gay Rodeo Is Branching Out to Women, Straight Competitors While Staying True to Its Inclusive Roots

Jennifer Brown

If you have a digital edition of this book, please click on the link below to access the article:

https://coloradosun.com/2019/07/11/rocky-mountain-gay-rodeo/

If you have a print edition of this book, please use your cell phone to scan the QR code below to access the article:

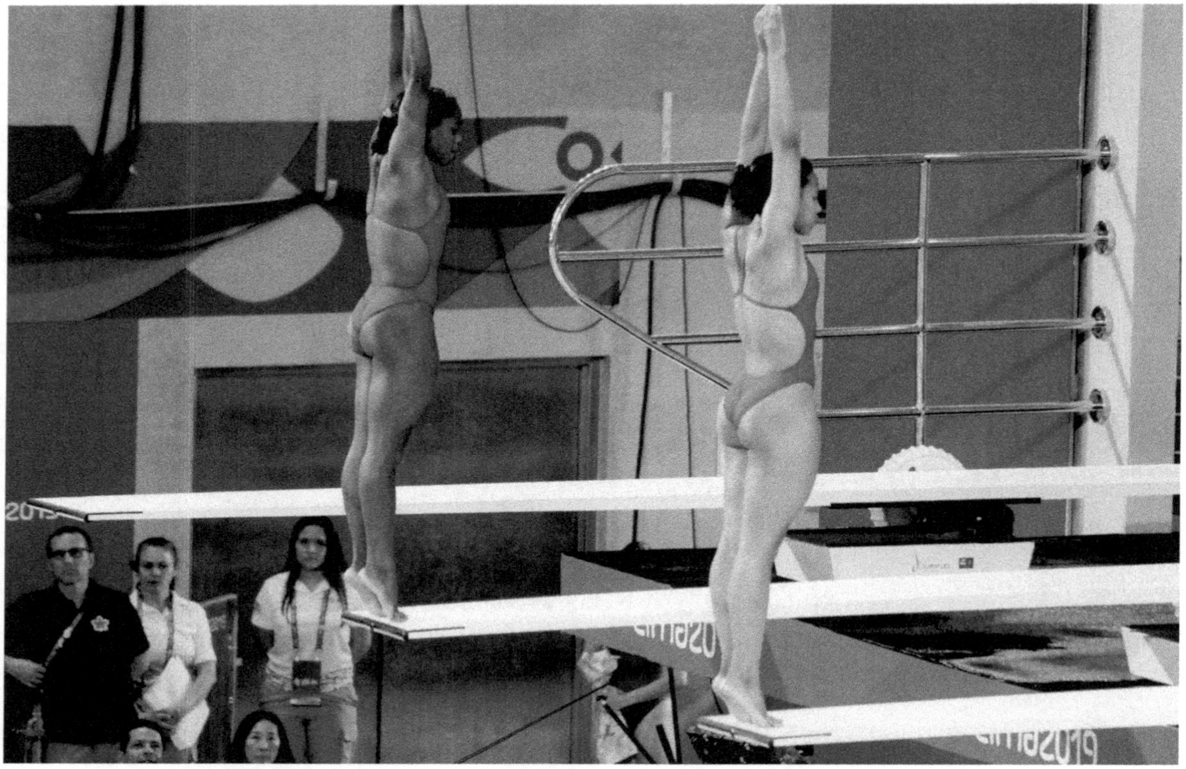

CHAPTER 9
BODY IMAGE

In sport and society, it is nearly impossible to ignore all of the media references to body image. Whether we are watching a televised sports event such as the Olympics or commercials during late-night television, media consumers are continuously exposed to an overabundance of images celebrating the "ideal" body image in sport and society. For women, that image requires them to adhere to appearing appropriately feminine, with toned bodies that are much thinner than the average woman. These images can contribute to disordered eating know as **anorexia nervosa** and **bulimia nervosa**. For men, the body image has a body-fat percentage that is below 9 percent; it is far more muscular than the average man and can be seen in hyper-masculine settings. Men suffer from both of the previously mentioned eating disorders, as well as **muscle dysmorphia**, the concern that they are too small and cannot appreciate the physique they have. In sport, these physiques for men and women have become the standard set by the media, celebrated by fans, and reinforced through social pressures from coaches and teammates. These documents examine the danger associated with this obsession.

What does the "ideal" body look like in sport? A simple response might be lean and muscular for women and big and bulky for men. However, body image is much more complicated than those simple descriptors, depending on the sport. For athletes in wrestling, distance running, and diving, like the women photographed for this chapter, a lean and muscular physique is essential. For some power and performance sports that have more physical contact, a larger and muscular frame might appear to be better. Body image in US society is socially constructed like many other identities. The "ideal" body for a woman is socially constructed to be thin, toned, with an "appropriately" feminine look, while men must be big and muscular, with chest and bicep size appearing most important when photographed. These images are introduced at an early age to girls with Barbie and boys with their superhero (pick any one of more than two dozen from the Marvel Cinematic Universe films since 2000). In both cases, children grow up with this image as the ideal body, or, at the very least, an unobtainable standard.

20

BODY IMAGE AND FEMALE STUDENT-ATHLETES

Jennifer M. Miles

Women enroll in college for a number of reasons. Initially, women may decide to pursue college degrees for career preparation and for the sake of learning. The years in college, however, also offer women opportunities for personal growth and development. Because women represent over half of the current student population, the experience of female college students is becoming increasingly significant. They arrive on campus seeking to identify who they are as individuals and as a group.

Student-athletes enter college for additional reasons. These reasons can vary based on a variety of factors, including the student's athletic ability, the athletic division of the institution, the student's reliance on scholarships, and the influence of family, friends, and coaches. At institutions with less competitive athletic programs, students may decide to participate on an athletic team after being accepted to the institution. In that instance, the student's college career is not dependent upon their success in the sport. In other cases, however, students are heavily recruited by many institutions. They may choose to attend an institution based on the team's national ranking or based on the experience of the coach. In those cases, the student's academic experience is inextricably linked to their experience on the team. For student-athletes, maintaining a minimum grade point average may be linked to scholarships. Student-athletes are not only at college to prepare for career or graduate or professional school, they are at that institution as a way to pay for college and/or because of skill and desire to compete.

An alarming number of women engage in self-destructive, unhealthy behaviors to conform to broad and societal-driven concepts of beauty. This is particularly true on college campuses (Levitt, 2004). Extensive research has been conducted regarding traditional-aged college students and body dissatisfaction (e.g., Forrest & Stuhldrehrer, 2007). Body image can affect how women see themselves and how they experience college. The years in college can be challenging, including new stressors and responsibilities as well as learning to manage time. Student-athletes must learn to balance the transition issues faced by all students and must, at the same time, learn to function as an effective member of a team. They are susceptible to the same influences of all students in terms of body image and the physical ideal, but must also balance needs in terms of fitness, weight, and health in order to perform as an athlete.

Body Image and Eating Disorders

Women change the way they see themselves throughout their college careers. The undergraduate experience includes learning both inside and outside of the classroom. When women enter college, they find themselves in a new culture. They need to adjust how they see themselves in relation to other students, faculty, and staff. They need to learn a new vocabulary and adjust to a new set of expectations. The students must learn to use technology, to study, and to make a place for themselves. These experiences and challenges can be an opportunity for women to reinvent themselves. Consistent with Rudd and Lennon (2000), Trautmann, Worthy, and Lokken (2007) found that individuals may attempt to conform to a culture's physical ideal through diet, exercise, clothing choices, and surgery.

Body image can be defined as how an individual perceives her body (Cash & Pruzinsky, 1990, 2002). Regardless of how the societal definition of physical beauty has been developed, many college women seek conformity with the pages of magazines (Hawkins, Richards, Granley, & Stein, 2004). Hawkins et al. (2004) found that viewing images of the thin-ideal in magazines caused an increase in body dissatisfaction, negative mood states, and eating disorder symptoms. They also determined that viewing the images was associated with a decreased sense of self-esteem.

In the quest for some vision of beauty, college women may exercise excessively, to almost unhealthy levels, and develop eating disorders. Other women may decide that the images they see are physical impossibilities. Instead of working to conform to what they see as unattainable, these women may choose to abandon healthy lifestyles completely. Without proper nutrition and exercise, women may develop lower self-esteem, be unsatisfied with their physical appearance, and may not have the energy needed to pursue their desired lifestyles. This lack of satisfaction could affect all of their roles, including those of students, campus, and community leaders, friends, daughters, sisters, mothers, wives, employees, mentors, and athletes.

College women are at risk of developing eating disorders because of a variety of factors, including excessive exercise, social isolation, body dissatisfaction, high levels of anxiety, and disturbed eating and dieting patterns (Levitt, 2004). Body image disturbance has been associated with developing eating disorders (Bergstrom & Neighbors, 2006). Risks associated with developing an eating disorder may arise from overestimation of personal size and dissatisfaction with weight (Striegel-Moore et al., 2004). Additional risk factors include fear of fat, fear of failure, and a poor body image (Beals & Manore, 1994; Leon, 1991; Williams, Sargent, & Durstine, 2003).

An eating disorder is diagnosed when specific criteria are present. Psychopathlogy and psychological distress are included. The terms "subclinical eating disorders," however, and "disordered eating" are used to describe various abnormal behaviors that do not fulfill that diagnosis. These women may share symptoms of an eating disorder, but do not meet all of the criteria (Williams et al., 2003). A poor body image may or may not lead to an eating disorder meeting a clinical diagnosis; disordered eating, however, can still be problematic.

Body Image and Female Student-Athletes

Etzel, Watson, Visek, and Maniar (2006) defined college student-athletes as "predominantly undergraduate students enrolled in colleges and universities across the United States who participate in institutionally sponsored, competitive sporting activities, not including club or intramural sports" (p. 519). Student-athletes participate in athletics sponsored by organizations including the National Collegiate Athletic Association, the National Association of Intercollegiate Athletics, the National Junior College Association, and the National Christian College Association (Etzel et al., 2006).

The enactment of Title IX of the Education Amendments Act in 1972 increased opportunities for women in college and university sports. Title IX prohibits discrimination on the basis of sex in any education program or activity that receives federal funding. Increased opportunities and societal acceptance has resulted in more women participating in intercollegiate athletics (Malinauskas, Cucchiara, Aeby, & Bruening, 2007). In addition to increased participation from students and financial commitments from institutions, the enforcement of this act has also led to athletic departments reassessing their structure and purpose (Gerdy, 2006).

Student-athletes represent a diverse and visible student population with their own needs and expectations (Parham, 1996). They are faced with the same developmental challenges as nonathletes, but must also deal with challenges associated with athletics (Etzel et al., 2006). As they try to fulfill the requirements associated with the roles of student and athlete, they are faced with specific pressures. Some of these pressures include separation from family and friends, academic expectations, injuries, and career preparation (Pinkerton, Hinz, & Barrow, 1989; Selby, Weinstein, & Bird, 1990; Williams et al., 2003).

Although athletes are considered emotionally healthy (Powers & Johnson, 1996), the additional pressures they confront can make them susceptible to health problems, including both psychological and physical problems (Etzel et al., 2006). Major health problems of student-athletes include alcohol use, eating disorders and dysfunctional eating behaviors, and coping with injury or stress (Selby et al., 1990). Mood and self-esteem can be affected by the student's weight (Seime & Damer, 1991).

In a study of subclinical eating disorders in female student-athletes, students were asked to indicate reasons for dieting and controlling their weight. The study included 587 female student-athletes from nine institutions and represented 13 sports. All institutions were in the state of Virginia. The sports included cross-country, diving, basketball, crew, gymnastics, golf, field hockey, lacrosse, swimming, volleyball, soccer, softball, and tennis. The reasons reported included enhancing performance, enhancing appearance, improving health, and because someone recommended they diet. The students who gave improving appearance as a reason for dieting represented 12 sports including diving, basketball, crew, gymnastics, golf, field hockey, lacrosse, swimming, volleyball, soccer, softball, and tennis. All sports except for cross-country had over 50% of the student reporting dieting or other methods to control their weight (Williams et al., 2003).

The "female athlete triad" is a three-part syndrome found in female student-athletes (American College of Sports Medicine, 1997). The triad includes disordered eating, amenorrhea, and osteoporosis (Etzel et al., 2006). In the short term, disordered eating can lead to lower weight and improved performance, but long-term effects may include major complications such as organ failure (Seime & Damer, 1991).

Low body fat can enhance an athlete's performance. This can place pressure on the athlete to reduce fat, specifically in sports where a specific weight is deemed critical for performance or appearance (Williams et al., 2003). Weigh-ins are sometimes a requirement to being a member of an athletic team (Willams et al., 2003). Female athletes may become preoccupied with food and may develop eating disorders (Beals & Manore, 2002; Wichmann & Martin, 1993). At the same time, adequate nutrition is necessary for a student-athlete to perform at his or her best (Williams et al., 2003). In response to disordered eating and health problems in student-athletes, athletic departments have developed eating disorder policies and prevention programs (Thompson & Sherman, 1993). Coaches and family members have been found to play a role regarding whether or not a student-athlete develops an eating disorder (Beals & Manore, 1994).

Implications for Student Affairs

Divisions of student affairs are responsible for creating a safe environment in which students can learn. This learning occurs both inside and outside the classroom. Student affairs is also charged with providing resources for students to help them succeed. Functional area assignments vary from institution to institution, especially regarding size of the institution and institutional mission. Some of the functions of divisions of student affairs customarily include housing, health centers, counseling, wellness, residence life, fraternity and sorority affairs, and leadership development.

One of the themes seen in student affairs involves assisting students with transitions. New student orientation programs are in place to assist students with the transition to college. The students learn about residence life, tutoring, course registration, and social opportunities. Career development centers provide assistance regarding transitioning from the role of student to employee. Students can receive help with resumé writing, interview preparation, and salary negotiation.

Moving from a high school student-athlete to a college student-athlete is another transition. Student affairs professionals are uniquely qualified to assist students with this transition. They oversee areas designed to ease transitions, such as counseling and health centers. Student-athletes also represent a specific subpopulation. Student affairs is charged with serving all populations of students and creating environments designed for success. Body image can affect all students. While in college, students feel a need to conform and fit in with the community. Student affairs personnel are uniquely positioned to help all students through the transition.

In a study examining help-seeking preferences in college women, Prouty, Protinsky, and Canady (2002) found that college women prefer to seek help from friends instead of professionals. There is a need for programs in which student leaders can learn the symptoms of eating disorders. Training may be provided by college counselors. Counselors can also provide training to faculty, staff, and coaches. This training may fall under the purview of a division of student affairs. University physicians should be trained to screen students for disordered eating. Campus awareness is a vital component in helping women with eating disorders find appropriate treatment (Meyer, 2005).

Professionals in sports medicine look at more than just physical health, but also mental health issues, including anxiety, depression, substance abuse, and grief (Brown & Blanton, 2002; Hinkle, 1996). Student affairs can be instrumental in helping athletes with these problems (Etzel et al., 2006). The isolation of student-athlete departments from the rest of the student population may encourage coaches and athletic staff to handle problems within their program or off campus (Etzel et al., 2006). Given their in-depth knowledge regarding student development, student affairs professionals are in the unique position to collaborate effectively with coaches and trainers to provide appropriate and timely interventions and programs to the students.

Communication between student affairs and administrators and coaches, as well as regular confidential meetings between student-athletes and student affairs staff, may prevent serious health problems from occurring or escalating (Etzel et al., 2006). Student-athletes face additional and special stressors as they balance responsibilities of students and athletes. Student-athletes are exposed to different health risks than nonathletes (Etzel et al., 2006). Student affairs professionals would benefit from familiarizing themselves with the health issues of this student population (Etzel et al., 2006).

Discussion

Women attend college to further themselves through education, but are confronted with traditional concepts of beauty and stereotypes regarding physical appearance. College and university women also receive mixed messages regarding their value as students and the importance of attractiveness. For many women, college is a paradox between the serious nature of intellectual curiosity and the pull to conform to societal expectations. These expectations can be powerful forces as they define themselves mentally and physically. This quest for recognition of a physical definition presents many problems, particularly as female students attempt to conform to often distorted views of beauty and self-image (Bergstrom & Neighbors, 2006).

Like all students, student-athletes must learn how to function as a member of a new community. In addition to the transitional issues experienced by all college students, student-athletes must also cope and adjust to the pressures of serving on an athletic team. Involvement in athletics may also involve increased expectations for successful academic performance. These increased expectations may come from coaches, academic advisors, teammates, and the students themselves. The success of a college or university's athletic program is tied to wins and losses, television appearances, championships, and revenue generated (Gerdy, 2006). Student-athletes may feel pressure to perform to contribute to the success of their institution.

Concern with body image starts well before the college years. In a study of middle school boys and girls, Wiseman, Peltzman, Halmi, and Sunday (2004) found that a relationship exists between a drive for thinness and self-esteem in girls. This relationship could put them at risk to develop eating disorders. The researchers have also examined body dissatisfaction, the drive for thinness, and self-esteem in middle school students. When children first begin to participate in athletics, measures can be taken to avoid negative consequences seen in older athletes. Coaches and parents can assist by becoming aware of the positive and negative psychological effects associated with athletics (Etzel et al., 2006).

Female athletes are subject to the pressures on all athletes to maintain a certain weight and fitness level. Student-athletes may diet to improve their performance, their appearance, or their overall health. Student-athletes who have heard others comment on their body weight were more likely to develop subclinical eating disorders (Williams et al., 2003). Preventive education is important for coaches and athletes (Williams et al., 2003).

Female student-athletes are faced with the pressures placed on all women to be thin. The ideal woman portrayed in the media is slim (Maliauskas et al., 2007), but that body type may not be ideal or healthy for a female athlete to excel at her particular sport. This pressure and mixed messages may lead female student-athletes to pursue an unrealistic body size (Beals & Manore, 1994). This preoccupation with an unattainable ideal may affect a student's athletic performance, academic performance, and overall success as a student.

References

American College of Sports Medicine. (1997). ACSM position on female athlete triad. *Medicine and Science in Sports and Exercise, 29*(5), i–ix.

Beals, K. A., & Manore, M. M. (1994). The prevalence and consequences of subclinical eating disorders in female athletes. *International Journal of Sport Nutrition, 4*(2), 175–195.

Beals, K. A., & Manore, M. M. (2002). Disorders of the female athlete triad among collegiate athletes. *International Journal Sport Nutrition and Exercise Metabolism, 12*(3), 281–293.

Bergstrom, R. L., & Neighbors, C. (2006). Body image disturbance and the social norms approach: An integrative review of the literature. *Journal of Social and Clinical Psychology, 25*(9), 975–1000.

Brown, D., & Blanton, C. (2002). Physical activity, sports participation, and suicidal behavior among college students. *Medicine and Science in Sports and Exercise, 34*(7), 1087–1096.

Cash, T. F., & Pruzinsky, T. (Eds.). (1990). *Body images: Development, deviance, and change.* New York: Guilford Press.

Cash, T. F., & Pruzinsky, T. (Eds.). (2002). *Body image: A handbook of theory, research, and clinical practice.* New York: Guilford Press.

Etzel, E. F., Watson, J. C., Visek, A. J., & Maniar, S. D. (2006). Understanding and promoting college student-athlete health: Essential issues for student affairs professionals. *NASPA Journal, 43*(3), 518–546.

Forrest, K. Y. Z., & Stuhldreher, W. L. (2007). Patterns and correlates of body image dissatisfaction and distortion among college students. *American Journal of Health Studies, 22*(1), 18–25.

Gerdy, J. R. (2006). *Air ball: American education's failed experiment with elite athletics.* Jackson: University Press of Mississippi.

Hawkins, N., Richards, P. S., Granley, H. M., & Stein, D. M. (2004). The impact of exposure to the thin-ideal media image on women. *Eating Disorders, 12,* 35–50.

Hinkle, J. (1996). Depression, adjustment disorder, generalized anxiety, and substance abuse: An overview for sports professionals working with student athletes. In E. F. Etzel, A. P. Ferrante, & J. W. Pinkney (Eds.), *Counseling college student-athletes: Issues and interventions* (2nd ed., pp. 109–136). Morgantown, WV: Fitness Information Technology.

Leon, G. R. (1991). Eating disorders in female athletes. *Sports Medicine, 12*(4), 219–227.

Levitt, D. H. (2004). Drive for thinness and fear of fat among college women: Implications for practice and assessment. *Journal of College Counseling, 7,* 109–117.

Maliauskas, B. M., Cucchiara, A. J., Aeby, V. G., & Bruening, C. C. (2007). Physical activity, disordered eating risk, and anthropometric measurement: A comparison of college female athletes and non athletes. *College Student Journal, 41*(1), 217–222.

Meyer, D. F. (2005). Psychological correlates of help seeking for eating-disorder symptoms in female students, *Journal of College Counseling, 8,* 20–30.

Parham, W. (1996). Diversity within intercollegiate athletics: Current profile and welcomed opportunities. In E. F. Etzel, A. P. Ferrante, & J. W. Pinkney (Eds.), *Counseling college student-athletes: Issues and interventions* (2nd ed., pp. 26–49). Morgantown, WV: Fitness Information Technology.

Pinkerton, R. S., Hinz, L. D., & Barrow, J. C. (1989). The college student-athlete: Pschological considerations and interventions. *Journal of American College Health, 37*(5), 218–226.

Powers, P. S., & Johnson, C. (1996). Small victories: Prevention of eating disorders among athletes. *Eating Disorders, 4*(4), 364–377.

Prouty, A. M., Protinsky, H. O., & Canady, D. (2002). College women: Eating behaviors and help-seeking preferences. *Adolescence, 37,* 353–363.

Rudd, N. A., & Lennon, S. J. (2000). Body image and appearance-management behaviors in college women. *Clothing and Textiles Research Journal, 18*(3), 152–162.

Seime, R., & Damer, D. (1991). Identification and treatment of the athlete with an eating disorder. In E. F. Etzel, A. P. Ferrante, & J. W. Pinkney (Eds.), *Counseling college student-athletes: Issues and interventions* (pp. 175–198), Morgantown, WV: Fitness information Technology.

Selby, R., Weinstein, H. M., & Bird, T. S. (1990). The health of university athletes: Attitudes, behaviors, and stressors. *Journal of American College Health, 39*(1), 11–18.

Striegel-Moore, R. H., Franko, D. L., Thompson, D., Barton, B., Schreiber, G. G., & Daniels, S. R. (2004). Changes in weight and body image over time in women with eating disorders. *International Journal of Eating Disorders, 36*, 315–327.

Thompson, R., & Sherman, R. (1993). *Helping athletes with eating disorders.* Champaign, IL: Human Kinetics.

Trautmann, J., Worthy, S. L., & Lokken, K. L. (2007). Body dissatisfaction, bulimic symptoms, and clothing practices among college women. *Journal of Psychology, 141*(5), 485–498.

Wichmann, S., & Martin, D. R. (1993). Eating disoreders in athletes: Weighing the risks. *Physician and Sportsmedicine, 21*(5), 126–135.

Williams, P. L., Sargent, R. G., & Durstine, L. J. (2003). Prevalence of subclinical eating disorders in collegiate female athletes. *Women in Sport and Physical Activity Journal, 12*(2), 127–145.

Wiseman, C. V., Peltzman, B., Halmi, K. A., & Sunday, S. R. (2004). Risk factors for eating disorders: Surprising similarities between middle school boys and girls. *Eating Disorders, 12*, 315–320.

EATING DISORDERS AND DISORDERED EATING

Abigail J. Larson and Kary Woodruff

Introduction

Eating disorders are mental health disorders that can be extremely detrimental to physical and psychological well-being. If left untreated, the consequences of these disorders can last a lifetime. Exercise professionals should be able to identify signs and symptoms of disordered eating and eating disorders because early identification leads to earlier treatment, and improves long-term prognosis. The following information is not intended for diagnostic purposes, rather it is intended to help coaches, trainers, and other exercise professionals recognize the unique signs, symptoms, and consequences of various eating disorders as well as how to reduce risk of eating disorders among athletes through fostering healthy eating and training practices.

Classifications of Clinical Eating Disorders

Clinical eating disorders include anorexia nervosa, hallmarked by severe food restriction and excessive weight loss; bulimia nervosa, characterized by a cycle of bingeing and compensatory behaviors such as self-induced vomiting, laxative abuse, and/or excessive exercise; binge eating disorder, defined as recurrent episodes of consuming large quantities of food without compensatory behaviors seen in those with bulimia nervosa; and Other Specified Feeding or Eating Disorder (OSFED), which includes eating and feeding disorders of clinical severity but do not meet the diagnostic criteria of the other three categories. While most exercise professionals do not need to know specific diagnostic criteria, it is important to be familiar with risks of developing an eating disorder, and able to identify signs and symptoms associated with these life-threatening diseases.

Eating Disorder Risk Factors

Eating disorders and disordered eating are more common among athletes compared to nonathletic peer groups. Unfortunately, there are many athletes who intentionally engage in unhealthy eating behaviors to achieve a perceived ideal body weight, or a weight he or she associates with optimal performance. Any athlete can develop an eating disorder, male or female, underweight, normal weight, or overweight; coaches and athletic trainers who only look for potential eating disorder behaviors in low body weight athletes can potentially misidentify someone who is just naturally thin as well as miss helping other at-risk athletes.

In general, athletes in weight-sensitive sports are at greatest risk for developing disordered eating and/or exercise behaviors. Weight-sensitive sports include those that emphasize a low body weight for a maximum power-to-weight ratio (distance running, cycling, rock climbing, cross-country skiing, and ski jumping), those that emphasize aesthetics and a small physique (gymnastics, figure skating, diving, and various dancing events), and weight-class sports (rowing, weight lifting, wrestling, and boxing). Athletes in these sports may feel pressure to achieve or maintain a low body weight because he or she believes it will improve performance. These pressures may be perceived to come from coaches, teammates, and/or parents, or may be entirely self-imposed. Other characteristics such as perfectionism, high-achievement orientation, and early start of sport-specific training are other specific traits, often seen as positive attributes of an athlete, known to increase risk of disordered eating behaviors (Sundgot-Borgen et al. 2013). Whatever the source(s), the pressure to lose excess body fat and/or to maintain a low body weight can cause occasional dieting efforts to progress into chronic behaviors that can last a lifetime.

In some weight-class sports there is also a *culture* of accepted extreme *making-weight* practices such as using saunas and excessive exercise to lose water weight or to consume very few calories for several days prior to a competition. While these behaviors may be temporary, they increase the risk of an athlete progressing to more chronic dieting behaviors that can promote the development of disordered eating/eating disorders. Exercise professionals and parents can help prevent the adoption of unhealthy eating practices by focusing on athletes' physical performance and health and not excessively focusing on body weight and/or composition. A coach or parent should never encourage an athlete to lose weight, but if an athlete chooses to do so, he or she should be referred to a sports dietitian for an appropriate strategy.

Key Points

Eating disorders are serious and potentially life-threatening conditions that include anorexia nervosa, bulimia nervosa, binge eating disorder, and other specified feeding or eating disorders. Athletes are at greater risk than their nonathletic peers, and weight-dependent sport athletes are particularly at risk. Parents and coaches should not base risk off of weight alone as athletes of all body shapes can struggle with an eating disorder.

Eating Disorder Signs and Symptoms

Disordered eating behaviors can be viewed on a spectrum of dietary and exercise behaviors. On one end of the spectrum are behaviors that allow for healthy and balanced eating and training habits as well as an overall sense of comfort with food, exercise, and one's body. Individuals whose behaviors fall on this end of the spectrum consume adequate calories to meet their energy needs for training and overall health and have a healthy relationship with food. The opposite end of this spectrum includes behaviors such as severe restriction of caloric intake, fasting, eliminating certain food groups from the diet, self-induced vomiting, and excessive exercise intended to compensate for real or perceived over-consumption of calories. Alone or in combination, these practices can progress into the development of a clinically diagnosed eating disorder. Somewhere within the mid-section of the eating disorder spectrum are behaviors that are not necessarily indicative of an eating disorder but, taken too far, can become problematic; such behaviors include engaging in fad diets, repeated weight cycling, compromised body image, and having an excessive preoccupation with food, body weight, and exercise.

Specific eating disorders have unique and identifiable characteristics. In the case of anorexia nervosa, individuals have an intense fear of gaining weight and become obsessed with maintaining a low body weight. Other characteristics of this disorder include dramatic weight loss (or failure to gain weight during a period of growth), preoccupation with food and its contents (i.e., calories, fat grams, carbohydrates, and added sugars), preoccupation with one's weight, and an unrealistic perception of actual body size (i.e., *feeling* fat). Eating-related anxieties and desire to hide atypical eating behaviors may also lead to social isolation, thereby intensifying associated behaviors. Bulimia nervosa includes warning signs such as frequent fluctuations in body weight, avoidance of food-related social events, making highly critical comments regarding body shape and size, and evidence of vomiting behaviors including frequent trips to the restroom after eating, and swollen parotid glands around the cheeks. Individuals who suffer from bulimia report a sense of lack of control over eating and may consume extremely large amounts of food in a short period of time which is followed by self-induced vomiting, excessive laxative use, and/or excessive exercise. Individuals with bulimia nervosa can remain undiagnosed for long periods of time because they do not look emaciated and related behaviors are hidden because of intense shame regarding binging and purging habits. Physical symptoms to look for include swelling of the cheeks or jaw area, calluses on the back of the hands and knuckles, and tooth erosion. Signs and symptoms of binge eating disorder include those associated with bulimia nervosa (i.e., eating large amounts of food in a short period of time, feeling a loss of sense of control over one's eating, and secretive eating behaviors), but there is no evidence of compensatory behaviors and binging behaviors are accompanied by excessive weight gain. If any of these warning signs are identified, an individual should be referred to an expert for further assessment and treatment options.

Consequences of Eating Disorders

Behaviors associated with eating disorders can have dangerous health-related complications. A common complication of self-induced dehydration, purging, excessive laxative use, and/or severe caloric restriction includes clinical electrolyte imbalances which result in irregular heartbeats and possibly heart failure and death. Dehydration can also result in heat exhaustion or even heat stroke which ultimately can be life-threatening, and even moderate dehydration can reduce cardiovascular capacity and ability to thermoregulate. Self-induced vomiting can result in inflammation and potential rupture of the esophagus; and laxative abuse can result in chronic constipation. Individuals with anorexia nervosa often experience slowed heart rate (<55 beats per minute) and very low blood pressure (<100/60 mm Hg) due to hypothalamic-induced reductions in sympathetic nervous system output. Extreme self-starvation can eventually result in heart failure. Even moderate caloric restriction among teenage girls can cause decreased hormonal output which causes a reduction in peak bone mineral density and increases risk of bone injury and ultimately osteoporosis.

Proper nutrition and hydration practices are essential for growing athletes in particular because unhealthy eating habits can delay pubertal development and ultimately may stunt growth, physical maturation, and peak bone density. In a chronically undernourished athlete, maximal force production, power production, speed, mental acuity, and agility are impaired. Not only does performance suffer but the overall health of the athlete is compromised. Chronically undernourished athletes are at risk for nutrient deficiencies, chronic fatigue, increased incidence of illness and infection, anemia, muscle atrophy, general weakness, fainting, and intolerance to cold. Many athletes with prolonged patterns of disordered eating may fail to achieve peak height and bone mass and could face other risks including chronic injuries and stress fractures. These disorders should not be taken lightly and need to be addressed immediately once identified.

Prevention and Treatment of Eating Disorders

Early identification and early treatment of eating disorders and/or eating disorder behaviors is essential for successful long-term recovery. Ideally all eating disorder behaviors could be prevented through fostering a healthy environment and good self-esteem, but in susceptible individuals, prevention tactics may not prove effective. If and when issues do arise, early intervention is of the utmost importance for the individual as well as for the team as there is evidence to suggest that disordered eating behaviors can be socially *contagious*.

Athletes identified as having an eating disorder should be considered an *injured athlete* and should not participate in sport while engaging in unhealthy eating behaviors. In order to return to training and competition, the athlete should be medically cleared by a doctor as well as commit to an eating disorder treatment plan. Such a plan includes working with a sports physician to address any medical concerns, a registered dietitian (ideally a sports dietitian) to ensure adequate energy intake, a licensed psychologist or psychiatrist (preferably one who specializes in eating disorders) to work through psychological causes of the eating disorder, and possibly an exercise specialist or physical therapist if existing injuries are present.

Even when an individual reaches an acceptable body weight or ceases to engage in eating disorder-related behaviors, underlying feelings of inadequacies and anxiety are likely to linger. Relapse is common among those who suffer from eating disorders and is most likely to occur in the midst of dramatic life-changing events. To prevent relapse, underlying mental health conditions must also be treated in order to ensure long-term recovery as evidence suggests that the vast majority of those who are diagnosed also suffer from other mental disorders such as depression, obsessive compulsive disorder, attention-deficit/hyperactivity disorder (ADHD), and bipolar disorder. Often treatment of an eating disorder is a long journey with bumps and setbacks along the road to recovery.

Key Points

Coaches, parents, and staff who work with athletes should be familiar with the signs and symptoms of disordered eating and eating disorders, as well as the health consequences related to eating disorders. Athletes who have been identified with disordered eating or an eating disorder should be referred to a treatment team that at minimum consists of a sports physician, sports dietitian, and therapist.

The Female Athlete Triad

The *female athlete triad* is an increasingly common condition in female athletes. The Triad is a cluster of symptoms that include inadequate energy intake (also known as inadequate energy availability) with or without an eating disorder, missed menstrual cycles (also called amenorrhea), and decreased bone density. It is important to understand that low energy availability, that is, inadequate energy intake, is the cornerstone of the Triad and is what causes the other two components. Adequate energy availability means that an athlete is consuming enough calories to meet her energy demands for sport, activities of daily living, and basic metabolic functions such as respiration, circulation, digestion, and reproduction. If a female athlete has low energy availability because of restricted energy intake or very high levels of physical activity, the body will respond by decreasing estrogen production, thereby decreasing likelihood of a pregnancy for which there is no energy to support. Low estrogen production is evidenced by missed menstrual cycles, delayed menarche, and/or amenorrhea. Decreases in estrogen have also been associated with decreases in bone mass and/or lower peak bone density. This is especially troubling because low energy intake is often found in conjunction with low nutrient intake which further decreases osteoblast (bone-building) activity and causes an even lower peak bone mineral density. While not all female athletes have all three components of the Triad, even having one component indicates a strong likelihood of risk for or presence of the other two Triad members, even if not yet apparent. Thus, identifying an athlete that has one component and providing treatment can prevent the progression of the other two components. See Figure 21.1 for a schematic of the female athlete triad.

It is important to note that in some female athletes, low energy availability results from intentional restrictive intake intended to facilitate achieving or maintaining a low body weight for performance reasons. However, there are also athletes who are simply unaware of their energy needs (how many calories their bodies actually require to support health and exercise) and underconsume calories without intentionally restricting intake. Thus, the female athlete Triad may or *may not* include disordered eating or an eating disorder. Regardless, in either scenario, the cornerstone of treatment for the Triad will include increasing caloric intake, reducing energy expenditure, or a combination of both. Increased energy intake and/or reduced energy expenditure allows for positive energy availability,

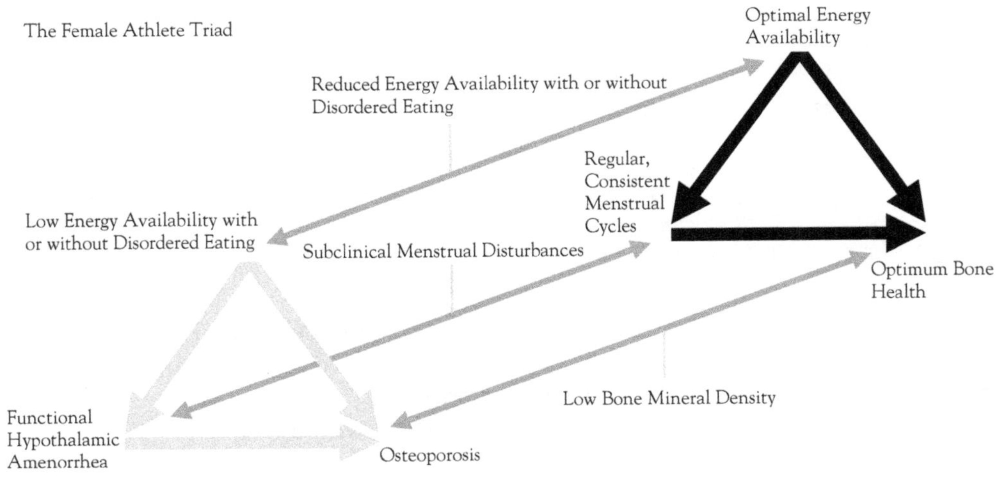

FIGURE 21.1 Female Athlete Triad Spectrum Schemata.

which will help stimulate estrogen production, and thus improve menstrual dysfunction and possibly bone mineral density.

Bottom line: When a young woman is not consuming enough energy (kcals) and micronutrients (vitamins and minerals) to meet the energy demand of physical activity and normal biological functioning, she will experience a decrease in estrogen production *which sets the stage for stress fractures now and osteoporosis later.* Female athletes with the Triad also experience more overuse injuries and have lower immune function compared to their healthy peers. If an athlete is experiencing symptoms associated with the female athlete triad it is important to speak to a physician and a sports dietitian as soon as possible, as it may be a sign of a serious eating disorder and girls with eating disorders are at risk for serious and possibly irreversible bone loss.

It is important to note that while females are at greater risk for eating disorders and disordered eating, these eating patterns can also be seen among male athletes. For obvious reasons, the female athlete triad does not apply to males; however, low energy available *is* seen among some male athletes, particularly endurance athletes (cyclists), gravitational athletes (such as ski jumpers), and athletes in sports with weight classes. Although research in this area is sparse and further study is needed to fully understand the repercussions of low energy available among male athletes, we can assume that it increases risk for poor bone mineralization and possibly alters endocrine function. Importantly this includes reduced testosterone output which adversely affects the ability to gain muscle mass and recover from intense exercise. Treatment for male athletes with low energy availability include similar treatment approaches for women; increasing energy intake along with psychological counseling and medical management.

Key Points

As a health and fitness professional, it is important to help young athletes understand that not consuming enough energy (calories) or fluids can be very detrimental to performance. Eating disorders and disordered eating can have severe effects on performance and overall health. Exercise professionals can help prevent eating disorder behaviors by focusing on overall health, not an athlete's weight, and should refrain from commenting on an athlete's body weight. Athletes who are identified as having an eating disorder should be considered *injured* and only allowed to return to sport upon medical clearance and commitment to treatment of their eating disorder. Females are at a greater risk of developing eating disorders which are often associated with the female athlete triad. This is a serious condition that increases risk of stress fractures and poor bone development which leads to osteoporosis later in life.

References and Additional Readings

Beals KA. 2004. *Disordered Eating Among Athletes: A Comprehensive Guide for Health Professionals, 1st edition.* Champaign, IL. Human Kinetics.

Female Athlete Triad Coalition. http://www.femaleathletetriad.org/

National Eating Disorders Association. http://www.nationaleatingdisorders.org/

Sundgot-Borgen J, et al. 2013. How to minimise the health risks to athletes who compete in weight-sensitive sports review and position statement on behalf of the Ad Hoc Research working group on body composition, health and performance, under the auspices of the IOC Medical Commission. *Br J Sports Med.* 47, no. 16, pp. 1012–1022.

FURTHER READING

Bodybuilder, 39, Dies from Cancer Caused by Steroid Abuse

Sun

If you have a digital edition of this book, please click on the link below to access the article:

https://www.news.com.au/lifestyle/health/health-problems/bodybuilder-39-dies-from-cancer-caused-by-steroid-abuse/news-story/a4ef33c065cc7ce0570dc38243bb12b8

If you have a print edition of this book, please use your cell phone to scan the QR code below to access the article:

"Beasts" of Anorexia Nervosa, Bulimia Ravaged Gymnast's Body: Health: Christy Henrich was 22 and Weighed Less than 60 Pounds When She Died. Her Family Hopes Her Story Will Save Others.

Steve Wilstein

If you have a digital edition of this book, please click on the link below to access the article:

https://www.latimes.com/archives/la-xpm-1994-08-21-mn-29434-story.html

If you have a print edition of this book, please use your cell phone to scan the QR code below to access the article:

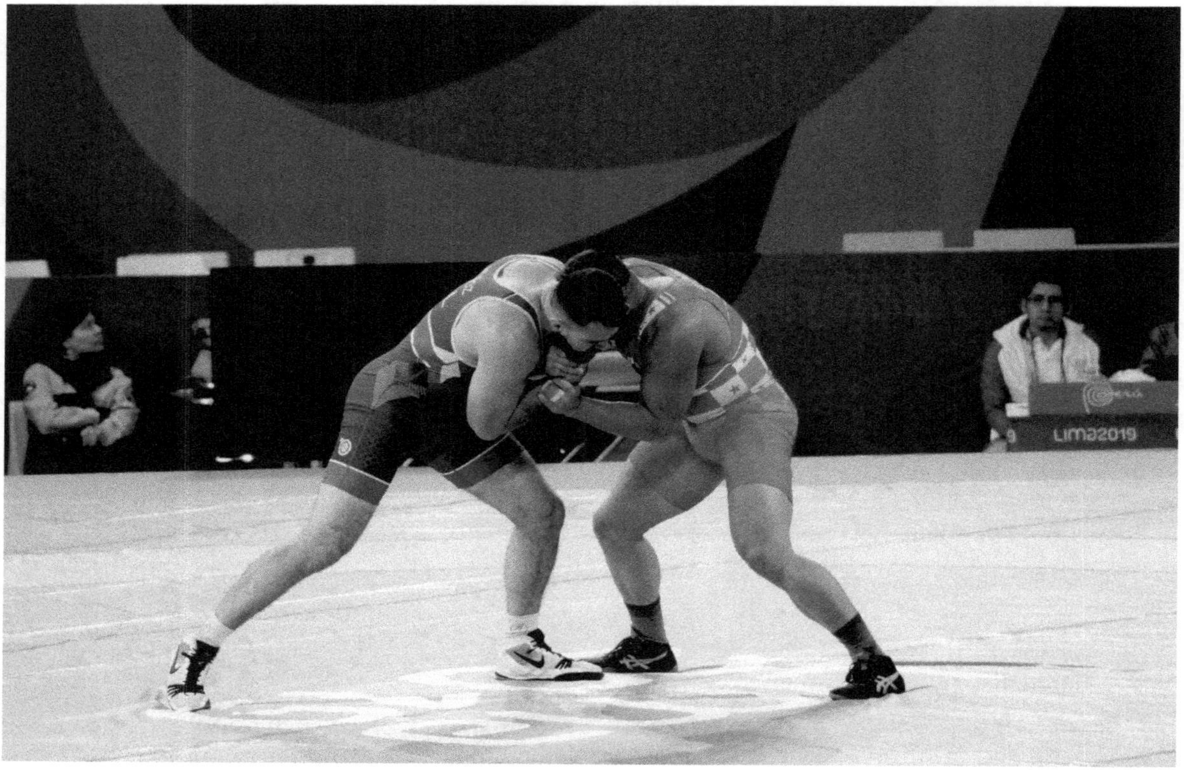
Lima2019

CHAPTER 10

TOXIC MASCULINITY AND VIOLENCE

Former college football tight end Brandon Vandenburg, 6 ft. 6 in. tall, walked into a Nashville, Tennessee, courtroom on August 25, 2017, requesting a new trial. The request was procedural because it laid the groundwork for an appeal. Vandenburg had served over one year of his seventeen-year prison term for his involvement with the rape of a woman in a dorm at his elite NCAA Division I university. The summer of 2013, Brandenburg embarked on the final chapter of his football playing career. Highly recruited by NCAA Division I universities, following a successful junior college career that earned him "the nation's No. 1 junior college tight end" title according to ESPN, Brandenburg had been on campus and practicing with the Vanderbilt University football team for only a few short weeks. On June 23, 2013, Vandenburg committed his heinous crime. It took two court cases, the first overturned because of a mistrial, but in the end the jury found Vandenburg guilty. A judge sentenced him to seventeen years in prison, and his first opportunity for parole will be after 85 percent of his sentencing is met in 2032.[1]

Many sport sociologists examine the connection between **toxic masculinity** and **violence** caused by male athletes off the field. Masculinity is so ingrained and rooted in the social world of sport that anything other than appearing big, strong, and tough is considered unacceptable. Moreover, the more **masculine capital** one can obtain, the more respect they feel they deserve from their peers. Masculine capital can be obtained by the sport you play (football appears to bring more masculine capital than gymnastics, and a player position such as defensive lineman might provide more masculine capital than being the kicker), and it can be obtained through violence on the field of play. In the image here, two Greco-Roman wrestlers battle on the wrestling mat with their large and muscular physiques exposed, providing the winner with additional masculine capital as the gold medal winner. The crowd consciously stands at attention for the winner, but spontaneously jumps to their feet when one athlete picks up and throws their competitor down to the mat, providing the crowd with the violence they came to see. This is at the core of toxic masculinity in sport. These beliefs and rewards can become so embedded in an athlete's understanding of their sport that it is difficult for them to participate in society without a continuous need to obtain more masculine capital. Gun violence, domestic abuse, and sexual assault are just a few of the many crimes brought on by toxic masculinity and violence.

1 Stacey Barchenger, "Judge Denies Brandon Vandenburg's Request for a New Trial," *USA Today*, August 25, 2017.

22

ATHLETES' INVOLVEMENT IN VIOLENCE AND AGGRESSION WITHIN THE CONTEXT OF SPORTS COMPETITION

Mihaela Rodica Mărăsescu

Introduction

Over the past decade, there has been increasing evidence describing athletes' perceptions and attitudes regarding aggression, athletes' perceptions of, and attitudes towards, aggressive behavior within competition, the conventions of aggression and violence that typify sports competition, and the interplay between characteristics of male athletes and factors associated with antisocial behavior. The aim of the present study is to examine and evaluate the athletes' personal perceptions of the team norm for aggression, sports-related spectator aggression, the violent strategies learned in sport, and sport participations' influence on aggressive tendencies in male athletes away from their respective fields of play. In the present paper, I focus on the relationship between team norm for aggression and players' self likelihood to aggress at the team level, the level and positive or negative nature of parental involvement in sport, the dynamics surrounding athlete violence beyond the sports context, and the link between male athletes and violence. My analysis complements the growing literature on the influence of game strategy efficacy on players' likelihood to aggress, the importance of parental involvement in youth sports, athletes' involvement in instances of aggression and violence, and the effects of sports participation on aggression in athletic contexts.

Mihaela Rodica Marasescu, "Athletes' Involvement in Violence and Aggression Within the Context of Sports Competition," *Contemporary Readings in Law and Social Justice*, vol. 5, no. 2, pp. 183-188.

The Effects of Sports Participation on Aggression in Athletic Contexts

Hyper-masculine sports dominate American sports culture and epitomize manliness. There is no way of determining whether sports breed aggressive characteristics, or aggressive individuals gravitate towards sports. (Stevens, 2012) Sports-related spectator aggression has transgressed into the everyday lives of our children. The personality characteristic that parents bring to their children's games (Bacalu, 2012) affects their situational tendencies or motivations. A cognitive-behavioral intervention (Popescu, 2013) might have positive psychosocial outcomes for the youth athletes. Defensiveness, emotional reactivity, anger, and subsequent aggression are influenced by one's control orientation, whereas having an autonomy orientation initially protects parents from being ego-defensive. (Goldstein and Iso-Ahola, 2008)

Parental involvement in youth's sports activities typically involves time and money. Parents influence their children's motivation to pursue sports in a variety of ways, and may play an important role in youth sports experiences through their own beliefs and practices (parents can be active promoters of youth's sports participation). The effects of parental involvement may vary as a function of parent and youth gender. High levels of perceived parental pressure can have important implications for youth performance anxiety. Parents may influence their youth sports experiences through their involvement as spectators. Spectator behavior may be more intense as the level of sports expertise increases (there are also significant differences in skill level between recreational and competitive hockey players). Competitive hockey matches draw more negative comments than recreational hockey matches. (Bowker et al., 2009)

The concept of passion may uncover some of the processes underlying aggressive behavior in sports. Instrumental aggression consists in causing a strategic nuisance to an opponent in a desire to hinder one's performance, whereas reactive aggression usually involves frustration or anger along with the intent to harm or injure another. Players with a predominant obsessive passion are more likely to behave with reactive aggression. Threatening the sense of competence attached to the passionate activity in obsessively-passionate athletes may trigger aggression. Obsessively-passionate players display higher levels of situational aggressive behavior than harmoniously-passionate players under self-threat. Athletes with a harmonious passion are less likely to engage in unnecessary aggressive behavior. (Donahue, Rip, and Vallerand, 2009) Power aggression in sport aims at dominating and subjugating a rival player or opposing team. It is possible to intend to hurt an opponent through sanctioned aggressive play. (Grange and Kerr, 2010)

The Culture of Hockey as an Instigating Mechanism of Male Violence

Not all athlete aggression is restricted to sports opponents. College athletes are overrepresented among those who are involved in aggressive and violent sexual behavior on college campuses. Many athletes are presented with the apparent dilemma of having to win at all costs and yet to adhere to moral and ethical sport behavior. Hockey players undergo a specialized socialization process (Manolache, 2013) in the production of a tough fighting unit. Fighting is a proactive means for not being easily intimidated and guarding against further aggression. Fans play an important role in the reinforcement of violence. The reinforcement through cheering and positive comments is appealing to the athletes. Hockey socialization and athletes' notions of masculinity combine to create a culture of aggression and violence (fighting plays a central role in hockey competition). Hockey players are likely to equate manliness with a willingness to engage in violent behavior. Hockey socialization has created a context within which violence and aggression are tolerated and encouraged. Referees do not intervene in professional hockey fights as long as only two players are involved. (Pappas, McKenry, and Skilken Catlett, 2004)

Fighting violates what it means to be a morally correct hockey athlete. Allowing players to fight defies the established code of ethics by demonstrating a lack of virtue. A fight out of evil intent violates what it means to be a moral athlete. By removing fighting, this will increase the number of moral hockey athletes. (Lewinson and Palma, 2012) Each sport is characterized by a particular web of relationships and roles that may have differing impacts on athletes. Ice hockey is known for its use of enforcers whose sole purpose is to aggress against the opponent. Aggressive behavior in ice hockey is a socialization process by which players learn to aggress via reinforcement and modeling. Players learn aggressive sport behaviors and become professionalized in their attitudes as length of sport participation increases. Players are socialized into the normative aggressive behaviors that define their sport. As ice hockey players increase in age and competitive level, there is a corresponding increasing trend in their perceived legitimacy of aggressive ice hockey behavior. Professional hockey players' perceptions of the legitimacy of aggressive on-ice behaviors differ from the perceptions of the younger players. Players' moral priorities become increasingly professionalized at higher levels of competitive hockey. Perceptions of the legitimacy of aggression and attitudes about sport may be a function of players' competitive levels. (Visek and Watson, 2005)

Coaches' Beliefs in Their Capabilities to Influence the Personal Development and Positive Attitude of Their Athletes

Coaches should be alert to the possibility of bullying and proactively seek to reduce it. Few clear collective norms exist within youth sports. Coaches are entrusted by parents and society (David, 2012) to support the growth of young athletes, but problems with coaches are not uncommon in youth sports. Sport cultures vary with regard to norms about behavior. There is much work to be done to build strong collective norms (Nica, 2013) around issues of fairness and respect. Learning skills of emotional self-regulation is key to improvement (Lăzăroiu, 2013), the concept of "good sport" is lacking sufficient behavioral specificity, and there is a strong desire on the part of parents and coaches to teach positive sport behaviors. (Light Shields, 2005)

Differences in gender and competitive age level (Paraschiv, 2013) are important variables to control for when examining moral behavior in sport. Previous experience in the sport and perceived ability relate to moral behavior. Athletes' personal attributes contribute to their views about aggression. The team norm for aggression is the strongest predictor of athletes' self likelihood to aggress scores. The moral atmosphere involves members' perceptions of their teammates' moral decisions (Pera, 2013) and coaches' beliefs and behaviors (the coach is influential in determining athletes' moral action). The coach serves as an influential significant other in the process of athletes' moral judgments. Coaches' attributes contribute to their players' aggressive tendencies. One likely social influence is their coach's behavior. One coach-related belief that may affect coaches' behavior is coaching efficacy. Character building efficacy may contribute to athletes' likelihood to commit unsportsmanlike behaviors. Coaches with high character building efficacy should be more likely to discourage antisocial behavior. Character building efficacy (Peters, 2013a; Peters, 2013b) is associated with athlete and team outcomes. Male coaches tend to have a higher sense of confidence in their game strategy abilities. Coaches' game strategy efficacy positively predicts their athletes' self likelihood to aggress, and the association with game strategy efficacy nearly approaches the magnitude of the team norm for aggression. Coaches' personal efficacy beliefs are strongly tied to their athletes' judgments regarding moral behavior. Coaches who have high game strategy efficacy may outright teach unfair tactics. Coaches high in game strategy efficacy may approve of and use unfair tactics. Game strategy efficacy emerges as a strong and positive predictor of players' likelihood to aggress. At higher competitive levels, athletes may be more likely to engage in aggressive behaviors. Character building efficacy is unrelated to athletes' self likelihood to aggress. Individual perceptions of the team norm for aggression predict athletes' likelihood to aggress. Coaches' playing experience positively predicts athletes' self likelihood to aggress. Aggressive tendencies reflect a negative aspect of morality. Teams having a higher norm for aggression are more likely to have aggressive players than teams having a lower norm for aggression. Coaches' confidence in their game strategy capabilities exerts a strong influence on their players' tendencies to aggress. (Chow, Murray, and Feltz, 2009)

Conclusions

The findings of this study have implications for moral behavior in sport, efforts to identify predictors of spectator aggression and violence, the links between sports participation and interpersonal violence, and the propensity for male athletes to express aggressive feelings and behavior outside of the sports domain. As a result of these earlier research findings, this study sought to determine athletes' tendencies to aggress, beliefs about what constitutes appropriate good sport behavior, the need to clarify the connections between athletic participation and violence, and the relationship between athletes' stage of moral development and aggression in youth sport. The overall results provide strong evidence for the problem of aggressive behavior in hockey, the role of individual factors as opposed to the culture of sport in producing violent behaviors, the actions and comments of parent and adult spectators at youth sporting events, and the pressure that hockey players feel from coaches who are perceived to promote aggression in their players. The current study has extended past research by elucidating the athlete-level factors of aggression, the nature of parental involvement, and its impact on children and adolescents, in a sports environment, attitudes or beliefs with regard to good sport behavior, and the culture of hockey as an instigating mechanism of male violence.

References

Bacalu, Filip (2012), "The Role of Learning in L2 Acquisition," *Linguistic and Philosophical Investigations* 11: 129–134.

Bowker, Anne, Belinda Boekhoven, Amanda Nolan, Stephanie Bauhaus, Paul Glover, Tamara Powell, and Shannon Taylor (2009), "Naturalistic Observations of Spectator Behavior at Youth Hockey Games," *The Sport Psychologist* 23: 301–316.

Chow, Graig M., Kristen E. Murray, and Deborah L. Feltz (2009), "Individual, Team, and Coach Predictors of Players' Likelihood to Aggress in Youth Soccer," *Journal of Sport and Exercise Psychology* 31: 425–443.

David, Bogdan (2012), "The Legal Construction of the Ethical Character of Society," *Analysis and Metaphysics* 11: 161–166.

Donahue, Eric G., Blanka Rip, and Robert J. Vallerand (2009), "When Winning Is Everything: On Passion, Identity, and Aggression in Sport," *Psychology of Sport and Exercise* 10: 526–534.

Goldstein, Jay D., and Seppo E. Iso-Ahola (2008), "Determinants of Parents' Sideline-Rage Emotions and Behaviors at Youth Soccer Games," *Journal of Applied Social Psychology* 38(6): 1442–1462.

Grange, Pippa, and John H. Kerr (2010), "Physical Aggression in Australian Football: A Qualitative Study of Elite Athletes," *Psychology of Sport and Exercise* 11: 36–43.

Lăzăroiu, George (2013), "Peters on the New Ecologies of Knowledge," *Review of Contemporary Philosophy* 12: 127–133.

Lewinson, Ryan T., and Oscar E. Palma (2012), "The Morality of Fighting in Ice Hockey: Should It Be Banned?," *Journal of Sport and Social Issues* 36(1): 106–112.

Light Shields, David, Brenda Light Bredemeier, Nicole M. LaVoi, and F. Clark Power (2005), "The Sport Behavior of Youth, Parents, and Coaches: The Good, the Bad, and the Ugly," *Journal of Research in Character Education* 3(1): 43–59.

Manolache, Elena (2013), "Transforming the Gendered Social Relations of Urban Space," *Journal of Research in Gender Studies* 3(1): 125–130.

Nica, Elvira (2013), "Organizational Culture in the Public Sector," *Economics, Management, and Financial Markets* 8(2): 179–184.

Paraschiv, Gavril (2013), "Gendered Decision-making Practices in the Juvenile Justice System," *Contemporary Readings in Law and Social Justice* 5(1): 76–81.

Pappas, Nick T., Patrick C. McKenry, and Beth Skilken Catlett (2004), "Athlete Aggression on the Rink and off the Ice: Athlete Violence and Aggression in Hockey and Interpersonal Relationships," *Men and Masculinities* 6(3): 291–312.

Pera, Aurel (2013), "The Social Aspects of Technology-enhanced Learning Situations," *Geopolitics, History, and International Relations* 5(2): 118–123.

Peters, Michael A. (2013a), "Managerialism and the Neoliberal University: Prospects for New Forms of 'Open Management' in Higher Education," *Contemporary Readings in Law and Social Justice* 5(1): 11–26.

Peters, Michael A. (2013b), "Prospects for Open Science," *Knowledge Cultures* 1(3): 118–130.

Popescu, Gheorghe H. (2013), "Partisan Differences in Evaluations of the Economy," *Economics, Management, and Financial Markets* 8(1): 130–135.

Stevens, Craig (2012), "Violence by Male Athletes: A Review of Literature," paper at the Center for the Study of Sport in Society, Northeastern University.

Visek, Amanda, and Jack Watson (2005), "Ice Hockey Players' Legitimacy of Aggression and Professionalization of Attitudes," *The Sport Psychologist* 19: 178–192.

A SISSY SPEAKS TO GYM TEACHERS

HOW I WAS FORMED AND DEFORMED BY TOXIC MASCULINITY

Jeff Sapp

That Was Then

I don't recall what happened in third grade, but I was suddenly different. In first and second grades, Philip, Danny, Rick, and I had been best friends. But not in third grade. In third grade I remember them isolating me. What had happened? Why was it different now? Was it because they all wore their baseball caps to school that autumn from their summer little league teams?

In fifth grade I wrote a poem about Easter, and my teacher, Mrs. Porter, printed it and gave a copy to each student in the entire class (see Appendix A). She raved and raved about how good it was and what a wonderful writer I was. I was so proud of that little poem that even today, decades later, I still have the purple ditto Easter poem tucked away in an old cigar box in a closet full of childhood memories. But I was clueless at ten years of age that being known for poetry instead of little league would be a bad thing. I also remember recess the day my poem hit the fifth-grade press. "Smear the Queer" was the playground focus and, since I was so obviously an Oscar Wilde, the boys came at me like the Green Bay Packers. This memory, too, is tucked away in an old memory box in a closet full of childhood remembrances.

I remember drawing a wild rose for the school art contest (see Appendix B). It connected to our science lessons on Appalachian wildflowers and I was proud that I had made an academic connection in my art project. I won a blue ribbon. Yes, it was for participation, but it was still an honor, as I had never won anything before this. I still have that piece of art framed and hanging on my bedroom wall today as a way to honor my elementary years even though I am many years away from them today. I think it is good to have a part of sixth-grade with you always. It reminds you of things. My sixth-grade teacher, Miss Gibbs, also had us learn about the medicinal properties of wildflowers as well as their edible parts. We had to demonstrate our culinary knowledge to the class and I remember making jam out of the petals of the same wild roses I had drawn for my art project. Can you imagine how my popularity grew? First a poet, next an artist, and finally a chef! To the other boys, it was like I had leprosy. I remember being called so many names by my boy peers during my school years. First a queer, next a homo, and finally a fag. School is an absolute torture for those of us boys who do not fit into the narrow constructs of gender and masculinity that have been spoon fed to us since we were born.

Remember the gym rope in sixth grade? I can feel the eyes of all the other sixth-grade boys watching me try to pull the full weight of my own 86 pounds up to the ceiling. It's true that most are not paying attention. Several particularly insightful and self-confident peers are cheering me on. "Come on Jeff! I know you can do it! Just a little more! You're half way there!" A couple are giggling, knowing I'll give up like I did last gym period—and the one before that. The gym teacher is among those that smirk. How have my ears been so trained to hear those soft, un-encouraging giggles and not hear those loud cries of support?

I have such a great memory for detail that it actually shocks me that I can't remember this next teacher's name. I know it started with a "W" but that is all my memory can squeeze out. Mr. W was my seventh-grade shop teacher. He was also the middle school football coach and he had coached each one of my three older brothers, introducing them to the manly sport of football. And, today, so many years after he pinned me to the shop class wall and threatened and terrorized me, I find myself writing about him because my experience with him seems unresolved.

I was scared to death of shop class in the first place. Being raised by a single mother in the 50s, I hadn't had the luxury of a father who would have given me the prerequisites I needed for shop class. The only tools I'd known were the garden tools I'd used to weed the pansies in my flower garden. Anyway, what remains unresolved for me is why he targeted me and, seemingly, not other classmates. He came at me nice enough the first week of school.

"I've had all the Sapp boys in football," he said. "I take it you'll be joining the team too?"

I have no idea how I said "No" but I did, and he was enraged. He actually pinned me against the wall and said in a low, quiet mafia voice, "You *will* join the team." After that, he asked me every class period, growing more and more angry each time. And, finally, once the actual football season started he stopped speaking to me and only threw wrenches at me. It was his classroom management style to throw wrenches at those students who weren't paying attention to him. To my knowledge he never actually hit anyone with a wrench. No, his tactic was simply to terrorize you with fear in hopes, I guess, that you'd saw your finger off or something like that.

Today my adult-self holds the quivering, sweaty hand of that little boy and asks: "Why is he picking on us?"

There are only two rational answers my adult-self can come up with. One, my brothers or my mom had spoken with Mr. W and told him that I grew pansies in my flower garden and that I needed to be hit regularly by ninth-graders to rid myself of my flower fetish. Or, two, Mr. W was not really a teacher at all, but a terrorist. But, surely they don't allow terrorists to teach children in school...or do they?

When is it that you realize that you are a sissy? What age? What grade? Who lets you know that you aren't like the other boys?

High school gym class petrified me. I'm serious. I mean absolutely petrified me. I'd have rather faced the living dead and fought zombies then dress out for gym class and, once again, be reminded of how I wasn't like the other boys. I remember that I eventually just started hiding in the library, among books that for some reason comforted me. And I carefully forged absent slips from my mom that addressed my horrible illness, an illness so terrible that I should not be allowed to exercise. And even though I used different colored ink to forge my mom's name for the different days I had missed, I wasn't quite as clever as I'd thought and I was busted for skipping class. The gym teacher was so disgusted at me, the same gym teacher that used gender as motivation. "Okay girls," he'd say to the all-male class, "Surely you can do more pushups than that?"

It's no wonder I had such a difficult academic time in my public-school years as a child. The truth is, I had entirely too much curriculum to negotiate: learning to read and write, classifying plants and animals, doing reports on state history, negotiating gender norming roles, deciphering why I was attracted to boys, passing as a heterosexual, and trying to fend off the bullies who saw my difference as weakness. It felt as if I was swimming upstream while everyone else seemed to be going with the current. I was simply too exhausted by the time I got to sentence diagramming and long division to concentrate on it. My grades suffered. And my sense of self suffered even more. It still affects me today. I have a daughter now and when we are at a play date and the other fathers are in the living room watching and bonding over a soccer game, I do not join them. I hate sports, for the most part. I do not for a second want to use sports as a way to bond. And, so, I remain on the outside of the father club, still a spectator. It still feels exactly like that summer going into third grade when the other boys—strutting the school in their baseball caps—wouldn't speak to me.

Toxic Masculinity

Perhaps nowhere on a school campus is the construction of masculinities more apparent than in the physical education class and its extracurricular counterpart of school athletics. Pascoe (2012) notes that schools are a major socializing institution in the life of children and, sadly, it is a dominant place where boys learn heteronormative and homophobic discourses, practices, and interactions and internalize them into adulthood. Boys often lay claim to their own masculine identities by hurling homophobic epithets at other boys and engaging in misogynistic discussions of girls' bodies, too. I am not the first to write about the toxic terrain of physical education in the school setting (Davison, 2004; Kehler & Atkinson, 2010) and I won't be the last. As a matter of fact, all one needs to do to learn about the devastating and lasting impact of toxic masculinity as a result of physical education classes is to ask about men's memories of it in any personal circle. Toxic masculinity—the socially constructed attitudes that describe expressions of maleness as violent, unemotional, aggressive, domineering, and controlling—is harmful to everyone.

The Gym Teacher I Wish I Had

As a former child terrorized by gym class and now as a veteran teacher educator, what is it that I wish I'd had in a physical educator? What kind of space would I have flourished in as a timid sissy-child? What could have occurred that would have had me fall in love with health and fitness as a way of life? Here are three overarching pedagogies I urge physical educators to be aware of and implement. You don't have to be a physical educator to implement these strategies. We all have children in our lives and these three ways of being with children can work anywhere, not just in a gym class. Stop telling young boy children they are "studs" and young girl children they are such a "pretty princess" and begin complementing boys on their kind spirit and girls on their fierce strength. Anyone can use the following three ways of being with children. Anyone. Anywhere. Any time.

Be explicitly safe. First and foremost, there must be a cornerstone of building relationships and trust within the class (Fitzpatrick, 2010). I encourage physical education professionals to begin their school year by discussing issues of gender, masculinities, and homophobia. Tell students what is appropriate and what is inappropriate and take a stand for the social and mental wellbeing, as well as the physical wellbeing, of your students. Lay out exactly what kind of a climate you want in your class and remain diligently consistent in modeling and guiding students towards it. Do not privileged athletes who, because of their athletic performances, often reside in schools with positions of power and prestige? Instead, enlist them as team leaders and train them about your classroom climate, having them to model true leadership as those who make physical fitness spaces safe for all students. Give athletes responsibilities to be exemplary leaders within the school community who aid you in making your gym class the most popular and safe space on campus. Not a gym teacher? Okay, then have as many conversations as you can about gender with children. Challenge gender norms, policing, and stereotyping.

Be explicitly pro-feminist. Understand there are societal and institutional forces against your being a loving, caring male. All too often sexism and homophobia walk comfortably hand-in-hand (Pharr, 1997). When you are anti-woman in any form it communicates to boys in your class that sexism is okay. When you are homophobic it typically is in a form that disparages the feminine (e.g., "You throw like a girl!") and this communicates that anything associated with the feminine is negative and less-than. Being pro-feminist is effort well spent for all males (hooks, 2004). Gorski (2008) states five reasons it is important for men to be pro-feminist. First, violence against women in all of its forms—sexual harassment, rape, domestic violence—is a form of terrorism. Secondly, hyper-masculinity contributes to other forms of violence in the world. Thirdly, patriarchal gender roles limit everyone's ability to live and contribute fully to society. Fourth of all, male privilege perpetuates a system of oppression. Gorski's fifth reason is a powerful one as well. His fifth reason is his grandmother. Think of the womyn[1] in your own life as well. And then reflect on whether your day-to-day interactions are anti-sexist and anti-oppressive. Go further and become a student of all things gender related in school cultures (Butler-Wall et al., 2016) and model excellence to the boys you're bringing into manhood.

Be explicitly non-toxic in your masculinity. Of course, this means that each individual educator must work through their own internalized issues around gender constructs so that they can comfortably teach these topics in a genuine and authentic manner. Just this very week I had students in my teaching credential course speak about their most memorable teachers. Two physical educators spoke of the same gym teacher they had in high school and how he really was tough on them and made them "man up." Honestly, the teacher they were speaking of sounded like a horrible bully to me. My two students shared their pride in surviving his masculinity and hazing and how it made them the men they were today. I could only think of how they were going to treat students in the same brutalizing manner to make "boys into men." I am struck by a Quaker tenet I heard once at a school I'd written about (Sapp, 2005) when I wrote an article on holistic education—teaching to body, mind, and spirit. The tenet was, "Strong women, gentle men." I see strong womyn all around me but, honestly, I rarely ever see gentle men. Fight against toxic masculinity in all its forms. Be better than the shallow Hollywood portrayals of men that are consumed daily in the media. Be gentle. To this day, I am always stunned by heterosexual men who are comfortable in their own sexuality and are not threatened by a queer man in their presence; it is more unusual than you would think to have men of strength reach out and be kind and loving to queer men in their midst. I recently reunited with a former student of mine from twenty years ago named Matt. Matt was amazing even as a young college man and I remember him once grabbing my hand and walking across a school campus holding it. When I saw him recently it was with his wife and two children and he still held my hand, kissed my cheek, and wept with emotion at seeing his mentor. He brought me a gift. He had his high school students—students in another state who have never met me—write me notes of appreciation for being the teacher who had impacted and shaped him the most. It was so touching. Matt reminds me that there are gentle men out in the world who have rejected toxic masculinity and are safe and kind. Be like Matt.

1 Some feminists use the word "womyn" or "womxn" to avoid using the suffix "-men" at the end of the term.

Be explicitly on the lookout for gender non-conforming students in your classroom. I suspect if you do the three above pedagogical practices that there will be less need for you to actually look and monitor those students that were like myself, kids that didn't fit the gender norms. Still, though, look for us. And look out for us. I do not mean to "look out after us" in a patriarchal manner where you are an overseer, but in a way that demonstrates your ethic of caring. Seek us out and be our leaders as well, even though we're not your best students and don't exhibit physical prowess. We will try harder if you know our names and we feel like we have our own personal connections with you as a teacher and a leader. Your kindness can inspire us to involve ourselves in fitness for life, and isn't that your goal? Again, if you're not in a classroom, just notice the children around you with eyes that see them for their character and not for the way they perform gender.

This Is Now

I find an odd joy in being a teacher educator that has future physical education teachers in my teacher credential courses today. There they sit. Terrorists. And I stand before them now as a veteran of many years in teaching and speak to them of becoming a teacher. Of becoming a caring teacher. Of becoming an aware teacher. Of becoming.

The first thing I tell them is that I wish I'd learned "fitness as a way of life" in gym class. Instead, I learned that I was a worthless sissy that was always to be picked last for any team. I struggled with health and wellbeing in my adulthood as a result of this. I became an athlete later in life ... a runner, a swimmer, and an accomplished 20-year career veteran lifeguard and lifeguard instructor. But I grieve not running track in high school; it's one of the few regrets I have in life. How will those adults who model fitness and health embrace and encourage the sissy who would rather be in the library than in the gym class? Will the rewards only be for those gifted athletes who come equipped with the physical skills for success? How will teams be picked? Who will be the captains? Will you stand guard against homophobia or will you let *The Lord of the Flies* attitudes take over? Will gender violence be given a shoulder shrug and a boys-will-be-boys wink?

I remember a time when I hated waking up for school. I hated hearing the alarm go off. I hated seeing the light invade the perimeter of the blinds. I hated leaving the familiar blankets wrapped around me like a cocoon. I hated that I would have to spend another entire day trying to figure out what teachers and peers were telling me about gender and why I felt so incredibly alone in a school full of thousands of children the same age as I was. I hated that I was the sissy boy that was always picked last for gym class. To this day, I hate waking up in the morning, but I am suddenly struck by how much I missed because I slept far too long.

Appendix A

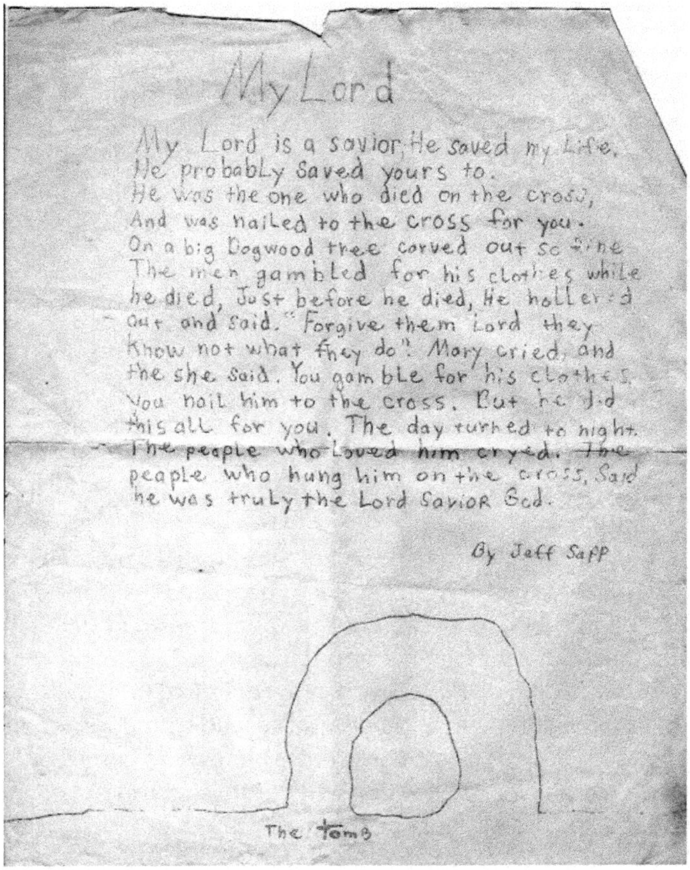

My Lord

My Lord is a savior, He saved my Life,
He probabLy saved yours to.
He was the one who died on the cross,
And was nailed to the cross for you.
On a big Dogwood tree corved out so fine
The men gambled for his clothes while
he died, Just before he died, He hollered
out and said. "Forgive them Lord they
Know not what they do". Mary cried, and
the she said. You gamble for his clothes.
You nail him to the cross. But he did
this all for you. The day turned to night.
The people who Loved him cryed. The
peaple who hung him on the cross, Said
he was truLy the Lord SavioR God.

By Jeff Sapp

Appendix B

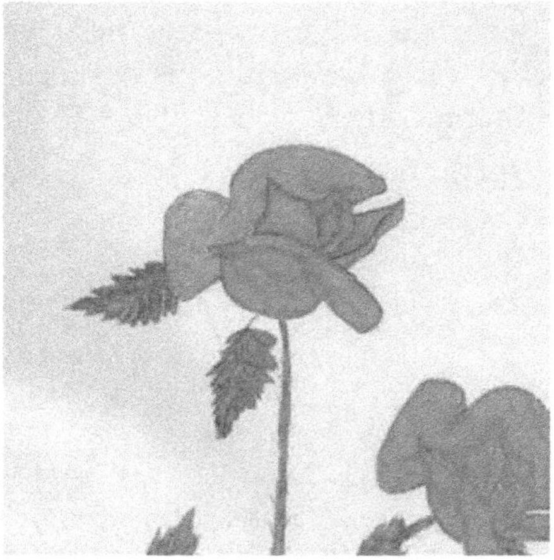

References

Butler-Wall, A., Cosier, K., Harper, R. L. S., Sapp, J., Sokolower, J., & Bollow Tempel, M. (2016). *Rethinking sexism, gender, and sexuality.* Milwaukee, WI: Rethinking Schools.

Davison, K. G. (2004). Texting gender and body as a distant/ced memory: An autobiographical account of bodies, masculinities and schooling. *The Journal of Curriculum Theorizing, 20*(3), 129–149. http://hdl.handle.net/10379/5229

Fitzpatrick, K. (2010). A critical multicultural approach to physical education: Challenging discourses of physicality and building resistant practices in schools. In S. May & C. E. Sleeter (Eds.) *Critical multicultural theory and praxis* (pp. 177–190). New York, NY: Routledge.

Gorski, P. (2008). *The evolution of a pro-feminist.* Retrieved from http://www.edchange.org/publications/pro-feminist.pdf

hooks, b. (2004). *The will to change: Men, masculinity, and love.* New York, NY: Simon & Schuster.

Kehler, M., & Atkinson, M. (2010). *Boys' bodies: Speaking the unspoken.* New York, NY: Peter Lang Publishing.

Pascoe, C. J. (2012). *Dude, you're a fag: Masculinity and sexuality in high school.* Berkeley, CA: University of California Press.

Pharr, S. (1997). *Homophobia: A weapon of sexism.* Berkeley, CA: Chardon Press.

Sapp, J. (2005). Body, mind & spirit: Holistic educators seek authentic connections with students, subjects, colleagues and the world. *Teaching Tolerance Magazine, 27,* 24–29. Retrieved from http://www.tolerance.org/magazine/number-27-spring-2005/feature/body-mind-and-spirit

24

IVEY | Publishing

DOMESTIC VIOLENCE IN THE NFL

TIME FOR REAL CHANGE?[1]

Cara C. Maurer and Kyle Trahair

Kyle Trahair wrote this case under the supervision of Professor Cara Maurer solely to provide material for class discussion. The authors do not intend to illustrate either effective or ineffective handling of a managerial situation. The authors may have disguised certain names and other identifying information to protect confidentiality.

Introduction

Jerry Richardson sat rubbing his temples, having just returned to his office in Charlotte, North Carolina, from a ceremony to accept the "Award Against Violence" from the Echo Foundation. It was September 12, 2014, and the founder and principal owner of the Carolina Panthers (Panthers) National Football League (NFL) team was contemplating how to respond to domestic violence charges pressed against one of his star players, Greg Hardy. Hardy had been convicted on misdemeanour charges of communicating threats and assaulting a woman on July 15, 2014.[2]

1 This case has been written on the basis of published sources only. Consequently, the interpretation and perspectives presented in this case are not necessarily those of the National Football League or any of its employees or players.
2 "Timeline: Carolina Panthers Defensive End Greg Hardy," *Charlotte Observer*, October 31, 2014, www.charlotteobserver.com/sports/nfl/carolina-panthers/article9226367.html, accessed November, 10, 2014.

He had appealed the charges and was waiting for a jury trial, which was expected to take place at the end of the 2014/15 NFL season.

The mood in the NFL surrounding domestic violence had shifted dramatically in the past week. A video had surfaced that depicted Ray Rice, the Baltimore Ravens running back, punching his fiancée, Janay Palmer unconscious in an elevator (see http://www.cnn.com/2014/09/09/us/ray-rice-timeline/, assessed April, 20, 2015). The strong public reaction to this incident came on the heels of two months of inaction on the part of the Panthers with respect to Hardy. Richardson thought back to his remarks during his award ceremony:

> Standing before you tonight, I would be remiss if I did not acknowledge an issue weighing heavily on our sport and our society. When it comes to domestic violence, my stance is not one of indifference. ... I stand firmly against domestic violence, plain and simple.... To those who would suggest that we've been too slow to act, I ask that you consider not to be too quick to judge. Over the course of our 20 years, we have worked extremely hard to build an organization of integrity and earn the trust of our community. I will work hard to continue to earn your trust.[3]

At the same time, performance expectations for the Panthers were high. Richardson's goal was nothing less than winning the 2014 Super Bowl Championship. This year could offer one of his last opportunities to cement his legacy as his retirement neared. The Panthers had just played their first game of the season with Hardy and had not yet taken any disciplinary action towards him.

Overview of the NFL

Origin and History

Professional football was first played in the United States in the 1890s, but there was no central organization responsible for coordinating team schedules or creating a uniform version of rules to play by until 1920. This disorganization not only inhibited the growth of professional football across the country but also cost owners large sums of money due to rapidly increasing player salaries as teams poached players from one another. In 1920, several owners of various football clubs joined to create the American Professional Football Association (APFA).[4]

The mission of the APFA was to solve scheduling and player salary issues so that football would scale profitably across the United States.[5] In its early stages, the league consisted of 18 teams, but it did not experience much success. Fan attendance reached an average of only 4,241 per game compared to college football games that experienced attendance of up to 100,000 fans. In 1922, the team owners decided that the league needed a president with more business acumen and brought in Joe Carr, the owner of the Columbus Panhandles (one of the APFA teams at the time). One of his first actions as president was to change the name to the National Football League.[6]

3 Michael Amato, "Panthers Owner Jerry Richardson Condemns Domestic Violence After Accepting Award," The Score, September 10, 2014, www.thescore.com/nfl/news/575446, accessed October 15, 2014.

4 Christopher Klein, "The Birth of the National Football League," History in the Headlines, September 4, 2014, www.history.com/news/the-birth-of-the-national-football-league, accessed October, 15, 2014.

5 Ibid.

6 According to Robert W. Peterson, *Pigskin: The Early Years of Pro Football*, Oxford University Press, New York, 1997, accessed October 15, 2014.

The NFL's success greatly improved in the late 1950s, especially with the 1958 championship game, which was viewed by 45 million viewers on television. This rise in popularity led to the introduction of a competing professional football league in 1959, the American Football League (AFL). The AFL consisted of only eight teams and was therefore not perceived as much of a threat to the NFL. This perception changed, however, in 1966 when the AFL began poaching players from the NFL. Subsequent talks between the leagues resulted in an agreement to merge in 1966 and brought about the first Super Bowl, played between the NFL and AFL champions. League operations and schedules were not fully merged until 1970, at which point it was agreed that the NFL would absorb the AFL and split the teams into two conferences, the American Football Conference and the National Football Conference.[7]

Current Structure and Appeal

The current NFL structure came to be in 2002 with the introduction of the league's 32nd team, the Houston Texans. This opportunity enabled the league to alter its format from six divisions (three in each conference) to eight divisions (four divisions of four teams in each 16-team conference).[8]

Each NFL team played 16 games during the regular season, and the teams with the best record in their division as well the two teams in each conference with the best records that did not win their division (the wild card teams) advanced to the playoffs. The top two teams from each conference received a buy into the divisional round, while the other eight teams were seeded (ranked) and matched up to play a single elimination game, determining the team that would advance to the divisional round. The divisional round consisted of eight teams, which played a single elimination game to determine which four teams would advance to the conference championships. The two winners of their respective conference championship games would advance to the Super Bowl to play for the league championship.[9]

Football was the most popular sport in the United States, and the NFL had the highest average per game attendance of all international sports leagues. In 2013, the top 26 most viewed sporting events in the United States were all NFL games, led by the Super Bowl, which was viewed by over 108 million people. The closest domestic competitors were the National Basketball Association (NBA) and Major League Baseball (MLB), which had 26.32 million and 19.18 million viewers, respectively, in their final games.[10] Average attendance was over 66,000 people per game, almost double the average attendance in top international soccer leagues, including the English Premier League, which had an average of 36,156 people in attendance.[11]

Organizational Structure

The NFL was an unincorporated non-profit association, considered a trade association, made up of the 32 teams. Its organizational structure was very simple at the league level. The commissioner,

7 "NFL and AFL Announce Merger," This Day in History, www.history.com/this-day-in-history/nfl-and-afl-announce-merger, accessed October 15, 2014.

8 Ibid.

9 Ibid.

10 Paulsen, "2013 Ratings Wrap: NFL Dominates List of Most-Watched Sporting Events," Sports Media Watch, December 31, 2013, www.sportsmediawatch.com/2013/12/2013-ratings-wrap-nfl-dominates-list-of-most-watched-sporting-events/#thelist, accessed November 10, 2014.

11 "Statistics," www.espnfc.us/barclays-premier-league/23/statistics/performance, accessed November, 10, 2014.

Roger Goodell, was the principal executive officer and there was one president for each conference (the AFC and NFC).

The commissioner was elected by the team owners (this required at least two-thirds of the vote) and had very broad powers including the ability to suspend individuals, issue a fine of up to $500,000,[12] cancel contracts with the league and award or strip teams of draft picks. What made the commissioner much more powerful than his or her counterpart in the NBA or MLB was that there was no independent review of the NFL commissioner's actions, allowing nearly unlimited disciplinary power.[13]

All of the teams except the Green Bay Packers were private, for-profit organizations. The key decision-making parties in a typical NFL team were the owner, general manager and head coach. The owner had the largest financial stake in the team and had ultimate veto power. The general manager reported directly to the owner and made the final call on all front-end personnel related decisions.[14] The head coach was responsible for all on-the-field issues and reported to the general manager to assist in decisions relating to player acquisition and retention. The power balance between these three parties varied widely from franchise to franchise. For example, the degree of involvement among NFL owners varied widely, with some delegating almost all of their responsibilities and others encroaching on the responsibilities of the general manager.[15]

NFL Performance

The NFL was the highest grossing sports league in the world, with earnings of $9.5 billion in 2013.[16] In comparison, Premier League Football revenue totaled $4.19 billion in revenue over the same period of time.[17] The Super Bowl led the way for the NFL as the highest grossing single-day sporting event, making an estimated $420 million in revenue. This was almost double the 2008 Beijing Summer Olympic games and was well above the 2010 FIFA World Cup, which earned an average of $230 million and $120 million per day respectively.[18]

The four main sources of revenue in the NFL were broadcasting deals, ticket sales, sponsorships and licensing and merchandising. Broadcasting deals were by far the largest source of revenue, totaling $4.9 billion in the 2014/15 season.[19] Broadcasting revenues were split evenly between the teams, projected to amount to over $150 million per team in the 2014/15 season. Licensing and merchandising was the next largest source of revenue, totaling $2.1 billion for the league in 2010 and was also split

12 All currency in U.S. dollars unless otherwise specified.

13 Adriano Pacifici, "Scope and Authority of League Commissioner Disciplinary Power: Bounty and Beyond," Berkeley *Journal of Entertainment and Sports Law* 3.1, May 2014, http://scholarship.law.berkeley.edu/cgi/viewcontent.cgi?article=1041&context=bjesl, accessed January 10, 2015.

14 Paul Thelen, "What Exactly Does Each Member of an NFL Team's Front Office Do?," Bleacher Report, June 8, 2013, http://bleacherreport.com/articles/1666258-what-exactly-does-each-member-of-a-teams-front-office-do/page/2, accessed March 10, 2015.

15 Albert Breer, "Who's Really in Charge?: Power Structures for All 32 NFL Teams," June 10, 2013, www.nfl.com/news/story/0ap1000000210536/printable/whos-ireallyi-in-charge-power-structures-for-all-32-nfl-teams, accessed March 10, 2015.

16 "Total Revenue of All National Football League Teams from 2001 to 2013," Statista, www.statista.com/statistics/193457/total-league-revenue-of-the-nfl-since-2005, accessed February 10, 2015.

17 James Masters, "And the Richest Soccer Team in the World Is ... ," CNN, June 5, 2014, http://edition.cnn.com/2014/06/05/sport/football/football-deloitte-money-report/, accessed February 10, 2015.

18 Peter J. Schwarz, "The World's Top Sports Events," *Forbes*, March 5, 2010, www.forbes.com/global/2010/0315/ companies-olympics-superbowl-daytona-worlds-top-sports-events.html, accessed December 10, 2014.

19 Howard Bloom, "NFL Revenue Sharing Model Good For Business," *Sporting News*, September 5, 2014, www.sportingnews.com/nfl/story/2014-09-05/nfl-revenue-sharing-television-contracts-2014-season-business-model-nba-nhl-mlb-comparison-salary-cap, accessed February 10, 2015.

evenly among the teams.[20] League sponsorships were another large source of revenue for the league at $1.07 billion in 2013, up 5.7 per cent from the previous season.[21] Teams additionally had their own sponsors and corresponding revenue. The final source of revenue was ticket sales, which generated an average of $51 million per team per year.[22]

The average NFL team was worth $1.43 billion in 2014, up 23 per cent from 2013. This was the largest year over year increase since 1999. The average NFL team made $299 million in revenue and $53 million in operating income in the 2013 season.[23]

Jerry Richardson[24]

Richardson was born in Spring Hope, North Carolina, on July 18, 1936. He grew up in Fayetteville, a self-proclaimed football town and excelled academically and athletically due to his work ethic. Richardson's talent as a receiver became evident when he played on his high school football team, which ultimately led to his ability to attend Wyfford College on a $250 athletic scholarship.

Richardson graduated with a degree in psychology and was drafted to the world champion Baltimore Colts (Colts) of the NFL in the 13th round of the draft as the 153rd player overall. He was a long-shot to make the team but overcame this challenge and sealed the 1959 NHL Championship for the Colts by catching a touchdown pass in the 4th quarter.

Richardson cut his NFL career short, retiring after two years to join a friend from college, Charlie Bradshaw, in a new business venture. He invested his entire NFL earnings with Bradshaw to open the first franchised Hardee's Hamburger restaurant in Spartanburg, South Carolina in 1961. Richardson was known for working inside his restaurants and quickly gained a reputation for his hands-on, no-nonsense approach to management.

Richardson and Bradshaw's company, then named Spartan Foods, was listed on the NYSE on June 22, 1976; three years later, they sold it to Transworld Corporation for $80 million. Transworld soon became Flagstar Corporation, where Richardson assumed a leadership role. In 1995, Flagstar had interests in over 2,500 restaurants and over 100,000 employees, making it the largest publicly held company based in South Carolina.

In 1993, Richardson and his investment team successfully bid $210 million for the rights to create the Carolina Panthers, the 29th NFL franchise. Richardson retired from Flagstar in 1995 to focus on the team.

Richardson was the only person to have been inducted into both the North and South Carolina Business and Athletic Halls of Fame.[25] In addition to this, he had also been honoured with the highest civic recognition the State of South Carolina could bestow, the Order of the Palmetto.

20 Pellegrino, "Top Five Revenue Sources That Drive Value for the NFL," February 22, 2013, www.pellegrinoandassociates.com/top-five-revenue-sources-that-drive-value-for-the-nfl/, accessed February 10, 2015.

21 Ike Ejiochi, "How the NFL Makes the Most Money of Any Pro Sport, CNBC, September 4, 2014, www.cnbc.com/id/101884818, accessed February 10, 2015.

22 Pellegrino, op.cit. Tickets sales were split 60 per cent for the home team, 40 per cent for the away team per game.

23 Mike Ozanian, "The NFL's Most Valuable Teams," Forbes, October 20, 2014, www.forbes.com/sites/mikeozanian/2014/08/20/the-nfls-most-valuable-teams/, accessed January, 10, 2015.

24 www.woffordterriers.com/sports/2011/10/31/FB_1031114021.aspx?id=265, accessed March 10, 2015.

25 "Staff: Jerry Richardson," www.panthers.com/team/staff/jerry-richardson/4bcc4b2e-0a78-468a-a00c-bdc925d797a9, accessed January 10, 2015.

The Carolina Panthers

The Carolina Panthers (see Exhibit 1) were one of the NFL's most successful expansion franchises. In its first year, the team accumulated a record of seven wins and nine losses, an NFL record for wins by an expansion team,[26] followed by a much-improved second season that had them finishing first in their division with 12 wins and four losses. The Panthers had yet to win a Super Bowl, but their performance had been improving steadily over the last five years, to the point that they were considered to be championship contenders (see Exhibit 2). Richardson's role and influence in the NFL had continued to expand as well, exemplified by his role as co-chairman of the NFL Executive Committee.

The Panthers were the 17th most valuable franchise in the NFL, at an estimated $1.25 billion (up 18 per cent year over year). In 2013, they earned $283 million in revenue and $55.6 million in operating income.[27] Their largest sponsor was the Bank of America, with a 20-year $140 million agreement signed in 2004.[28] The bank had been recognized as one of the top employers in the country for women and was one of *Working Mother* magazine's 100 Best Companies.[29] While the Bank of America had not made any public statement about the state of the sponsorship agreement, one of the Panther's other sponsors, Harris Teeter Supermarkets, had commented on Hardy's conviction by noting that they "remain a sponsor ... but continue to follow the story closely."[30] Exhibit 3 shows the Panthers' financial projections for the 2014/15 season.

Domestic Abuse in the NFL

Since 2000, there had been 85 domestic violence-related arrests in the NFL. Since 2006, about 60 per cent of the domestic violence cases reported had resulted in league discipline.[31] Only one woman, Dewan Smith Williams, had spoken publicly about her abuse as the significant other of a former NFL player. She indicated that other women may have been concerned about negatively influencing their partner's career as a player by speaking out, stating, "They use [the NFL's current policies] as leverage against you. There's abuse on every team. Everybody knows, but you know not to tell."[32]

The video that portrayed NFL player Rice knocking his fiancée unconscious in an elevator became public on September 8, 2014.[33] The incident put the NFL under a high degree of scrutiny for its way of historically dealing with these issues as well as for placing a two game ban on Rice before the release of the video, which was deemed by many to be too mild a punishment.[34] In the past, cases were often dismissed because witnesses had rarely testified against the NFL,[35] but this incident was fundamen-

26 "Team History: Carolina Panthers," www.profootballhof.com/history/team/carolina-panthers/, accessed January 10, 2015.

27 "NFL Team Values: The Business of Football," *Forbes*, August 2014, www.forbes.com/nfl-valuations/#page:2_sort:0_direction:asc_search, accessed January 10, 2015.

28 Erik Spanberg and Adam O'Daniel, "No Audibles for Carolina Panthers Sponsors—Yet—Concerning Greg Hardy," *Charlotte Business Journal*, September 16, 2014, www.bizjournals.com/charlotte/blog/queen_city_agenda/2014/09/no-audibles-for-carolina-panthers-sponsors-yet.html?page=all, accessed February 10, 2015.

29 www.workingmother.com/2015-working-mother-100-best-companies-hub, accessed March 10, 2015.

30 Ibid.

31 "NFL Player Arrests," *USA Today*, www.usatoday.com/sports/nfl/arrests/, accessed January 10, 2015.

32 Simone Sebastian and Ines Bebea, "For Battered NFL Wives, a Messages from the Cops and the League: Keep Quiet," Washington Post, October 17, 2014, www.washingtonpost.com/posteverything/wp/2014/10/17/for-battered-nfl-wives-a-message-from-the-cops-and-the-league-keep-quiet/, accessed January 10, 2015.

33 www.huffingtonpost.com/2014/09/08/ray-rice-punch-video_n_5783380.html, accessed November 10, 2014.

34 Ibid.

35 http://thinkprogress.org/sports/2015/02/11/3621698/nfls-latest-domestic-violence-case-victims-dont-testify, accessed March 10, 2015.

tally different because of the now-public nature of the video. The league initially suspended Rice for two games, but was expected to revise this decision as a result of the backlash. Up until the beginning of the 2014/15 season, the traditional response in the NFL to domestic violence concerns had been a combination of suspensions, fines and mandatory counseling.[36]

Attention on Hardy's conviction increased as a result of the NFL's alleged mishandling of the Rice situation. Hardy was in the process of appealing the court ruling and a resolution was not expected until the end of the current season. Hardy was set to earn $13.11 million over the course of the season at which point his contract was going to expire, and he could sign with any other team in the league at that point.

Richardson had to consider the perspectives of many parties when addressing Hardy's situation. Some of these individuals had made their opinions public. Head Coach Ron Rivera:

> There's a lot to be looked at, measured and weighed. The climate has changed. And we have to most certainly look at things the right way because we really do have to get this right. I get that part of it. Believe me… . We have a young man (Hardy) who is going through a very difficult time as well. Just don't forget that, OK? And there's a lot of people involved. There's a lot of other people who are going through some difficult times as well. Just don't forget that, either. It's a very serious issue and we're trying to treat it with as much dignity as possible.[37]
>
> If you play him and you win, then you don't have a conscience; and if you play him and you lose, he's a distraction.[38]

General Manager Dave Gettleman:

> Q: Why did you let him play in Week 1?
>
> A: Because at that time we felt it was the right thing to do. It's constantly changing. There's no rulebook for this. There's no magic list that we can hit checkboxes with and for that to bring us to the right answer. Again, through this whole process since it started back in May, we've tried to be as thoughtful and as intentional as possible with everybody that's involved. This is hard, now. This is not easy. We're constantly trying to do the right thing.[39]

Teammate Josh Norman:

> A guy of that caliber, we need him, I mean, hands down I would welcome him back, and relish the chance to play with that guy again. He's that guy that takes us to a whole other level ... at the end of the day the man's got to make a living. He's got to work. He's got a job to do.[40]

36 http://abcnews.go.com/US/nfl-punished-players-arrested-domestic-violence-goodell-era/story?id=25534452, accessed November 10, 2014; and www.cnn.com/2014/09/09/us/nfl-players-domestic-violence-accusations, accessed November 10, 2014.

37 Jim Corbett, "Ron Rivera: Greg Hardy Will Play Again But Sitting Him Was in Panthers' 'Best Interest,'" *USA Today*, September 14, 2014, www.usatoday.com/story/sports/nfl/panthers/2014/09/14/greg-hardy-future-ron-rivera-jerry-richardson/15639937, accessed November 10, 2014.

38 Steve Reed, "Carolina Panthers Coach: Unsure if Hardy Will Play vs. Steelers, Team Hasn't Considered Releasing Defensive End," *Herald Sports*, September 15, 2014, http://thechronicleherald.ca/sports/1236631-carolina-panthers-coach-unsure-if-hardy-will-play-vs-steelers-team-hasn-t-considered-, accessed January 10, 2015.

39 Bill Voth, "TRANSCRIPT: Panthers GM Dave Gettleman on Greg Hardy's 'Leave of Absence,'" Black and Blue Review, September 17, 2014, http://blackandbluereview.com/gettleman-hardy-absence-panthers/, accessed November 10, 2014.

40 "Panthers' Teammates Want to See Greg Hardy Back," Fox Sports, January 11, 2015, www.foxsports.com/nfl/story/panthers-team-mates-want-to-see-greg-hardy-back-011115, accessed February 10, 2015.

Teammate Antione Cason:

> It is tough because being in this locker room and being a teammate, we say we're a band of brothers. Who knows what he is going through? I can't imagine the type of feelings he is going through. So for me it's just support him and let him know that I'm your teammate and I'm here for you.[41]

Domestic Abuse in the NBA and MLB

The NBA and MLB offered relevant comparisons for the NFL's performance in the context of domestic abuse. The NBA under its commissioner, Adam Silver, had recently begun approaching domestic violence proactively, whereas the MLB showed a model of inaction.

Silver had spoken out on behalf of the NBA saying, "In addition to its profound impact on victims, domestic violence committed by any member of the NBA family causes damage to the league and undermines the public's confidence in it." Beyond this, he had taken action that supported this assertion. The most recent example of this had been in his dealing with Jeff Taylor, a player for the Charlotte Hornets. Taylor had been arrested on domestic violence charges in 2014. The league responded quickly and transparently, ultimately handing down one of the longest unpaid suspensions in its history and ensuring Taylor was required to do community service directed at victims of domestic abuse.[42]

Given the nature of his suspension, Taylor could have appealed the punishment handed down by the commissioner, but he chose not to, stating publicly that he would be uncomfortable making an appeal knowing his actions were wrong.[43] The team additionally issued a statement supporting the decision of the commissioner.

Silver summarized the response to the issue by saying: "While the suspension is significantly longer than prior suspensions for incidents of domestic violence by NBA players, it is appropriate in light of Mr. Taylor's conduct, the need to deter similar conduct going forward, and the evolving social consensus—with which we fully concur—that professional sports leagues like the NBA must respond to such incidents in a more rigorous way."[44]

On the other hand, the approach taken in the MLB showed what a model with a dismissive stance on domestic violence looked like. In the past 25 years, there had not been a single instance of a commissioner-level sanctioning of a player for domestic violence, and almost all teams followed this pattern of inaction.[45] In 2005, Milton Bradley, an MLB player on the Los Angeles Dodgers, was visited by police three times on domestic violence calls. There was no discipline handed down from the team or the league, and Bradley went on to be nominated by the Dodgers for the Robert Clemente Award that year. In a separate incident in January 2000, Colorado Rockies pitcher Pedro Astacio pleaded

41 Steve Reed, "Carolina Panthers' Greg Hardy Will Not Play Until Domestic Violence Case Resolved, Team Says," *National Post*, September 17, 2014, http://news.nationalpost.com/sports/nfl/carolina-panthers-greg-hardy-will-not-play-until-domestic-violence-case-resolved-team-says, accessed November 10, 2014.

42 Smriti Sinha, "The NBA Just Showed the NFL How to Handle Domestic Violence Cases," Vice Sports, November 26, 2014, https://sports.vice.com/article/the-nba-just-showed-the-nfl-how-to-handle-domestic-violence-cases, accessed January 10, 2015.

43 Ibid.

44 Ibid.

45 Mike Bates, "MLB's Record on Domestic Violence Worse than NFL's," SB Nation, July 28, 2014, www.sbnation.com/mlb/2014/7/28/5936835/ray-rice-chuck-knoblauch-minnesota-twins-mlb-domestic-abuse-violence, accessed December 10, 2014.

guilty to a misdemeanour charge of punching his pregnant wife and went on to start for the Colorado Rockies on the opening day of their season.[46]

Richardson's Dilemma

Domestic violence was a national issue in the United States. The National Intimate Partner and Sexual Violence Survey estimated that 10 million individuals were victims of physical assault by an intimate partner each year and that more than one in three women are victims at some point in their life.[47]

Richardson knew that whatever decisions he made would be closely scrutinized by multiple parties. He had to decide whether or not to suspend Hardy and what approach to take with Hardy's salary. In the longer term, his focus was on whether or not to try to re-sign Hardy to the Panthers and what approach to take regarding the team's culture. Richardson knew that he had little time to make a public statement and that whatever he did would have profound implications for his legacy.

EXHIBIT 1: Organizational Chart

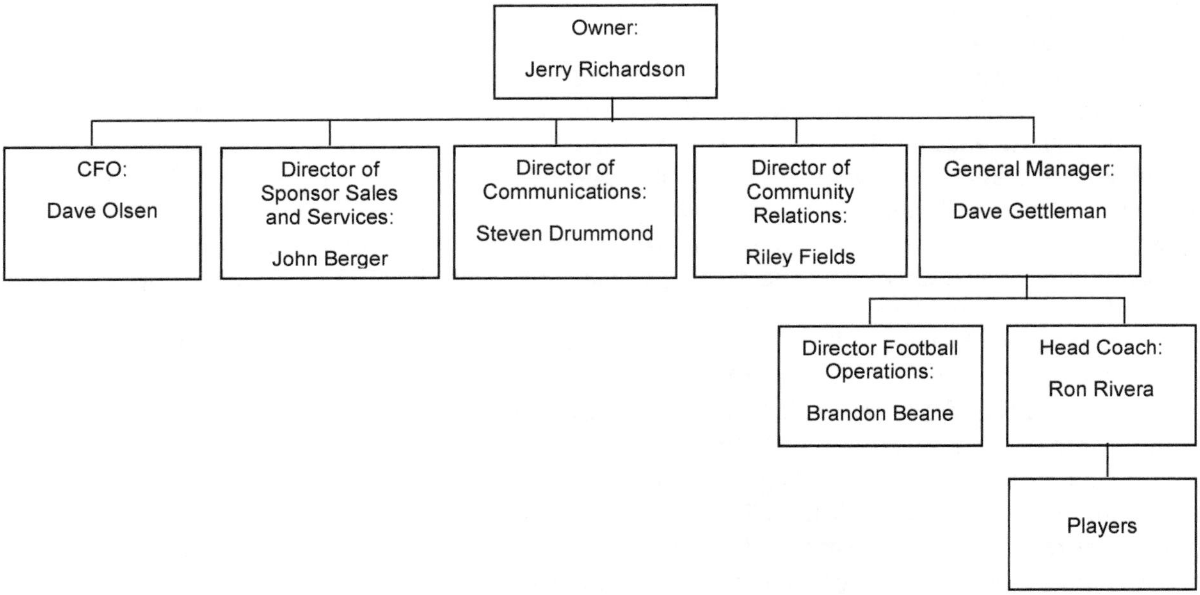

Source: Created by case writer based on information available at www.panthers.com/team/staff.html, accessed January, 10, 2015.

46 Ibid. The Robert Clemente Award was an award given annually to the MLB player who "best exemplifies the game of baseball, sportsmanship, community involvement and the individual's contribution to his team" and is voted on by members of the media and fans.

47 The National Intimate Partner and Sexual Violence Survey, Centers for Disease Control and Protection, www.cdc.gov/violenceprevention/nisvs/ and www.cdc.gov/violenceprevention/pdf/nisvs_executive_summary-a.pdf, accessed February 10, 2015.

EXHIBIT 2: Carolina Panthers Season Records

Season	Regular Season Record (wins – losses)	Season Result
2013	12 – 4	Lost Divisional Round
2012	7 – 9	Missed Playoffs
2011	6 – 10	Missed Playoffs
2010	2 – 14	Missed Playoffs
2009	8 – 8	Missed Playoffs
2008	12 – 4	Lost Divisional Round
2007	7 – 9	Missed Playoffs
2006	8 – 8	Missed Playoffs
2005	11 – 5	Lost NFC Championship
2004	7 – 9	Missed Playoffs
2003	11 – 5	Lost Super Bowl

Source: www.nfl.com/standings, accessed January, 10, 2015.

EXHIBIT 3: Carolina Panthers Projected Revenue 2014/2015 Season (In Millions)

Revenue:	
Broadcasting	$153
NFL Sponsorships	$35
Panthers Sponsorships	$10
Merchandise	$65
Ticket Sales	$51
Total Revenue	**$314**
Player Salary Expense	$133
Other Expenses	$119
Operating Income	**$62**

Note: The NFL salary cap limited teams from spending more than $143 million on player salaries for the 2014/2015 season.

Sources: www.pellegrinoandassociates.com/top-five-revenue-sources-that-drive-value-for-the-nfl/; http://overthecap.com/salary-cap/carolina-panthers/; www.forbes.com/nfl-valuations, accessed February, 10, 2015.

FURTHER READING

On-field Violence, Off-field Deaths: We Need a More Realistic Version of Masculinity

Sean Wales

If you have a digital edition of this book, please click on the link below to access the article:

https://www.theguardian.com/commentisfree/2017/may/28/on-field-violence-off-field-deaths-we-need-a-more-realistic-version-of-masculinity

If you have a print edition of this book, please use your cell phone to scan the QR code below to access the article:

Toxic Masculinity in Sport

Lizz Darcy

If you have a digital edition of this book, please click on the link below to access the article:

https://unbalanced.media/toxic-masculinity-in-sports

If you have a print edition of this book, please use your cell phone to scan the QR code below to access the article:

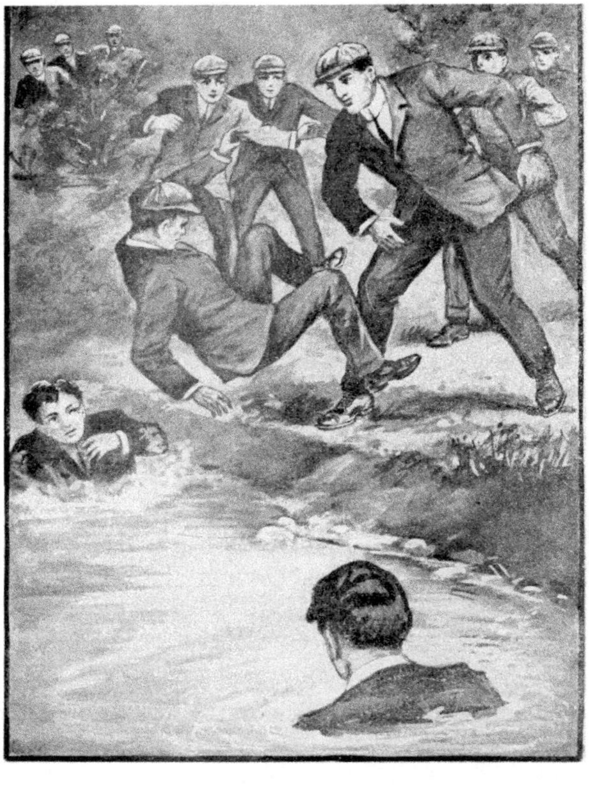

CHAPTER 11
HAZING

Lake Zurich High School paid over $50,000 in legal fees within the first five weeks of an alleged **hazing** incident, eventually settling a lawsuit for $399,000.[1] The financial burden for off-the-field transgressions for institutions that oversee sporting teams—high schools, colleges, club teams—can suspend or eliminate an entire program. The boys, girls, men, and women participating in these organizations can do so for as little as one season, most often for four years, and in some cases slightly longer, while coaches, administrators, alumni, and community members often revere these teams for decades, entire careers, or a lifetime. The mistakes of a few members can harm a program with over 100 years of history and tradition. The consequences not only impact those directly responsible, but they can also end the careers of individuals overseeing these sporting programs. In April 2018, community members of Richland 44 School District in South Dakota saw the departure of school superintendent Tim Godfrey, high school principal Bruce Anderson, and athletic director John Freeman after an investigation revealed student-athletes conducted a hazing ritual.[2]

Athletes often conflate on-the-field traditions with off-the-field initiations. Initiation activities are common among social groups. In sport, athletic teams go through a continuous maturation cycle of a rookie to a captain to retirement. In the image here in Chapter 11 is a group of college football players hazing freshman recruits in 1911. Within this cycle, new team members are expected to perform initiation acts argued to be based on tradition, team bonding, and trust. However, when does an initiation activity become hazing? It begins when a power dynamic is created in a group and a subordinate member conforms to the requirements outlined by members in power. While collecting data on hazing is difficult, the data regarding deaths associated with hazing are challenging to ignore. According to CBS News correspondent Tony Dokoupil, since 1961 there has been at least one hazing death in the United States each year.[3]

Hazing is a multifarious problem in our society and survives because of power dynamics within an organization. The members within the group who have the most power are revered by the subordinate members, reinforcing the power dynamic that is left unquestioned by new members. These organizations studied can have their own belief system and definition of hazing

1 Bob Susnjara, "Lake Zurich Football Hazing Attorney Tab Nearly $51,000 for One Month," *Daily Herald*, February 6, 2017; and Doug T. Graham, "Lake Zurich High School Football Hazing Lawsuit Settled for $399,000," *Daily Herald*, December 22, 2017.

2 Kim Hyatt, "Report Alleges Ongoing 'Rape Game' at Richland 44 School District," *Bemidji Pioneer*, April 6, 2018.

3 "Andrew Coffey's Family Calls for 'Accountability and Education' After Alleged FSU Hazing Death," *CBS News*, cbsnews.com, March 13, 2018, accessed May 12, 2018, https://www.cbsnews.com/news/andrew-coffey-florida-state-fraternity-death-parents-push-federal-hazing-law/

and separate it from what they view as harmless initiation rituals. The problem with the "tradition" or ritual of hazing is that it has become normalized because it is symbolic of and/or resembles other standard practices in our society with similar power dynamics. In the military, willing volunteers endure hours of harsh training overseen by a senior drill sergeant. The recruit is provided a pocket-sized training manual in addition to the unwritten rules of this formal process and an understanding that they must follow both in order to be successful. Embedded in our society is a hierarchical system that, at times, appears to include ritual or tradition to advance. The authoritative power and control over these young people in sport reinforce and normalize dominant and submissive relationships found in fraternities and sororities, on sports teams, and in the US military.

Figure Credit

Fig. 11.1: Source: https://commons.wikimedia.org/wiki/File:The_winning_touch_down_-_a_story_of_college_football_(1911)_(14566294718).jpg.

25

DEFINING HIGH SCHOOL HAZING

CONTROL THROUGH CLARITY

Krzysztof Tokar and Craig Stewart

The need to belong is a strong human trait that motivates individuals in many ways. Major names in psychology such as Freud (1930) and Maslow (1968) have presented their views on that essential human characteristic (as cited in Baumeister and Leary, 1995). In those early works the desire to belong was second only to drives like safety, hunger and reproduction. According to Baumeister, Brewer, Tice and Twenge (2007) human behavior is often heavily influenced by the need for membership in a social or cultural group and the threat of exclusion can manifest itself in strong behavioral reactions. These behavioral reactions are frequently discernable in groups of all ages that will either perpetuate or participate in initiation rites that are prerequisites to group membership. Keating, et al. (2005) stated that threatening practices such as hazing sustain and preserve groups by reinforcing collective skills and attitudes, supporting a group hierarchy, and developing a social dependency among members. In some cases these authors found that the more severe the ritual the greater the association between the victim and the group. It did not matter if the hazing were physical, mental, or emotional abuse.

In sport the definition of *hazing* can reflect many behaviors. Those behaviors vary from positive actions like requiring new athletes to attend meetings or special study halls to dangerous, often life-threatening actions such as branding or consuming large quantities of alcohol in binging rituals. That variability is reflected in the evolution of definitions from Olmerts (1993) in which hazing was vaguely defined as *a formal introduction of beginners into some position in which knowledge has been bestowed* through Hoover's (1999) where the activity was defined as *any requirement that humiliates, degrades, abuses or endangers individuals regardless of their willingness to participate.* As legal bodies became involved, the definitions of hazing grew both in detail and difficulty of interpretation and enforcement. Those definitions increased specificity of negative behaviors, but also included additional vague terms that can easily create problems of identification and compliance. One state legislature (253 N.Y. S 2nd 9, 1964) included wearing clothing such as 'beanie caps' with behaviors that result in permanent disfigurement, while the Texas legislature (Reagins-Lilly, 2007) used the qualification of any behaviors that were of 'unreasonable' risk or harm or that would adversely affect a person's mental or physical health.

Krzysztof Tokar and Craig Stewart, "Defining High School Hazing: Control Through Clarity," *Physical Educator*, vol. 67, no. 4, pp. 204-208.

More recently, other organizations have taken steps to clarify the exact meaning of hazing. Authors on the very popular website, Character Counts, define hazing as:

> Any activity expected of someone joining a group that humiliates, degrades, abuses or endangers, regardless of the person's willingness to participate. This does not include activities such as rookies carrying the balls, team parties with community games, or going out with your teammates, unless an atmosphere of humiliation, degradation, abuse or danger arises (http://charactercounts.com).

Others such as the Mothers Against School Hazing (MASH) organization, (2005) defined hazing as:

> ... a broad term encompassing any action or activity which does not contribute to the positive development of a person; which inflicts or intends to cause physical or mental harm or anxieties; which may demean, degrade, or disgrace any person regardless of location, intent or consent of participants. Hazing can also be defined as any action or situation, which intentionally or *unintentionally* endangers a student for admission into or affiliation with any student organization (http://www.mashinc.org).

One can see by contrasting those that the definition in Character Counts is much more specific than that by MASH. The MASH definition would allow extensive subjective interpretation as to what behavior does and does not 'positively contributes to the development of a human being, as well as includes any act that is unintentional. In that subjectivity lays a danger of overuse and possible abuse as dangerous as the act itself. Even a more contemporary definition by anti-hazing author and researcher, Hank Nuwer, "an all-encompassing term that covers silly, potentially risky, or degrading tasks required for acceptance by a group of full-fledged members" (p. xiv) allows for the inclusion of 'silly tasks' with those labeled as 'risky or dangerous'.

In the extensive work on hazing completed at Alfred University, over 1500 high school students responded to a national survey, and the lack of clarity and agreement on what constitutes hazing was reflected. In their results the researchers found that although only 14 percent of the subjects said they were hazed, 48 percent said they participated in activities that were defined as hazing, and 29 percent said they did things that were potentially illegal in order to join a group (http://www.alfred.edu/hs%5Fhazing/executive_summary.html).

Behaviors that put people at risk are intolerable and should be eliminated from sport. The tragedies that continue to occur are unacceptable. However, to combat the negative aspects of this practice, every effort should be taken to clarify the specific behaviors that are considered intolerable. There are many behaviors listed in even the most specific definitions of hazing that are not only harmless, but are a historical foundation of building team cohesion and camaraderie. The purpose of this study was to initiate that objectification of hazing in hopes that specific guidelines could be created to assist in the elimination of all negative actions.

Method

Over the period of two years, 189 students in introduction to coaching classes completed a survey in which they determined in what 'hazing' behaviors they were forced to participate during high school. Participation by the 96 females and 93 males was both voluntary and anonymous.

Measures

The survey was developed by the nonprofit organization, Josephson Institute of Ethics (http://www.josephsoninstitute.org/), whose mission is "to improve the ethical quality of society by changing personal and organizational decision making and behavior" (http://charactercounts.org). The close-ended questions/phrases were divided into three categories according to the intensity of potential hazing incidents. While no statistical data were reported on this instrument, the face validity of the statements is evident.

The first grouping of eight questions (see Table 25.1) related to positive team activities such as *'completing a ropes course or team trip 'attending a skit night or team roast', or 'attending pre-season training'.* The second grouping included questions that were more negative hazing behaviors, such as, *'being yelled,*

TABLE 25.1 Percent of Participants Involved in 'Hazing' Behaviors

Behaviors:	Total (n=189)	Female (n=96)	Male (n=93)
Grouping 1:	%	%	%
Attending pre-season training	69	71	67
Testing for skill, endurance, or performance in a sport	74	72	75
Keeping a specific grade point average	90	89	91
Dressing up for team funcions (besides uniforms)	90	89	92
Attending a skit night or team roast	47	36	57
Doing volunteer community service	38	32	43
Taking an oath or signing a contract of standards	73	70	75
Completing a ropes course or team trip	29	29	28
Grouping 2:			
Being yelled, cursed, or sworn at	54	42	68
Tattooing, piercing, head shaving, or branding	6	1	12
Being forced to wear embarrassing clothing	9	13	5
Participating in calisthenics not related to a sport	18	20	16
Associating with specific people, not others	11	9	13
Being forced to deprive oneself of food, sleep, or hygiene	5	1	9
Acting as personal servant to players off the field, court	8	7	1
Consuming extremely spicy/disgusting concoctions	5	1	1
Grouping 3:			
Making prank calls or harassing others	2	0	4
Destroying or stealing property	2	2	2
Engaging in or simulating sexual acts	1	0	1
Being tied up, taped, or confined in small spaces	6	0	12
Being paddled, whipped, beaten, kicked; beating others	9	0	18
Being kidnapped or transported and abandoned	3	0	5

cursed, or sworn at', *'being forced to wear embarrassing clothing'*, or *'acting as personal servant to players off the field, court'*. The third grouping was the most extreme in severity such as *'destroying or stealing property'*, *'engaging in or simulating sexual acts'*, or *'being paddled, whipped, beaten, kicked; beating others'*.

A final open-response question allowed students to furnish any additional statements desired. Earlier, demographic data had been gathered that allowed the determination, among other information, of how many (the vast majority) students had participated in high school sports.

Results

Descriptive statistics were used to illustrate the extent and types of hazing reported by these students (Table 25.1). The highest level of participation by students occurred in the first set of behaviors. For example, 89% of the female subjects and 91% of male subjects were required to maintain a specific grade point average to participate in their sport. Similarly, 89% of female subjects and 91% of male subjects reported being required to dress up for team functions. In contrast, there was diminished participation in the second groupings of behaviors. For example, male subjects (68%) and their female counterparts (42%) admitted to being subjected to yelling, cursing, or swearing by others, and 20% of the females and 16% of the males were forced to do calisthenics that were unrelated to their sports.

The third, more negative, behaviors were even fewer in occurrence. Only 12% of male subjects reported "being tied up, taped, or confined in small spaces" and 18% *"being paddled, whipped, beaten, kicked; or beating others"*. Similarly, females reported being involved in *'destroying or stealing property'* only 2% of the time. There was no reported involvement by female students in the other behavioral categories in the third grouping.

Discussion

In the concluding sections of the extensive report on hazing completed at Alfred University (http://www.alfred.edu/hs%5Fhazing/recommendations.html), the authors included in their recommendations that every effort be made to discuss in detail among diverse groups what hazing is and is not. In addition, there was an expectation that each high school group continue to provide initiation rites that are meaningful and challenging. In a similar observation, Nuwer (2007) wrote that often too much emotion and too little serious debate has occurred in the legislation concerning hazing. He wrote:

> I'd urge lawmakers to be very much in agreement on a definition of hazing before passing this or any other bill that calls for punishment of hazers. Evidence presented by Alfred University researchers Norm Pollard and Nadine Hoover demonstrates that student athletes usually are unclear when hazing has occurred. The Initiation Rites and Athletics national survey found that 80 percent of all athletes acknowledged going through hazing behaviors, while only 12 percent believed they had experienced hazing (http://www.stophazing.org/nuwer/federal-bill.htm.)

No one can argue in favor of hazing that results in any negative results. However, responsible adults who are charged with the elimination of hazing must know exactly what they are looking for. There are behaviors that have been mislabeled as hazing and the results of that error can be almost as damaging as the negative acts themselves. In this study, students reported anonymously the behaviors in which they were involved as athletes that could be construed as 'hazing' by some. The vast majority of involvement, however, was in behaviors that would be considered either positive, *'community service, maintaining grades, completing team activities, etc.'* or neutral at worse. In the second grouping of behaviors, the only behavior that athletes consistently reported was *'being yelled, cursed, or sworn at'*. While that action is unacceptable as written, one must exert care in the interpretation of the results. Swearing at or cursing athletes is an unacceptable behavior in any circumstance. However, the interpretation by young athletes as to what constitutes *'being yelled at'* is very subjective. It is not uncommon to have young athletes misinterpret some enthusiastic, but acceptable coaching behaviors as *'being yelled at'*. Likewise, the second most frequently reported behavior *'participation in calisthenics not related to a sport'*, is also very subjective. A common coaching error is the failure to thoroughly explain the reason for doing a certain exercise or activity. However, the magnitude of that error should not be defined as *'hazing '*.

The interpretation of results of this study is in no way intended to downplay the seriousness of hazing behaviors that are intended to mentally or physically harm athletes. The intent, however, is to direct those responsible for identifying and eliminating *'hazing'* that the first step in elimination is to define the term in concrete, observable terms. By specifically defining *'hazing'*, those adults will also ensure that harmless and often positive actions that are used to build team cohesiveness and ensure quality performances of athletes on and off the field will continue.

References

Baumeister, R.F., Brewer, L. E., Tice, D. M. & Twenge, J. M. (2007). Thwarting the need to belong: understanding the interpersonal and inner effects of social exclusion. *Social and Personality Psychology Compass*, 1/1, 506–520.

Baumeister, R.F. and Leary, M.R. (1995). The need to belong: Desire for interpersonal attachment as a fundamental human motivation. *Psychology Bulletin*, 117, 3, 497–529.

Definition of hazing (2007). Character Counts website. Retrieved November 20, 2007, http://charactercounts.com

Hoover, N. C. & Pollard, N. J. (2000). Initiation rites in American high schools: A national survey. Retrieved October 12, 2006, from http ://www.alfred.edu/hs%5Fhazing/

Keating, C.F., Pomerantz, J., Pommer, S.D., Ritt, S.J.H., Miller, L.M., & McCormick, J. (2005) Going to college and unpacking hazing: A functional approach to decrypting initiation practices among undergraduates. *Group Dynamics: Theory, Research, and Practice*, 9, 104–126.

Josephson Institute mission statement (2007). Website. Retrieved November 15, 2007, from http://charactercounts.com

Lipkins, S. (2006). *Preventing Hazing: How Parents, Teachers, and Coaches Can Stop the Violence, Harassment, and Humiliation*. San Francisco: Jossey-Bass

McGlone, C. (Ed.). (2005). *Hazing in N.C.A.A. Division I Women's Athletics: An Exploratory Analysis*. A Doctoral Dissertation.

Mothers Against School Hazing (2007). Website. Retrieved October, 2006 from http://www.mashinc.org/

Nuwer, H. (Ed.). (2004). *The Hazing Reader*. Bloomington, IN: Indiana University Press.

Nuwer, H. (2008). New federal proposal needs input. Website. Retrieved August, 2008, from http://www.stophazing.org/nuwer/federal-bill.htm

Peluso, A. R. (2006). Hazing in sports: The effects and legal ramifications. [Electronic version]. *The Sport Journal*, 9(1). Retrieved October 15, 2006, from http://www.thesportjoumal.org/2006Joumal/Vol9-No1/Peluso.asp

Reagins-Lilly, S. (2007) Texas hazing statute summary. Retrieved January, 2008 from http://deanofstudents.utexas.edu/events/downloads/HazingMemorandum.pdf

What is hazing? (2006) Retrieved October 15, 2006, from http://www.mashinc.org/ resources-whatis.html

26

BULLYING AND HAZING IN SPORT TEAMS

Leslee A. Fisher and Lars Dzikus

What are bullying and hazing in sport? Should sport psychology consultants be concerned with these behaviors? If so, what role should sport psychology consultants play in dealing with abusive relationships in sport? These questions are the major issues we explore in this chapter. We understand bullying and hazing as abusive behaviors related to group dynamics that occur within teams and also when team members harass, bully, or haze non-team members.

The Role That Power and Power Dynamics Play in Sport

As Fisher, Butryn, and Roper (2003) observed, power is a concept not frequently discussed in the field of sport psychology nor in sport psychology consultation. Although sport studies scholars frequently examine power and the power dynamics inherent in sport, only a few sport psychology researchers and practitioners have done so (e.g., Schinke & Hanrahan, 2009). Recently, Fisher, Roper, and Butryn (2009) suggested that such an analysis could provide a meaningful understanding of athlete's experience and welfare. This type of understanding seems critical for sport psychology consultants, coaches, parents, and administrators who work with athletes and care about their overall well-being.

Brackenridge (2008) summarized over 600 cases of sexual abuse and exploitation in sport. Most relevant for this discussion, Brackenridge proposed that there are several aspects of sport that may allow for the exploitation of athletes to occur: we believe these aspects include not only harassment but bullying and hazing as well. In particular, Brackenridge (2001) posited that

> the male-dominated nature of sport, prevalence of high-ranking sport positions populated by men, adherence to hegemonic masculinity, and emphasis on the physical body are each significant contributors to the development and maintenance of a culture of violence and objectification of sport women and men.
>
> (p. 44)

Further, although most sport participants see exploitation and abuse as personally perpetrated and personally experienced, Brackenridge revealed a complex network of stakeholders in abusive and exploitive situations that included coaches, teachers, team managers, trainers, sport organizations, the media, and even peer athletes, parents, and sport scientists. Sport psychology consultants could play an important role in educating such stakeholders about sexually transgressive and other abusive behaviors. At the minimum, consultants could engage stakeholders in discussions about how bullying and hazing are defined. At most, consultants might find themselves in the position of being the first person an athlete tells about being a victim of these behaviors.

In 2003, Fisher *et al.* described how the power dynamics in sport contexts can encourage homophobic, heteronormative, racialized, and classist "accepted" behaviors. To combat such practices, consultants should be aware of how sexuality, race, gender, and class may be "viewed not as simple categories, but as relations of power, as spaces where individuals negotiate for greater agency within the existing power structure" (p. 396). Further, consultants should

> acknowledge gender-biased and homophobic behaviors within the hyper-masculine structure of many sports, as well as to confront ways that consultants, whether male or female, have the potential to be both perpetrators and victims of discriminatory practices themselves.
>
> (p. 393)

Power dynamics are at the heart of many sport behaviors that occur in locker rooms, sport club settings, coaches' houses, and on the field. In these spaces, more experienced athletes and coaches often work hard to maintain their control and power over less experienced participants (Curry, 1991). Actions that are accepted in these contexts may be considered deviant in other spheres of society. For example, it is not unusual for "coaches to scream at athletes, belittle them, or challenge the masculinity of male athletes. At times, it appears only the most outrageous coaching behaviors lie outside the accepted norms" (Coakley, 2007, p. 152). Similarly, in many sports athletes use power via violence, aggression, and intimidation in ways that potentially would be considered criminal behaviors outside the boundaries of sport. Also, the dynamics of bullying and hazing in sport are often not the same as in schools or the workplace (Institute for Global Ethics, 2007).

Some bullying and hazing behaviors in sport may also be rooted in overconformity to what Coakley (2007) referred to as the *sport ethic*. The norms in the sport ethic include athletes' unwavering dedication to their sports, striving for distinction, accepting risks and pain, and overcoming many obstacles in the pursuit of their goals. Bullies often attack those whom they define as outside the range of what they consider acceptable or "normal" in terms of appearance, behavior, musical preference, interests, friends, and so forth (Kimmel & Mahler, 2003). Because athletes often learn to use power strategically in sport via aggression and intimidation and may receive positive feedback for their aggressive behaviors (Coakley, 2007), athletes who bully and haze non-athletes may overconform to notions such as striving for distinction and accepting risks and pains. Similarly, some coach bullying and hazing behaviors could be brought into the locker room because coaches are overconforming to the accepted norm of using intimidation in their sports.

Sport psychology consultants are in a critical position in their work with athletes. Many espouse an athlete-centered approach where athlete welfare is first and foremost (Fisher *et al.*, 2009). As Brackenridge (2008) pointed out, however, practitioners need to also be concerned with sport environments and whether they are safe for those who participate in them. Because of the close relationships developed between consultants and athletes, athletes might reveal incidents of bullying and hazing to consultants before telling others. Therefore, consultants need to develop the necessary skills to educate themselves, athletes, and teams about appropriate and inappropriate sport behaviors including hazing and bullying. They can also develop skills to help athletes once they have been bullied or hazed.

What are Bullying and Hazing in Sport?

Bullying

Bullying in sport is a historical and international problem that affects a broad range of individuals. For example, bullying was a daily occurrence in English public schools from the eighteenth century through to the present. Early forms of student-organized rugby football games became a means for older, stronger boys to exercise control over younger boys (Dunning & Sheard, 2005).

Bullying has been defined as "a conscious, willful, deliberate and repeated hostile activity marked by an imbalance of power, intent to harm, and/or a threat of aggression" (Government of Alberta, 2005, p. 1). Many theorists regard the continued, systematic abuse of power as a defining aspect of bullying; bullying often includes the systematic harassment of weaker individuals via humiliation and torment (Lines, 2008). Specific forms of bulling can occur before, during, and after sport-related events in the form of verbal taunts, social exclusion, physical attacks, and cyber harassment. More specifically, sport bullying could include:

> (a) unwarranted yelling and screaming directed at the [athlete]; (b) continually criticizing the [athlete's] abilities; (c) blaming the [athlete] for mistakes; (d) making unreasonable demands related to performance; (e) repeated insults or put downs of the [athlete]; (f) repeated threats to remove or restrict opportunities or privileges; (g) denying or discounting the [athlete's] accomplishments; (h) threats of, and actual, physical violence; and (i) emails or instant messages containing insults or threats.
>
> (Government of Alberta, 2005, p. 1)

Many insults or put downs of athletes are homophobic, focusing on personal attacks related to athletes' sexual orientation, femininity, or masculinity.

Hazing

Historically, hazing has occurred in universities since medieval times, in the American fraternity and sorority systems, in high school and university athletic settings, and in modern sports (Trota & Johnson, 2004). In recent times, research has been conducted related to hazing in professional hockey (Robidoux, 2001), military combat units (Malszecki, 2004), and even in sport reporting (Nuwer, 2004). Hazing has been defined as "a rite of passage wherein youths, neophytes, or rookies are taken through traditional practices by more senior members in order to initiate them into the next stage of their cultural, religious, academic, or athletic lives" (Trota & Johnson, p. x). Allan and DeAngelis (2004) suggested that based on a United States National Collegiate Athletic Association (NCAA) survey (see Hoover, 1999), hazing can be further delineated into three major categories:

> (a) *questionable behaviors*: Humiliating or degrading activities, but not dangerous or potentially illegal activities; (b) *alcohol-related [behaviors]*: Drinking contests, exclusive of other dangerous or potentially illegal activities; or (c) *unacceptable and potentially illegal behaviors*: Activities carrying a high probability of danger or injury, or which could result in criminal charges. (p. 63)[1]

Both bullying and hazing can refer to either the actions of an individual or a group or team. Although definitions vary in the degree of specificity regarding individual versus group acts, the systematic and deliberate abuse of power is a main theme in each. Nevertheless, the inclusion of intent in both definitions can often be confusing for those in sport to interpret (Lines, 2008). For example, sport participants may believe that belligerent coaches do not intentionally hurt their athletes; they might believe that coaches intend to bring out "better" performances. In addition, cultural values specific to sports in certain countries may promote an "ends justify the means" approach to sport bullying and hazing. American basketball coach Bob Knight is often discussed in the context of the "potential positive effects of strategic bullying behavior on unit or team performance [including a] ... short-term increase in productivity [and] underperforming employees [voluntarily deciding to leave an organization]" (Ferris, Zinko, Brouer, Buckley, & Harvey, 2007, pp. 202–203). Although Knight's treatment of players has long been controversial and has often been used as an example of bullying in sports (Myers, 2000), because Knight was one of the most successful coaches in American men's collegiate basketball, many appear to have championed his style of strategic assertive bullying. Such a positive view of bullying (and by extension, hazing) is obviously problematic because it may justify and encourage the use of coach bullying and hazing within sport teams.

Therefore, it is crucial to educate coaches, athletes, consultants, and other stakeholders about how bullying and hazing in sport may make teams appear to perform better in the short term but can have long-term damaging consequences. In addition, given sport psychology consultants' ethical codes and laws related to reporting abuse, once consultants are educated about sport bullying and hazing definitions, they may be in a position to report incidents of bullying and hazing before others can (Brackenridge, 2001, 2008; Fisher *et al.*, 2009). Although ethical codes apply to all sport psychology consultants, legal ramifications pertain especially to registered/licensed psychologists. What complicates matters further is that psychologists are bound to confidentiality if a client reveals information in confidence and in the privacy of a one-on-one consultation.

Ethical Codes Related to Sport Psychology and Athlete Welfare

Several national and international professional organizations in sport psychology have ethical codes concerned with the welfare of athletes. Two are reviewed here: the International Society of Sport Psychology (ISSP, n.d.) and the Association of Applied Sport Psychology (AASP, 2005). The ISSP code states that among sport psychology consultants' tasks is the protection of athletes' welfare and the guarding of sport in general "against any dangerous threats to morality" (para. 1). The challenges for consultants are not only to enhance the performance of athletes but also to help "formulate ethical guidelines for conduct of athletic programs" and to "develop means by which athletes are protected against psychological and moral damage" (para. 3). Consultants could contribute their professional

1 Although Hoover (1999) examined NCAA athlete hazing behaviors, the NCAA itself has discussed hazing issues but has yet to put any policies in place that we know about as of 2009.

expertise to these efforts, focusing on a wide range of stakeholders including athletes, administrators, coaches, parents, physicians, and trainers.

The primary goal of AASP's (2005) code of ethics is "the welfare and protection of the individuals and groups with whom AASP members work" (para. 6). Thus, members of organizations such as ISSP and AASP are called upon to encourage ethical conduct among their members, colleagues, students, and those constituencies with whom they work. Members of these professional bodies can help sports organizations develop and implement their own codes of ethics and policies regarding bullying and hazing. Consultants can partner with athletes, coaches, parents, and administrators to prevent harmful bullying and hazing behaviors as well as help those who have already been hurt.

Specific Suggestions for Change

As a starting point, we believe that sports teams and clubs at all levels of competition should adopt anti-bullying and hazing policies if they have not done so already. There are several components that should be built into an anti-bullying and hazing policy, including definitions of bullying and hazing, what the punishments for both are, how to report offenders, how to respond to these behaviors when they occur, and, in the case of hazing, how to develop alternative ways to initiate or bond with other athletes (see Crow & Phillips, 2004). Regardless of whether an organization has a policy in place or not, consultants should have an understanding about how to work with athletes who have been bullied, those who bully others, how to work with teams/coaches/parents on these issues, and also how to refer out to a qualified specialist if the situation is beyond their expertise.

Working with Athletes Who Have Been Bullied

There may be times when athletes come to sport psychology consultants first before telling anyone else that they have been bullied. According to the website for the U.S. Department of Health and Human Services' Health Resources and Services Administration Department (2009), those who are qualified mental health professionals (such as consultants who hold licensure as clinical or counseling psychologists) should help give those who have been bullied:

> (a) permission and support to tell what has happened to them and to talk about their feelings; (b) protection from continued bullying through adult supervision, consequences for those who bully, and adults taking reports of bullying seriously; (c) strong, positive relationships with adults and peers; (d) assistance from peers in feeling that they belong; (e) assistance in not blaming themselves for the bullying; and (f) support with post-traumatic stress symptoms, in some cases, even after the bullying has been stopped.
>
> (HRSA, 2009)

Working with Athletes Who Have Bullied Others

There may also be times when those same consultants are working with athletes who are bullying others. According to HRSA (2009), qualified mental health professionals should:

(a) help them see the consequences or the cost of bullying behavior and consider alternatives; (b) hold them fully accountable for their actions by confronting excuses that minimize the behavior or externalize the cause of the behavior; (c) help them fully acknowledge their behavior; (d) support authority figures in holding them accountable for their actions and not suggesting or allowing rationalizations; (e) once they are able to recognize problems with their behavior, help them set and work toward goals for change (e.g., channeling aggression into leadership), help them track their progress toward new behaviors, and feel pride about those changes; and (f) help them build genuine empathy and conscience; after learning that their own actions can cause them to get in trouble, they can begin to appreciate the impact of their actions on others.

Working with Teams

A recent report in *Sports Illustrated* highlighted the involvement of high school athletes in anti-bullying workshops in California (Roberts, 2008). By sharing their knowledge of sport cultures and moral behaviors, both athletes and consultants could support and facilitate such groups. Consultants could begin by holding workshops to educate athletes about how to critically examine otherwise "accepted" sport behaviors and norms such as overconformity and the concept of the "sport ethic" (Coakley, 2007). They could also help athletes learn to *not* praise overconforming teammates and elevate them to the status of role models for others. Such an approach would not just target bullying and hazing behaviors but could also help teams question behaviors such as athletes playing hurt or practising excessively, above and beyond expectations.

Consultants can also work to educate athletes about what they can do to prevent bullying and hazing on their teams. The Government of Alberta's (2005, p. 2) bullying prevention program tells athletes:

- Trust your instincts. If someone's behavior is making you feel uncomfortable or threatened, don't ignore it. You have the right to be treated respectfully.
- Talk to someone you trust—a parent, friend, coach, manager or another player. Remember to keep speaking up until someone helps you.
- Stay calm. Bullies love a reaction, so don't give them one.
- Project confidence. Hold your head up and stand up straight. Bullies pick on people who they think are afraid. Show them you're not.
- Don't reply to messages from cyberbullies. If you're receiving threatening text messages or emails don't reply, but keep the messages as evidence. The police and your internet service provider and/or telephone company can use these messages to help you.

Consultants can also encourage athletes to interfere when they witness bullying. Instead of fighting the bully physically, speaking up, getting help, and helping the target are appropriate reactions. Quiet bystanders give bullies the audience they want. Once athletes understand bullying and its negative effects, they are more likely to speak up against it. Athletes also need to learn about alcohol responsibility, because many hazing events are fueled by the overconsumption of alcohol. Consultants could then help athletes construct alternative initiations, team-building, or bonding rituals that are not humiliating, degrading, or toxic (Johnson & Donnelly, 2004).

Working with Coaches

Once policies have been established related to sport bullying and hazing, coaches should have thorough knowledge about and understanding of those policies, and then provide strong leadership for the athletes with whom they come into contact (Johnson & Donnelly, 2004). These steps require first noticing sport bullying and hazing, then interpreting these behaviors as problems. Next, coaches must recognize their own and others' responsibilities to change a bullying/hazing culture and acquire the skills necessary to make such a change. Finally, they must take action to eliminate bullying/hazing on their teams (see Allan & DeAngelis, 2004, as related to Berkowitz's [1994] five-step model for educating males about sexual violence).

To facilitate these steps, consultants could hold workshops to educate coaches about bullying and hazing and help them learn how to model and reinforce positive behaviors. Coaches' responsibilities include creating "a safe and respectful sport environment by not engaging in, allowing, condoning, or ignoring behavior that constitutes, or could be perceived as, bullying" (Government of Alberta, 2005, p. 2). Consultants can teach coaches how to establish positive communication patterns between all parties involved and how to provide and receive constructive criticism. Most important, such workshops can help coaches become critically reflective practitioners who examine their own behaviors.

Consultants could also help established coaching certification programs to empower coaches to think critically about the structure of their sport programs and encourage them to make changes to the same (Coakley, 2007). Because most coaching certification programs tend to be geared toward helping coaches become "sport efficiency experts rather than teachers who help young people become responsible and informed [about] ... who controls their sport lives and the contexts in which they play sports" (Coakley, p. 148), such workshops could provide a space for coaches to talk openly about pressures related to a focus on winning.

Working with Parents

At times, parents become bullies targeting their own children, players on opposing teams, referees, and coaches. Consultants could hold seminar workshops for parents addressing many of the aforementioned issues and strategies. In addition, interested consultants could work with parent sport education programs because parents have become increasingly involved and controlling when it comes to channeling their children into organized, competitive youth sports (Coakley, 2007).

The Consultant as Part of the Problem

Many of the suggestions listed above may appear easy to understand and, by extension, easy to implement. Nothing could be further from the truth for ending sport bullying and hazing. Consultants can be part of the "bystander effect" or "turning a blind eye" to what is occurring on the teams with whom they work. As Finley and Finley (2006) suggested, hazing is really about *groupthink* or when people act differently in groups versus when they are alone.

The hard reality is that groupthink includes sport psychology consultants who might, for example, quickly report incidents of sexual abuse in children with whom they are working but who are afraid to report incidents of bullying or hazing on sport teams. Consultants may choose not to report bullying or hazing for myriad reasons, including beliefs that: (a) they hold little power in the sport organizations or with the athletes they serve; (b) if they do challenge those in power about the "way things are done," they may find themselves quickly out of a job; (c) they will certainly lose money if the consulting job is lost; (d) they might feel more comfortable trying to effect change by working within the immediate system (e.g., with an individual athlete or team) versus challenging those higher up in the sport structure; and/or (e) they see change in sport organizations as slow and frustrating.

Deciding to report bullying and hazing for whatever reason is certainly difficult and complex. Similar to Brackenridge's (2001, p. 96) assertion about those who experience sexual exploitation in sport, those who know about bullying and hazing also face what seems like impossible choices:

> if [one] speaks out [one's] integrity remains intact but [one's] survival in elite competitive sport is hazarded. If [one] allows the abuse to continue without reporting it, [one's] personal ... integrity [is] violated but [one's] performance in the sport might be salvaged.

Non-reporting has a domino effect. If athletes see consultants and other stakeholders ignoring bullying and hazing, they may conclude that they will not be supported in reporting these behaviors themselves. We strongly suggest that consultants educate themselves about definitions of bullying and hazing and how to work with (or refer out) those who have been a part of these behaviors.

Conclusions

In this chapter, we have suggested that bullying and hazing in sport are serious, problematic behaviors that occur because of power dynamics in sport, sport cultural traditions, and overconformity to the sport ethic (Fisher *et al.*, 2009). We believe that although it will not be easy and will take time, sport psychology consultants can help create sport cultures where bullying and hazing no longer exist. If interested, consultants could play an integral role in changing coach education programs to include bullying and hazing definitions, creating policies related to athlete welfare and behavior, and also helping teams develop healthy and appropriate initiation or bonding alternatives (see Box 26.1). National and international psychology and sport psychology association codes related to the protection of athletes can serve as some guidance in these areas. Further, we believe that consultants could help coaches, athletes, and parents use the process of critical reflection to examine where they get their values about appropriate boundaries in relationships and how athletes should treat each other on teams (Brackenridge, 2008). Finally, as Brackenridge (2001) suggested, sport psychology consultants have specialized training and responsibilities to see that athletes get their psychological needs addressed and psychological injuries prevented.

References

Allan, E. J., & DeAngelis, G. (2004). Hazing, masculinity, and collision sports: (Un) becoming heroes. In J. Johnson & M. Holman (Eds.), *Making the team: Inside the world of sport initiations and hazing* (pp. 61–82). Toronto, ON, Canada: Canadian Scholars' Press.

Association for Applied Sport Psychology (2005). *Ethics code: AASP ethical principles and standards*. Retrieved from http://appliedsportpsych.org/about/ethics/code

Berkowitz, A. D. (Ed.). (1994). *Men and rape: Theory, research, and prevention programs in higher education*. San Francisco: Jossey-Bass.

Brackenridge, C. (2001). *Spoilsports: Understanding and preventing sexual exploitation in sport*. London: Routledge.
Brackenridge, C. (2008). Sex, lies, shock, and role: Sport psychologists as agents of athlete welfare. Presentation at the annual conference of the *Association for Applied Sport Psychology*, St. Louis.
Coakley, J. (2007). *Sports in society: Issues and controversies* (9th ed.). Boston: McGraw-Hill.
Crow, R. B., & Phillips, D. R. (2004). Hazing: What the law says. In J. Johnson & M. Holman (Eds.), *Making the team: Inside the world of sport initiations and hazing* (pp. 19–31). Toronto, ON, Canada: Canadian Scholars' Press.
Curry, T. (1991). Fraternal bonding in the locker room: A pro-feminist analysis of talk about competition and women. *Sociology of Sport Journal*, *8*, 119–135.
Dunning, E., & Sheard, K. (2005). *Barbarians, gentlemen and players: A sociological study of the development of rugby football* (2nd ed.). London: Routledge.
Ferris, G. R., Zinko, R., Brouer, R. L., Buckley, R. M., & Harvey, M. G. (2007). Strategic bullying as a supplementary, balance perspective on destructive leadership. *Leadership Quarterly*, *18*, 195–206.
Finley, P., & Finley, L. (2006). *The sports industry's war on athletes*. Westport, CT: Praeger.
Fisher, L. A., Butryn, T. M., & Roper, E. A. (2003). Diversifying (and politicizing) sport psychology through cultural studies: A promising perspective. *The Sport Psychologist*, *17*, 391–405.
Fisher, L. A., Roper, E. A., & Butryn, T. M. (2009). Engaging cultural studies and traditional sport psychology. In R. J. Schinke & S. J. Hanrahan (Eds.), *Cultural sport psychology* (pp. 23–34). Champaign, IL: Human Kinetics.
Government of Alberta. (2005). *Bullying prevention in sports*. Retrieved from http://www.bully freealberta.ca/pdf/Sports_FS.pdf
Hoover, N. (1999). *Initiation rites and athletics for NCAA sports teams: A national survey*. Retrieved on June 4, 2009 from http://www.alfred.edu/sports_hazing/
Institute for Global Ethics (2007). When the coach gets graphic, how important is winning? Retrieved from http://www.globalethics.org/newsline/2007/02/12/when-the-coach-gets-graphic-how-important-is-winning/
International Society of Sport Psychology (n.d.). *Statutes*. Retrieved from http://www.issponline.org/ab_statues.asp?ms=2&sms=2
Johnson, J., & Donnelly, P. (2004). In their own words: Athletic administrators, coaches, and athletes at two universities discuss hazing policy initiatives. In J. Johnson & M. Holman (Eds.), *Making the team: Inside the world of sport initiations and hazing* (pp. 132–154). Toronto, ON, Canada: Canadian Scholars' Press.
Kimmel, M. S., & Mahler, M. (2003). Adolescent masculinity, homophobia, and violence. *American Behavioral Scientist*, *46*, 1439–1458.
Lines, D. (2008). *The bullies: Understanding bullies and bullying*. London: Kingsley.

BOX 26.1

What sport psychology consultants can do to help prevent bullying and hazing

- Obtain and share information about the psycho-social conditions that contribute to abuse and exploitation in sport as well as the psychological effects of bullying and hazing.
- Support the adoption of anti-bullying and hazing policies.
- Facilitate workshops to educate coaches, athletes, and parents about bullying and hazing.
- Contribute to the development of coaching certification programs.
- Help teams develop healthy and appropriate initiation or bonding alternatives.
- Intervene by treating or referring out when observing abusive behavior.

Malszecki, G. (2004). "No mercy shown nor asked"—Toughness test or torture?: Hazing in military combat units and its "collateral damage." In J. Johnson & M. Holman (Eds.), *Making the team: Inside the world of sport initiations and hazing* (pp. 32–49). Toronto, ON, Canada: Canadian Scholars' Press.

Myers, B. (2000, March 26). Knight as a bully. *New York Times*, p. SP12.

Nuwer, H. (2004). How sportswriters contribute to a hazing culture in athletics. In J. Johnson & M. Holman (Eds.), *Making the team: Inside the world of sport initiations and hazing* (pp. 118–131). Toronto, ON, Canada: Canadian Scholars' Press.

Roberts, S. (2008, July 7). Jocks against bullies. *Sports Illustrated*, 109, 90.

Robidoux, M. (2001). *Men at play: A working understanding of professional hockey*. Montreal, QC, Canada: McGill-Queen's University Press.

Schinke, R. J., & Hanrahan, S. J. (2009). *Cultural sport psychology*. Champaign, IL: Human Kinetics.

Trota, B., & Johnson, J. (2004). Introduction: A brief history of hazing. In J. Johnson & M. Holman (Eds.), *Making the team: Inside the world of sport initiations and hazing* (pp. x–xvi). Toronto, ON, Canada: Canadian Scholars' Press.

U.S. Department of Health and Human Services, Health Resources and Services Administration Department (2009). *Stop bullying now*. Retrieved from http://www.education.com/partner/articles/stopbullying/

FURTHER READING

A Football Locker Room, a Broomstick, and a Sex Assault Case Roil a School

Dan Morse and Donna St. George

If you have a digital edition of this book, please click on the link below to access the article:

https://www.washingtonpost.com/local/crime/a-football-locker-room-a-broomstick-and-a-sex-
assault-case-roil-a-school/2019/03/29/01500f30-2fc8-11e9-8ad3-9a5b113ecd3c_story.htm-
l?utm_term=.f0872d8e2fc9

If you have a print edition of this book, please use your cell phone to scan the QR code below to access the article:

UC Davis Suspends Marching Band After Sacramento Bee Investigation of Raucous Culture, Hazing

Molly Sullivan and Ryan Sabalow

If you have a digital edition of this book, please click on the link below to access the article:

https://www.sacbee.com/news/investigations/article230956528.html

If you have a print edition of this book, please use your cell phone to scan the QR code below to access the article:

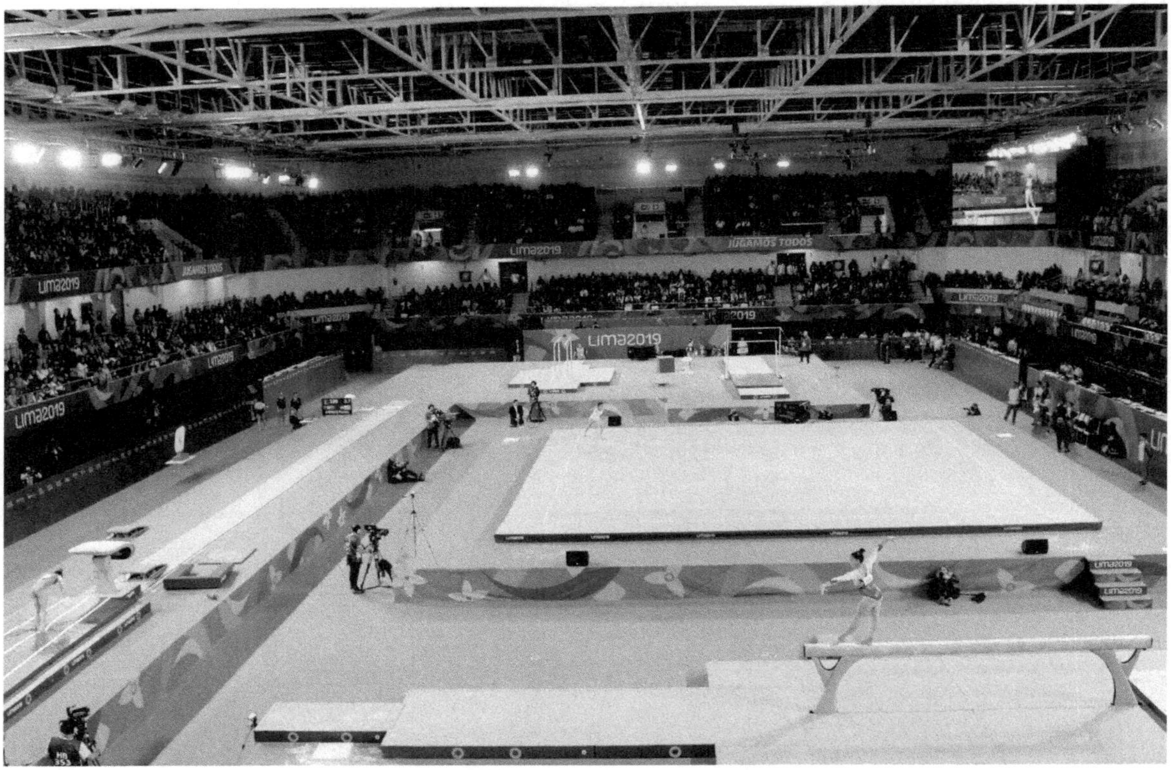
Lima2019
JUGAMOS TODOS

CHAPTER 12

ATHLETES, COACHES, AND ABUSE

During the summer of 2017, three women came forward to authorities reporting that their team physician had sexually abused them. A secret these women kept for years finally came out. By the end of the year, 224 women reported abuse by Larry Nassar while under his care with Team USA and while he was a physician at Michigan State University. Their stories and the stories of thousands of others often go unreported. Many factors contribute to victims withholding the truth about what happened to them. They range from fear, embarrassment, and a desire to forget about the experience. In the case of these women, the governing body of USA Gymnastics created a culture of fear and manipulation that silenced these women before they could share their abusive experience. Nassar continued this abuse for nearly three decades. In the end, Nassar was found guilty of 287 counts of rape and is serving 60 years in prison. As for the women, victims-turned-champions, they received the Arthur Ashe Award for Courage at the 2018 ESPN Espy Awards.

These documents examine the progression of abuse in sport. How does a culture of abuse come to fruition? Contributing factors include (1) **acceptance** of the "great sports myth," discussed in Chapter 1; (2) **emotional unity** within a sporting social world; (3) **detachment** from non-sporting groups; (4) **elitism** in sport; (5) the **pressure** for success at any cost; and (6) **ambivalence** toward responsibility. When examining systemic abuse within an organization, one finds nearly all of these factors are present. Over time, these issues become entwined, reinforcing a power dynamic in a social world that can foster a culture of abuse.

27

WORKING WITH ADULT ATHLETE SURVIVORS OF SEXUAL ABUSE

Trisha Leahy

The systematic documentation of sexual abuse of athletes within sport systems has begun to challenge the commonly accepted view of sport as an unproblematic site of youth empowerment and positive development (Leahy, 2010). Sport psychologists need to be equipped to be able to effectively help athletes through the recovery process without sacrificing their high-performance dreams and goals. Negotiating the complex dynamics of recovery work with profoundly traumatized athlete survivors of chronic sexual abuse poses a significant challenge to even the most skilled sport psychologist. Collaborative decisions about which path to take and which direction to turn, although crucial to an athlete's recovery, may not always be easy to assess from the rapidly evolving knowledge base (Leahy, Pretty, & Tenenbaum, 2003). In this chapter I will focus on the current standard of care guidelines regarding the treatment of survivors of chronic sexual abuse struggling with complex, dissociative posttraumatic conditions, with a particular emphasis on the social context of high-performance athletes.

Sexual Abuse and Trauma

Researchers and clinicians have for some time been applying a trauma framework to understand the effects of chronic and repeated sexual abuse. Central to this theoretical framework are the concepts of posttraumatic stress disorder (PTSD) and dissociation as key responses to traumatizing events. Core posttraumatic symptoms include re-experiencing, avoidance, and hyperarousal (American Psychiatric Association [APA], 2000). Symptoms related to re-experiencing and hyperarousal can include intrusive thoughts, physiological arousal, reactivity to trauma cues, and hypervigilance. Avoidant symptoms can include avoidance of thoughts, feelings, places, or people associated with the trauma (APA).

Dissociation is "a disruption in the usually integrated functions of consciousness" (APA, 2000, p. 477). Dissociative symptomatology (e.g., amnesia, derealisation, depersonalisation) involves a splitting between the "observing self" and the "experiencing self." During a traumatic experience,

Trisha Leahy, "Working with Adult Athlete Survivors of Sexual Abuse," *Routledge Handbook of Applied Sport Psychology: A Comprehensive Guide for Students and Practitioners*, ed. Stephanie Hanrahan and Mark Andersen, pp. 303-312.

dissociation provides protective detachment from overwhelming affect and pain, but it can result in severe disruption within the usually integrated functions of consciousness, memory, identity, or perception of the environment.

Seven areas of functioning are affected through prolonged and repeated abuse, particularly that perpetrated by those in positions of trust, guardianship, or authority (Courtois, 2004). These areas include affect dysregulation (inability to regulate the intensity of affective responses); alterations in attention and consciousness leading to dissociative symptoms; self-perception embedded in a sense of guilt, shame, and responsibility for the abuse; traumatized attachment to the perpetrator, incorporating his (or her) belief system; relational difficulties with trust and intimacy; somatization and medical conditions; and attributions centering on hopelessness and despair (Briere, 2004). Recently, the concept of "complex trauma" has been developed in an attempt to explain these convoluted and intertwined posttraumatic, dissociative, and related symptom clusters (Courtois, 2004). To date, only one group of researchers has investigated the long-term effects on athlete survivors of child abuse using a trauma framework, and their research provided evidence supporting the applicability of the concept of complex trauma to understanding athletes' needs for recovery (Leahy *et al.*, 2003; Leahy, Pretty, & Tenenbaum, 2008).

Sport Environment Issues

Effective abuse-related therapy must address the sociocultural context of the survivor's distress (Briere, 2004). Particularly evident from research reports across a number of countries is the manner in which certain aspects of the culture of competitive sport provide an environment that facilitates, rather than inhibits, the occurrence of sexual abuse in sport (Brackenridge, 2001). Two sport environment issues, perpetrator methodology and the bystander effect, require our understanding and attention if, as sport psychologists, we are to effectively engage in healing, therapeutic relationships with sexually abused athletes.

Perpetrator Methodology

Leahy, Pretty, and Tenenbaum (2004) published qualitative data describing specific perpetrator methodologies sexually abused athletes have experienced within sport. Two key dimensions of perpetrator methodology included strategies designed to simultaneously engender feelings of complete powerlessness in the athlete, and conversely, to present the perpetrator as omnipotent. What seemed to characterize the perpetrator's methodology, and was particularly obvious in cases where the abuse was prolonged and repeated, was the need to impose his version of reality on the athlete and to isolate the athlete within that reality. The perpetrator successfully maintained that reality by controlling the psychological environment, silencing, and isolating the athlete from potential sources of support. In addition to controlling the athlete's outer life, her/his inner life was controlled through direct emotional manipulation, psychological abuse, and the creation of a highly volatile, psychologically abusive training environment. The perpetrator's ability to successfully create and maintain such an environment may be related to the unique sociocultural context of competitive sport in some first-world countries. This context is one that has been criticized as being imbued with an intensely volatile ethos, and within which psychologically abusive coaching behaviors may be normalized as part of the winning strategy (Brackenridge, 2001; Leahy, 2010). This point brings us to the issue of the bystander effect.

The Bystander Effect

The bystander effect refers to the situation where the victim perceived that others, who knew about (or suspected) the sexual abuse, did not do anything about it (Leahy *et al.*, 2003). For example:

> He was in such a powerful position that no one interfered; I think no one questioned what he was doing. But now when I speak to people, they do say he stepped over the line with us, but ... they didn't say anything, they didn't want to interfere with him, Yeah, I'm a bit angry about that.
>
> (Leahy, 2010, p. 316)

Athletes' experiences of the bystander effect point to the apparent lack of systemically sanctioned accountability in relation to the power of the coach-perpetrator that allowed the abuse to continue for many years unchallenged by other adults in the system. These bystanders included coaching, sport psychology, and other support staff or volunteers who were not as senior in the competitive sport hierarchy as the perpetrator. The bystander effect was especially notable in the elite sport context: "No one ever interfered with us because we were so elite, and no one ever questioned what we were doing." (Leahy, 2010, p. 327).

For children, disclosure may be preempted if the child believes, or is aware that other adults know about the abuse (Palmer, Brown, Rae-Grant, and Loughlin, 1999). If observing adults take no action, the child may assume that the behavior is socially acceptable, or in the case of older children, as mentioned above, that the perpetrator's message that he is omnipotent is really true and that they really are trapped: "it never entered my mind that others could possibly be experiencing the same thing [pause]. ... This was something that was happening to me and it was between me and him and nobody else knew" (Leahy *et al.*, 2003, p. 532).

Disruptions in Attachment

Therapy is a trust-based relationship that requires not only authentic engagement but also vigilance in maintaining a healing dynamic within the therapeutic environment. One of the key difficulties in engaging in an effective therapeutic alliance with a chronically abused individual stems from alterations in the individual's capacity to develop and maintain healthy relationships, including the relationship with the therapist (Pearlman & Courtois, 2005). To understand this complex posttraumatic adaptation to prolonged and repeated abuse, particularly that which started from early childhood, we need to draw on attachment theory, and two related coping mechanisms: the locus of control shift, and traumatic attachment to the perpetrator.

Locus of Control Shift

Attachment theory proposes a biological drive in humans to attach. If attachment does not occur, a child will fail to thrive. Prolonged and repeated abuse by a trusted caregiver presents the child with an overwhelming challenge to the biological need to attach. The child cannot physically escape the abusive situation (e.g., if it is within the family) and cannot choose not to attach. The only developmentally available way of coping is an internal process of dissociating. Amnesia, however, is rarely total, even though specific abusive episodes may be dissociated, so the child has to try to understand why caregivers are hurting him/her. The meaning likely to be constructed at an early developmental stage, and arguably the only meaning capable of resolving the potential disruption of the attachment systems, is that it is the child who is causing the abuse (e.g., by being bad and, therefore, deserving of such treatment). This locus-of-control shift transfers responsibility for the abuse, or for inability to prevent it, onto the victim (Ross, 1997). This logic simultaneously preserves the idealized trusted caregiver (actively reinforced by the perpetrator methodology and the bystander effect) and allows the victim hope through the illusion of control. It also allows attachment systems to remain intact (Briere, 2004).

Traumatic Attachment to the Perpetrator

The outcome of the perpetrator methodology, described earlier, and the locus-of-control shift, is the development of a traumatized attachment to the perpetrator. This process has been repeatedly observed in not only chronically abused children but also in adolescents and adults in situations of prolonged traumatization (e.g., domestic violence, captivity; Herman, 1997; Ross, 1997). In these situations in which the victim is repeatedly rendered helpless and powerless, and the perpetrator is presented as omnipotent, with no alternative reference points, the victim becomes entrapped within the perpetrator's viewpoint (Herman, 1997).

In Leahy *et al.*'s (2004) study, the athletes' reports describe the perpetrator's unpredictable and volatile emotional reward–punishment cycle that pervaded the sports environment. Within such an environment, the isolated victim is likely to become increasingly dependent on the perpetrator both for information and emotional support (Herman, 1997). The unpredictable cycling of fear and reprieve, punishment and reward, in the relatively closed context of an elite competitive sports team can result in a feeling of extreme, almost "worshipful," dependence on the perceived omnipotent perpetrator (Herman, 1997). The more confused and frightened the victim becomes, the more need to cling to the one relationship that is permitted—the one with the perpetrator. A female athlete in the study said of the coach who sexually abused her over a number of years, "To us at that time, his word was like gospel" (Leahy *et al.*, 2004, p. 536).

Traumatized attachment to the perpetrator can continue long after the abuse has stopped, as illustrated in the following comment from an athlete also abused by her coach for many years (Leahy *et al.*, 2004, p. 536):

> I still remember I used to brag to my friends and my parents how great this guy was, how lucky I was, and how he was the best coach in the whole world, you know. I remember I used to say that to people, and he just made us believe that he was just absolutely brilliant and I did believe that. *Yeah, and I still think he's awesome ... and I still feel guilty that I did blow the whistle, and I made him lose his job.*

Where the locus-of-control shift and traumatized attachment are key coping strategies, disclosure simply does not happen, and common expectations of visible distress indicators may not be apparent. As the young person attempts to survive the toxic psychological environment, he or she may appear loving, needy, willing to please, and protective of the perpetrator. Silencing is an integral, not separate, part of the experience and is achieved through aspects of the perpetrator's methodology, which keeps the athlete in the state of traumatized entrapment, as a female athlete sexually abused by her coach described: "I didn't realize there was another way out [pause] or there was another option for me like [telling someone]." (Leahy *et al.*, 2003, p. 661).

Some clinicians view the dissociation-facilitated locus-of-control shift and traumatic attachment to the perpetrator as the core therapeutic considerations in working with survivors of chronic childhood sexual abuse (Herman, 1997; Ross, 1997). Failure to recognize these complex dynamics is a potentially therapy-ending error:

> I can't say that I had any thoughts of saying, "No" [to the perpetrator], which is hard to justify to someone who says you're old enough to say no .... and like the [sport psychologist] couldn't understand that, uhm at 17, or 16, I couldn't say no ... At the time it was crazy for me to try to explain how I felt, uhm, and so I actually said, "I can't do it" ... *I just didn't go back.*
>
> (Leahy *et al.*, 2003, p. 662)

Treatment Principles

Research on the efficacy of treatment for complex trauma is just emerging, much of it based on cognitive therapy approaches directed at stabilization of core PTSD and other symptoms (e.g., Reisick, Nishith, & Griffin, 2003). In general, however, there is insufficient evidence to categorically define the nature, longitudinal course, and relationship to PTSD treatment outcomes (Ford, Courtois, Steele, van der Hart, & Nijenhuis, 2005). Nevertheless, there is an evolving standard of care, and the current consensus model of treatment for chronic, complex traumatization is that a phase-oriented approach is necessary, in which treatment is clearly sequenced, tempered and task- and skill-focused (Courtois, 1999). Therapy must be empowering and collaborative and should normalize reactions to trauma. It is multi-modal and transtheoretical, employing a variety of therapeutic techniques tailored to the individual needs and requiring a range of linked biopsychosocial treatment approaches (Courtois, 2004).

Within this model, the basic principles of good therapeutic practice remain valid, and it is important that from the outset these are communicated and monitored. These principles include issues of informed consent, confidentiality, clarity of professional role and boundaries, client empowerment and responsibility, issues of safety, emergency procedures, and adjunctive treatment options such as medication and hospitalization, as necessary. Throughout the process of the treatment, care should be taken to ensure that clients are developing the necessary self- and symptom-management competencies to maintain a level of functioning consistent with their lifestyles. For high-performance athletes, this approach will include maximizing the ability to maintain training and performance levels. Finally, vigilance must be maintained to ensure effective management of transferential and countertransferential issues (see Chapter 17). The therapist will need to consciously model self-regulatory skills to manage vicarious trauma reactions while maintaining a therapeutic focus on providing a safe, authentic emotional presence with clear therapeutic boundaries (Pearlman & Courtois, 2005).

The pathway to recovery for complex posttraumatic conditions is likely to require a relatively long time-frame, be intensive in terms of frequency of sessions, and vary in length of each session. Dissociation, avoidance, and motivated forgetting are likely to be extensively used as defense and coping mechanisms to keep painful material, or even the therapist, at a distance. It is important that the psychotherapeutic process proceed slowly and cautiously to avoid prematurely dealing with material that may retraumatize, and overwhelm the individual's ability to cope and maintain daily functioning.

Phases of Treatment

The prevailing consensus model of treatment follows a three-phased macro-cycle, within a treatment framework cued to the symptom clusters of complex trauma described earlier. Treatment usually proceeds in a back-and-forth manner, more often taking the form of a recursive spiral, rather than a linear path (Courtois, 1999). The issues addressed in each phase will reemerge repeatedly as treatment progresses, and as the key survival coping mechanisms (dissociation, locus-of-control shift, and traumatic attachment) drive trauma-centric meaning attributions.

The First Phase

The first phase focuses on stabilization, the establishment of safety, the development of the therapeutic alliance, symptom management self-care, and skill building. Key tasks that have to be achieved include the development of personal safety strategies; education to demystify the psychotherapy process; education about the nature of trauma and its effects to normalize the often overwhelming trauma symptoms experienced by the client; self-management, and life stabilization skills; and building of social relationships and support systems. Affect regulation and modulation are key targets of skill building interventions, as are body awareness and self-care.

Sport psychology cognitive-behavioral mental skills interventions are applicable in this phase of building healthy coping strategies. For high-performance athletes, self-care will also include attending to the maintenance of proper nutrition, training recovery, and injury prevention. There can be severe physiological sequelae for athletes and their abilities to train and maintain the level of confidence necessary for elite performance. For example, an athlete violently sexually assaulted within her sport environment described how her attempts to cope with the overwhelming trauma psychologically and physically consumed all the energy she had previously directed towards training and competing:

> I was tired, sick. ... I had to really cut down my training because I'd break down [physically]. ... I used to really enjoy training and loved competing [long pause] ... like you know my sport has been the defining thing for me as a person [long pause, weeping].
>
> (Leahy *et al.*, 2003, p. 662)

The first phase also involves the establishment of the therapeutic alliance. Traumatic attachment processes may present significant challenges to this task. There may be recurrent testing of boundaries and the therapist's trustworthiness, along with fears of future betrayal and violation. If not properly managed by the therapist, these relational dynamics can compound harm by replicating the perpetrator dynamics within the therapeutic relationship. It is crucial that the therapist projects and models and makes available to the client, a stable, secure, reliable, well-bounded treatment relationship framework. This secure environment is the foundation upon which therapeutic work will proceed.

With the focus of the first phase work on skill building and self-management, significant improvements in clients' quality of life are likely to be experienced. For some clients at this juncture, termination or a break in therapy may be requested. Always ensure that an option to return to therapy at a later date remains open. For high-performance athletes, I have found it useful to try to use therapy "micro-cycles" to facilitate the athlete's competition goals, with priority tasks in each micro-cycle geared towards ensuring sufficient self-regulatory skills are in place to allow the athlete to continue to compete at key events. This strategy is important because it is not uncommon that survivors struggle with feelings of being "contaminated" by their traumatic experiences, with a sense of hopelessness about themselves and their lives. Being able to access the parts of their identities (e.g., elite sport performers) that are experienced as being free from this contamination provide an important reparative experience and counter the internalized negative perpetrator messages.

The Second Phase

In this phase, the therapist and client undertake a gradual, sequenced exposure to traumatic material. The trauma experience or experiences are directly processed to resolve posttraumatic symptoms and to integrate the trauma experiences into the survivor's life in such a way as to allow a forward self-development that is not solely defined by past trauma. This process includes coming to terms with overwhelming affect, gaining control of symptoms, and reducing the need for dissociative defenses to allow a coherent meaning to be constructed that can be lived with. Detailed exploration of traumatic material is not for the purposes of abreaction (release of emotional tension achieved through recalling a traumatic experience), which is not healing, and may simply retraumatize. It is to promote posttraumatic growth (Courtois, 2004).

Before entering this phase, the basic issues of informed consent, clarification of expectations, and demystification of the process must be again revisited. Stabilization skills must be in place, and pacing and intensity has to be planned so that the client leaves therapy sessions in control. I have found that it is during this phase that sessions may require a longer time than the usual therapy hour: up to ninety minutes to ensure this stabilization happens. If pacing and intensity are not managed well, there is a risk of decompensation and the resurgence of maladaptive trauma-based coping behaviors (e.g., self-injury, suicidality).

During this phase, when working with high-performance athletes, I have found guided imagery a useful technique, because athletes are often already familiar with it. Narrative recording, through written or oral presentation, or art and other expressive media, have also worked well. It is important that the therapist is able to be authentically present to acknowledge and normalize responses, and to provide a containing environment for this work. The therapist must also be ready to assist the processing of extremely intense emotions, such as rage, shame, grief, and mourning. Therapist dissociation or withdrawal from the traumatized person's sometimes overwhelming anger and grief are potentially harmful countertransferential responses. If a therapist is uncomfortable with anger or views anger or other negative affects as undesirable, then the practitioner may consciously or unconsciously encourage continued avoidance. Therapists also need to be knowledgeable about methods of safe expression and management of intense affect, to effectively facilitate the recovery of healthy affect regulation.

Common themes reoccurring during this phase will often center on the locus-of-control shift (i.e., the victim is responsible for the abuse) and traumatic attachment to the perpetrator, which can impede the expression and resolution of anger and grief and the development of empowered meaning attributions regarding the abuse. Acknowledging anger and grief is a major step to recovery, but it may be an intolerable step for the survivor unless traumatic attachment to the perpetrator is open for safe therapeutic exploration. Meaning attributions can reveal important underlying information about the locus of control shift and how traumatic attachment bonds are being maintained. The client, however, may perceive this information as unsafe to express if the superficial presentation (e.g., self-blaming attributions) appears to be unacceptable to the therapist who too quickly jumps in with, "It's not your fault" (Leahy *et al.*, 2003). As one athlete succinctly expressed, "Sometimes that makes me angry (pause) because it sounds like it's just a psychologist's spiel rather than sincere, uhm, helping me to understand my confusion." (p. 662). Rather than immediately challenging self-blaming attributions, and insisting that it is not the victim's fault, it may be more productive to respectfully explore the multi-layered construction of the attribution.

The second phase proceeds until PTSD symptoms become manageable. When processing is complete and memory is deconditioned, symptoms often cease and anguish recedes as trauma is integrated with other aspects of life, and clients develop more complete narratives of their lives than they had before (Ford *et al.*, 2005).

The Third Phase

The third phase involves reconnection with self and reintegration with social relationships and community networks. Therapeutic attention should still be maintained on issues of safety, self-care, and so forth. During this phase, issues related to the development of trusting relationships, intimacy, sexual functioning, vocational and career plans, and other life decisions are often the focus of ongoing work. This phase can also include the challenge of grieving for lost childhood. It may also involve decisions about ongoing relationships with abusive family members and perpetrators still within the client's social environment.

During this phase it is important to continue to facilitate the development of relational skills by modeling healthy negotiation of boundaries and dealing effectively with relational errors or misunderstandings. No therapist is perfect, and inevitably will fail to live up to idealistic projections, miss salient client cues, or fail to perceive accurately the survivors' needs. Modeling how healthy relationships can be preserved and repaired by good communication and emotional processing skills is an important therapist task through this phase to facilitate the development of present-day relationships that are not embedded in traumatized responses (Ford *et al.*, 2005).

Effectively managing the termination process is a challenge when working with traumatized survivors because feelings of abandonment, loss, and grief may re-emerge. Sport psychologists working on an ongoing basis with residential teams may be at an advantage at this point, because both the athlete and the sport psychologist remain in the same environment, allowing a gradual and closely monitored transition. It is helpful to allow for the possibility of return to therapy because future challenges my trigger distress or crises. Therapists should, therefore, be particularly vigilant with this vulnerable group of athletes to not have dual relationships, or post-termination relationships outside the therapy structure, because such involvements would prevent the possibility of a return to a therapy (Pearlman & Courtois, 2005).

Conclusions

> I spoke to the sport psychologist a couple of times but not once did [the sport psychologist] get it.
>
> (female athlete sexually abused by her coach for many years; Leahy, 2010, p. 316)

Research and clinical evidence indicates that athlete survivors of sexual abuse, whether perpetrated within sport or outside of sport, form a significant percentage of the athlete population with which sport psychologists will come into contact. Therefore, sport psychologists need to have the skills to be able to integrate effective treatment into the social context of the athlete's life. In this chapter I have described an introductory overview to the key treatment issues. This chapter is not enough to provide anyone with the competencies necessary to start engaging in an effective treatment relationship with traumatized athlete survivors of sexual abuse. Ongoing professional development training in this area should be undertaken before taking on the responsibility of facilitating recovery in this highly vulnerable group of athletes. Personal therapy may be useful to reveal therapist blind spots, and to protect from, or deal with, secondary traumatization. Finally, peer supervision is necessary to ensure the therapeutic process remains free of countertransferential errors that may be experienced by a traumatized athlete as harmful replications of perpetrator dynamics. See Box 27.1 for a summary of key points from this chapter.

BOX 27.1

Key points on working with adult athlete survivors of sexual abuse

- Effective therapy must address the client's sociocultural context. Sport psychologists are well-positioned to be able to facilitate recovery, without sacrificing athletes' sporting goals, by integrating treatment into the social context of the athlete's life.
- Therapy is a trust-based relationship that requires authentic engagement, but also vigilance in maintaining a well-bounded, healing dynamic within the therapeutic environment.
- Establishing an effective therapeutic alliance with athlete survivors of long-term sexual abuse is only possible if the therapist is sensitive to the possible alterations in the athlete's capacity to develop and maintain healthy, trusting relationships in light of the confounding influence of ongoing traumatic attachment to the perpetrator.
- Current standard of care guidelines follow a three-phased macro-cycle within a treatment framework cued to the symptoms of complex trauma.
- Collaborative decisions about therapeutic micro-cycles can help ensure the athlete's performance at key competition events is maintained.
- Treatment may take longer than usual therapy, individual sessions may require longer duration, and treatment is unlikely to be linear. Issues may repeatedly re-emerge in different forms as treatment progresses.
- Therapists should be vigilant about having access to ongoing peer-supervision and personal therapy as necessary to ensure the treatment process remains free from harmful transferential and countertransferential contamination.

References

American Psychiatric Association (2000). *Diagnostic and statistical manual of mental disorders* (4th ed., text Rev.). Washington, DC: American Psychiatric Association.

Brackenridge, C. H. (2001). *Spoilsports: Understanding and preventing sexual exploitation in sport*. London: Routledge.

Briere, J. (2004). *Psychological assessment of adult posttraumatic states: Phenomenology, diagnosis, and measurement* (2nd ed.). Washington, DC: American Psychological Association.

Courtois, C. A. (1999). *Recollections of sexual abuse: Treatment principles and guidelines*. New York: Norton.

Courtois, C. A. (2004). Complex trauma, complex reactions: Assessment and treatment. *Psychotherapy: Theory Research, Practice, Training*, *41*, 412–425.

Ford, J. D., Courtois, C. A., Steele, K., van der Hart, O., & Nijenhuis, E. R. S. (2005). Treatment of complex posttraumatic self-dysregulation. *Journal of Traumatic Stress*, *18*, 437–447.

Herman, J. L. (1997). *Trauma and recovery. From domestic abuse to political terror* (2nd ed.). New York: Basic Books.

Leahy, T. (2010). Sexual abuse in sport: Implications for the sport psychology profession. In T. V. Ryba, R. J. Schinke, & G. Tenenbaum (Eds.), *The cultural turn in sport psychology* (pp. 315–334). Morgantown. WV: Fitness Information Technology.

Leahy, T., Pretty, G., & Tenenbaum, G. (2003). Childhood sexual abuse narratives in clinically and non-clinically distressed adult survivors. *Professional Psychology: Research and Practice*, *34*, 657–665.

Leahy, T., Pretty, G., & Tenenbaum, G. (2004). Perpetrator methodology as a predictor of traumatic symptomatology in adult survivors of childhood sexual abuse. *Journal of Interpersonal Violence*, *19*, 521–540.

Leahy, T., Pretty, G., & Tenenbaum, G. (2008). A contextualised investigation of traumatic correlates of childhood sexual abuse in Australian athletes. *International Journal of Sport and Exercise Psychology*, *4*, 366–384.

Palmer, S. E., Brown, R. A., Rae-Grant, N. I., & Loughlin, M. J. (1999). Responding to children's disclosure of familial abuse: What survivors tell us. *Child Welfare*, *78*, 259–283.

Pearlman, L. A., & Courtois, C. A. (2005). Clinical applications of the attachment framework: Relational treatment of complex trauma. *Journal of Traumatic Stress*, *18*, 449–459.

Reisick, P., Nishith, P., & Griffin, M. (2003). How well does cognitive-behavioral therapy treat symptoms of PTSD? An examination of child sexual abuse survivors within a clinical trial. *CNS Spectrums*, *8*, 340–342, 351–355.

Ross. C. (1997). *Dissociative identity disorder: Diagnosis, clinical features, and treatment of multiple personality.* New York: Guilford Press.

28

THE PENN STATE SEX ABUSE SCANDAL

PERSONAL AND PSYCHOLOGICAL INSIGHTS

Russell Eisenman

I have both personal and psychological insights about the sex abuse scandal at Penn State that lasted for years as assistant football coach Jerry Sandusky sexually abused children. The personal insights come from twice applying for jobs there, including an on-campus interview as I was getting my doctorate. Also, the job I finally got, at Temple University, was in the same university system as Penn State, so I was somewhat aware of events there. Coach Joe Paterno took over the discipline of all Penn State football players, even though there was a separate university office for this. But, he never allowed that office to do its job, as he kept control of what was or was not done to his players. He was powerful enough to enforce his control here.

Interviews

My job interview at Penn State occurred as I was getting my doctorate in clinical psychology at the University of Georgia. Penn State is isolated from just about everything else. I had to take two planes and a long taxi cab ride to get to the campus. It is a major university in a rural setting, the great God of the area one could say. And many people in the geographic area who went to college went to Penn State, or worked there, or had some kind of ties to the university. The district attorney who, many years ago, first heard of charges against Jerry Sandusky and decided not to prosecute, had graduated from Penn State.

I did not get the job, although I had a good interview. In fact, one of my interviewers became a high-level administrator at a flagship state university and tried to recruit me to teach there. I was later told that the Penn State psychology department had already offered the job to someone else but that person took a long time to decide, so in the meantime they interviewed me. Finally, he accepted. I wonder if that is ethical: interviewing me when the job was already offered to someone else? It certainly is in their self-interest but is it ethical? I am not sure. But, even if it is not ethical, they can get away with things like that.

Russell Eisenman, "The Penn State Sex Abuse Scandal: Personal and Psychological Insights," *Journal of Information Ethics*, vol. 22, no. 1, pp. 8-10.

Years later, while at Temple, I applied for the job of Director of Clinical Training in the Psychology Department at Penn State. I did not get this job either, but instead it went to the Penn State faculty member who was head of the search committee. Is this ethical? It does not seem ethical to me, since the search committee head has an unfair advantage and thus should not be a candidate. But, again, Penn State is isolated and big and respected and can get away with a lot of things. Once in the habit of doing what one wants, the situation is ripe for more ethical abuses.

Psychological Insights

How could no one have seen that Jerry Sandusky was molesting kids when he was showering with children in the Penn State football building, etc.? Partly, they did not want to see because millions of football dollars were involved and the prestige of the school was at stake. Under these circumstances, many would turn a blind eye. This is mostly a conscious refusal to admit to bad things that are clearly there. Additionally, unconscious denial is a factor. People often are able to deny the obvious, as when parents cannot see that their child is using illegal drugs, even though the child leaves all kinds of drug stuff around the house.

Furthermore, there is the psychological reality of not believing that certain people can be child sex abusers or in some other hateful category. If someone has status in the community it might be very hard to comprehend that he is also doing something evil. It just does not compute in some people's minds. Coach Jerry Sandusky had high status while his victims often had low status, being poor, having no father, etc. A child sex abuser is often thought of as a dirty, low class person, in a raincoat, with an ugly face, and needing a shave. But the reality is that they can be judges, military officers, policemen, professors, et al.

Conclusions

Penn State is an isolated, respected institution that often has done what it wanted. It has the power to ignore ethical issues, at least at times. This is not unique to Penn State but would be true of many institutions and people with great power. Both conscious desires to make money and maintain prestige, and unconscious denial served to maintain a child abuser, Jerry Sandusky, as a football coach for many years, with many victims.

FURTHER READING

Silent No More: Inside the USA Gymnastics Sex Abuse Scandal

Tracy Connor, Sarah Fitzpatrick, and Kenzi Abou-Sabe

If you have a digital edition of this book, please click on the link below to access the article:

https://www.nbcnews.com/news/us-news/silent-no-more-inside-usa-gymnastics-sex-abuse-scandal-n868221

If you have a print edition of this book, please use your cell phone to scan the QR code below to access the article:

More Than 100 Former Ohio State Students Allege Sexual Misconduct

Catie Edmondson

If you have a digital edition of this book, please click on the link below to access the article:

https://www.nytimes.com/2018/07/20/us/politics/sexual-misconduct-ohio-state.html

If you have a print edition of this book, please use your cell phone to scan the QR code below to access the article:

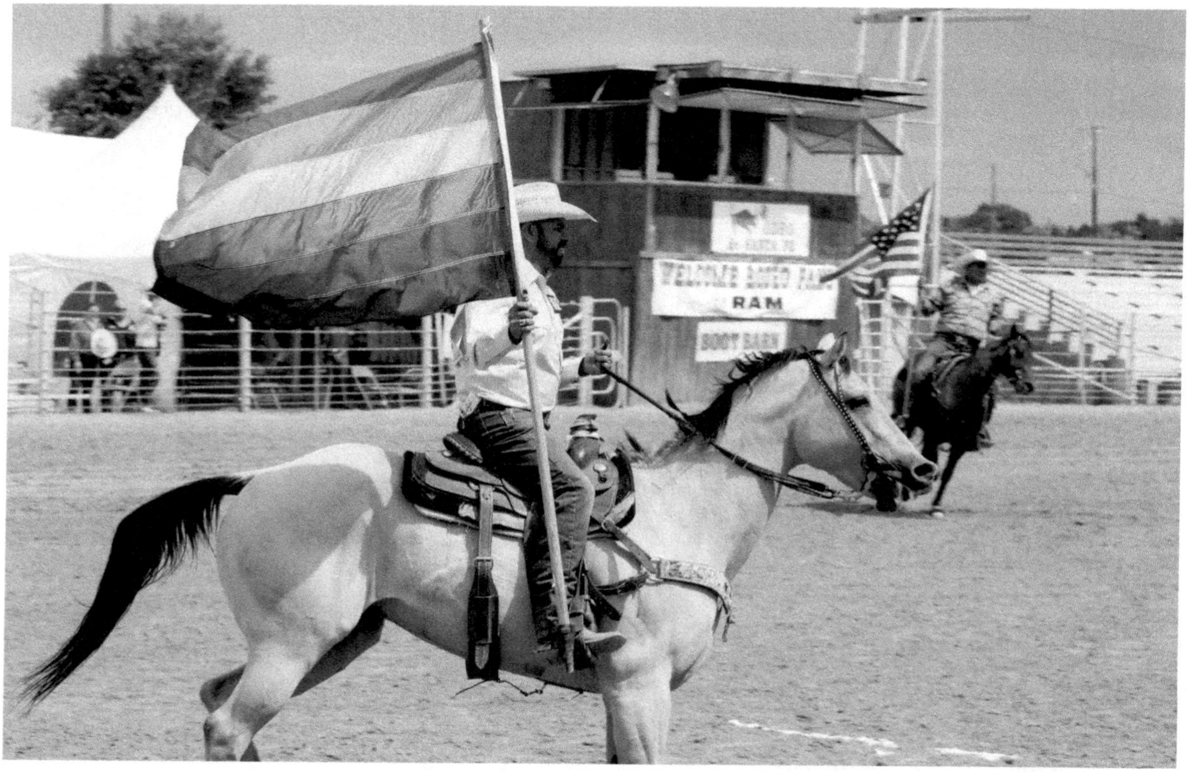
RAM

CHAPTER 13

SPORT FOR SOCIAL JUSTICE

Sport for **social justice** is the final goal of this text. For students who understand the need to see improvements made in terms of inclusion and equity in sport, they might find a need to engage athletes, coaches, and fans in the **social world of sport**. Featured here is Saul "Pepe" Lozada and his horse, Ponderosa Princess, during the Grand Entry Opening Ceremonies of the Zia Regional Rodeo in Santa Fe, New Mexico. The social world of rodeo is becoming more accepting of International Gay Rodeo Association athletes because cultural similarities create a bond. Many participants of both organizations are from rural towns and grew up on farms roping livestock. Mainstream rodeo competitors realize that there are more similarities between the LGBT participants and heterosexual cowboys and cowgirls than they originally believed.

Social worlds, for the most part, are fluid. A person may become part of a group and soon learn that the members all share similar cultural characteristics. For example, an NCAA Division I football recruit can visit six campuses and meet six different teams of athletes and coaches. At first glance, they all might appear to be similar social worlds. These young men may seem to share cultural attributes such as growing up in a Christian family, speaking English, and even find that these young men come from families with the same political affiliation. However, there are social worlds where group membership is restrictive, excluding people who do not strictly adhere to these cultural identifiers. For this recruit, it might not seem as apparent after their first few visits, but after signing and joining the team, they might realize these cultural traits are necessary for full inclusion. This becomes a problem when certain activities contradict their own personal values, and they are encouraged to conform and ignore actions, even when those actions go against their beliefs.

In the example of elite gymnastics, these pressures to become full members of this social world comes with its own price. Athletes might witness a teammate's disordered eating habits, but informing coaches, parents, or other athletes can jeopardize their social standing within the group. Once these social worlds become intensely secretive and isolating, an environment exists that privileges secrecy over whistleblowing, and an unwritten code becomes clear. First, win at any cost. Two, do not question authority. Three, "man up!" This final directive is the most dangerous in the world of sport: a gender ideology that places men and masculinity as superior and women as inferior subjects. Thus, women and girls in sport understand that there is a balancing act they need to successfully manage: be tough, like one of the guys; and be appropriately feminine, but not too "butch."

The isolation within this social world of elite sport prevents athletes from discussing many of the critical social issues they experience daily. If they could share the issues openly, they might shock a non-elite athlete, family members, and fans with their experiences. These final reading selections examine how athletes have taken it upon themselves to fight for inclusion in sport, break down barriers that exist, and encourage a healthier world of sport.

THE SPORT FOR DEVELOPMENT AND PEACE SECTOR

AN ANALYSIS OF ITS EMERGENCE, KEY INSTITUTIONS, AND SOCIAL POSSIBILITIES

Richard Giulianotti

Since the late 1990s, we have witnessed the emergence and exponential growth of what has become known as the Sport for Development and Peace (SDP) sector. SDP projects use sport as an interventionist tool to promote different types of social development and peaceful social relations across the world. While SDP projects are implemented in both the Global North and South, they tend to be sited in developing regions and in war-torn or post-conflict settings.

It is not possible to provide a complete picture or final calculation of SDP projects, but it might be reasonably estimated that there are now thousands of these initiatives across the world, varying greatly in scale, duration, and mission. The goals that are pursued across the SDP sector include poverty reduction; the education of young people; health promotion and disease prevention education; women's empowerment; and peace building, rehabilitation, and reconstruction in post-conflict contexts.

A substantial volume of academic research on the SDP sector has been undertaken since the late 1990s, particularly in the fields of anthropology, sociology, and political science, with sport studies providing an interdisciplinary foundation for this inquiry.[1] My own research and analysis with respect to SDP has been conducted over more than a decade, leading to the publication of

1 For example, see: Gary Armstrong, "The Lords of Misrule: Football and the Rights of the Child in Liberia, West Africa," *Sport in Society* 7, no. 3 (2004): 473–502; Gary Armstrong, "The Global Footballer and the Local War-Zone: George Weah and Transnational Networks in Liberia, West Africa," Global Networks 7, no. 2 (2007): 230–47; Fred Coalter, *A Wider Social Role for Sport* (London: Routledge, 2005); Simon Darnell, "Power, Politics and 'Sport for Development and Peace': Investigating the Utility of Sport for International Development," *Sociology of Sport Journal* 27, no. 1 (2010): 54–75; Patrick K. Gasser and Anders Levinsen, "Breaking Post-War Ice: Open Fun Football Schools in Bosnia and Herzegovina," Sport in Society 7, no. 3 (2004): 457–72; Hans Hognestad and Arvid Tollisen, "Playing Against Deprivation: Football and Development in Nairobi, Kenya," in Football in Africa, ed. Gary Armstrong and Richard Giulianotti (Basingstoke: Palgrave, 2004); Marion Keim, *Nation Building at Play: Sport as a Tool for Integration in Post-Apartheid South Africa* (Aachen: Meyer and Meyer, 2003); Paul Richards, "Soccer and Violence in War-Torn Africa: Soccer and Social Rehabilitation in Sierra Leone," in *Entering the Field: New Perspectives in World Football*, ed. Gary Armstrong and Richard Giulianotti (Oxford: Berg, 1997); Nico Schulenkorf, "Sport Events and Ethnic Reconciliation: Attempting to Create Social Change

Richard Giulianotti, "The Sport for Development and Peace Sector: An Analysis of its Emergence, Key Institutions, and Social Possibilities," *The Brown Journal of World Affairs*, vol. 18, no. 2, pp. 279-293.

papers in academic journals and books. This work has also included participation at the Sport and Development international conference, hosted by the Swiss Academy for Development in Magglingen, in February 2003, and the coproduction of the main text for the section "Peace 1: Sport, Violence and Crisis Situations," as part of the "Magglingen Declaration" at this event.[2]

This article draws on fieldwork and interview research undertaken in the Balkans, the Middle East, South Asia, and southern Africa, as well as in Germany, Switzerland, and the United Kingdom. A significant proportion of the research has examined how football is used by agencies for conflict resolution and peacemaking; however, this paper also considers the use of other sports for various SDP purposes.[3]

The article is divided into five main parts. First, I put forward some illustrative SDP activities and projects, highlighting their diverging missions and aims. Second, I set out four main categories of SDP institutions or agencies and consider the ways in which they are interrelated. Third, I outline why the different agencies are attracted to sports as a way to help them accomplish their missions. Fourth, I seek to challenge any tendencies within the SDP sector toward "sport evangelism" by examining sport's complex historical and sociopolitical relationships to violence, conflict, and peace. Finally, I identify some of the key features that are apparent in the more progressive SDP projects.

SDP Projects: Some Examples

It is useful to begin by providing some illustrations of the different types of SDP work that are undertaken. Some examples include:

- The United Nations Development Programme (UNDP) Match Against Poverty, which is regularly contested by the world's leading football players to raise money for the poor and to promote public awareness of the need to eradicate world poverty.[4]
- The "Segundo Tempo" project in Brazil, which promotes schooling among hundreds of thousands of poor young people through a mixture of after-hours sport, free meals, and additional school time.[5]
- The Grassroots Soccer program in Zimbabwe, which promotes HIV/AIDS education among young people.[6]

---

in War-Torn Sri Lanka," *International Review for the Sociology of Sport* 45, no. 3: 273–94; Geoffrey Whitfield, *Amity in the Middle East: How the World Sport Peace Project and the Passion for Football Brought Together Arab and Jewish Youngsters* (London: Alpha Press, 2006).

2 Richard Giulianotti, "Human Rights, Globalization and Sentimental Education: The Case of Sport," Sport in Society 7, no. 3 (2004): 355–69; Richard Giulianotti, "Sport, Peacemaking and Conflict Resolution: A Contextual Analysis and Modeling of the Sport, Development and Peace Sector," *Ethnic and Racial Studies* 34, no. 2 (2011): 207–28; Richard Giulianotti, "The Sport, Development and Peace Sector: A Model of Four Social Policy Domains," Journal of Social Policy 40, no. 4 (2011): 757–76; Richard Giulianotti, "Sport, Transnational Peace-Making and the Global Civil Society: Exploring the Reflective Discourses of 'Sport, Development and Peace' Project Officials," Journal of Sport and Social Issues 35, no. 1 (2011): 50–71; Richard Giulianotti and Gary Armstrong "Sport, The Military and Peacemaking," Third World Quarterly 32, no. 3 (2011): 379–94. See also: Richard Giulianotti, Gary Armstrong, and Hans Hognestad, "Sport and Peace: Playing the Game," Sport and Development: An International Conference (paper, Swiss Academy for Development: Magglingen, Switzerland, February 16–18, 2003).

3 As this paper will be reaching a largely North American audience, it is important to note that, though the sport is referred to as *soccer* in North America, it is known as *football* in most of the world.

4 "24,000 Fill Arena for Match Against Poverty," United Nations Development Program, http://www.beta.undp.org/undp/en/home/ourwork/goodwillambassadors/match_against_poverty.html.

5 "Segundo Tempo: Programas de Incentivo," Brazil.gov, http://www.brasil.gov.br/sobre/esporte/programas-de-incentivo/programa-segundo-tempo.

6 "Where We Work: Zimbabwe," Grassroots Soccer, http://www.grassrootsoccer.org/where-we-work/zimbabwe/.

- The work of the Elena NGO in Cameroon, which uses football to promote educational participation, empowerment, and domestic abuse prevention.[7]
- The UN Mission in Liberia's "Sport for Peace" initiative, which ran for five weeks across 15 counties in 2007.[8] The initiative aimed to encourage young people to use sport in order to build peace and promote development in the post-conflict context. Supported by the UN Mission in Liberia, the Liberian government, the International Olympic Committee (IOC), and various sport governing bodies and NGOs, the initiative saw sports events and tournaments staged across the country.

Clearly, these initiatives are focused on meeting key development and humanitarian needs. Such an approach is crystallized in the United Nations' Millennium Development Goals (MDGs) and, indeed, the UN considers sport to be "a viable and practical tool to assist in the achievement of the MDGs."[9]

However, it is important to recognize that the field of SDP work extends well beyond the MDGs. We need also to locate within the SDP sector those projects that are based in the Global North, as well as those that are focused on more political, legal, and normative issues relating to human development, such as social justice and human and civil rights. For example, Global North projects might include:

- The United Kingdom NGO Street League, which uses football as an interventionist tool to assist young people, particularly those involved in criminal activity, with employment, education, or training.[10]
- The Midnight Basketball initiative in the United States, founded in the late 1980s, which uses sport to draw young people away from criminal activity, particularly in inner-city African-American neighborhoods.[11]

Initiatives that focus on social justice and human/civil rights include:

- The United States Anti-Sweatshop Movement, which has developed campaigns against the exploitation of workers in developing nations by sports merchandise corporations.[12]
- The Play the Game NGO in Denmark, which is particularly critical of corruption in sport and is focused on transparency, good governance, and media freedom.[13]
- The Football Against Racism in Europe (FARE) network, which campaigns against racism, sexism, and homophobia in football.[14]
- Amnesty International and Human Rights Watch, each of which focused human rights campaigns on the hosting of the 2008 Olympic Games in Beijing.[15]

---

7 "Elena NGO: Cameroon," streetfootballworld, http://www.streetfootballworld.org/network/all-nwm/elena-ngo.

8 "United Nations Peacekeeping," United Nations Sport for Development and Peace, http://www.un.org/wcm/content/site/sport/home/unplayers/fundsprogrammesagencies/dpko.

9 "Sport and the UN Development Goals," United Nations Sport for Development and Peace, http://www.un.org/wcm/content/site/sport/sportandmdgs.

10 "Change Lives Through Football," Street League, http://www.streetleague.co.uk/.

11 Douglas Hartmann, "Notes on Midnight Basketball and the Cultural Politics of Recreation, Race and the Politics of At-Risk Urban Youth," Journal of Sport and Social Issues 25, no.4 (2001): 339–71.

12 "Nike Campus Activism," Campaign For Labor Rights, http://www.clrlabor.org/alerts/Da-teUnknown/nike_campus_activism.html.

13 "Playthegame.org," University of Aarhus Department of Sport Science, http://www.playthegame.org/.

14 We Are Football People, Fare Network, http://www.farenet.org/.

15 "Human Rights in China and the Beijing Olympics," Amnesty International, http://www.amnesty.org/en/china-olympics; "Beijing Olympics Basics," Human Rights Watch, http://china.hrw.org/press/faq/beijing_olympics_basics.

- Local community groups and national social movements, which campaign against the building of stadiums or hosting of sports mega-events in cities on the grounds of their high social costs, such as excessive expenditure of limited public monies, intensified surveillance and security, the forced removal or relocation of local people, the destruction of local communities, and the social exclusion of the poor.[16]

The SDP sector features initiatives and projects that have a diverse array of missions and objectives, and these in turn are underpinned by very different kinds of agencies and institutions, as I now explain.

SDP Agencies and Institutions: Four Categories

SDP institutions and agencies vary substantially with regard to their scale, location, objectives, policies, ideologies, and strategies. We may differentiate these agencies into four broad categories.

1. There are the *nongovernmental, nonprofit organizations*, which facilitate and/or implement SDP projects and come in many shapes and sizes. International NGOs that focus on SDP work include Right to Play, Street Football World, Football Against Racism in Europe, and Open Fun Football Schools. Other more established development NGOs such as Care and Action Aid have also used sport to promote their interests and agendas. At local and national levels, we find grassroots NGOs, such as the Sarvodaya movement in Sri Lanka, that are particularly well placed to implement SDP projects.
2. There are the *intergovernmental and governmental organizations*, which are particularly active in facilitating and overseeing SDP campaigns and projects, while also contributing to implementation. The United Nations plays a key role in this institutional category, having established its own SDP office (the UNOSDP), while as many as 26 UN associate agencies, such as UNDP and UNICEF, are active in SDP programs and campaigns.[17] Some international development departments and agencies that are linked to national governments have been active in SDP work—for example, the British Council, NORAD (Norway), and Canadian Heritage. National and international sport governing bodies, such as the Fédération Internationale de Football Association (FIFA) and the International Olympic Committee (IOC), might be placed within this category rather than in the NGO list as they function largely as governmental institutions while also seeking to grow their particular sporting interests at the international level.[18] These governing bodies are increasingly involved in SDP work; for example, FIFA established a large international Football for Hope initiative to run until 2015 and the Union of European Football Associations (UEFA), European football's governing body, has a significant "social responsibility" platform.
3. There is the *private sector*, which engages with the SDP sector mainly through voluntary initiatives that are themed around corporate social responsibility and principles of self-regulation within the marketplace. For example, Vodafone, Daimler, and Mercedes-Benz partner with

16 For example, see: "Sports Stadium News and Analysis," Field of Schemes, http://www.fieldofschemes.com/; Games Monitor: Debunking Olympics Myths, http://www.gamesmonitor.org.uk/; "Radical Africa," Bolekaja, http://bolekaja.wordpress.com/2010/06/14/the-kick-off-of-the-poor-peoples-world-cup-13-june-10-am/#more-306. On this subject, see also: Urban Studies, special issue on "Security and Surveillance at Sport Mega-Events" 48, no. 15 (2011); and Helen Lenskyj, Olympic Industry Resistance (New York: SUNY Press, 2008).
17 "Sport For Development and Peace," United Nations, http://www.un.org/wcm/content/site/sport/unoffice.
18 FIFA is world football's governing body; the IOC is the governing body of the Olympic movement.

Laureus, which organizes glitzy annual sports award ceremonies, and which also houses an SDP foundation that draws heavily on Laureus' association with celebrities in regard to public relations work. Additionally, sport manufacturers such as Nike have responded to campaigns against poor labor practices in their production plants by publishing self-reports of the industrial conditions and treatment of their workforce.

4. Finally, there are *radical NGOs and social movements*, which have more politicized approaches toward SDP and are more focused on promoting social justice and human and civil rights, as noted earlier. Invariably, this category of SDP agency tends to come into conflict with corporations, intergovernmental organizations, and some NGOs—as illustrated by their anti-Nike campaigns and protests against the 2008 Beijing Olympics.

These categories help to differentiate and to clarify the diverse SDP agencies, but inevitably some significant complications may arise in the classification of specific institutions. For example, in the NGO category, the Laureus model is relatively close to the "corporate social responsibility" field of activity that is associated with the *private sector*, while some smaller NGOs may be closer to the *radical NGO and social movement* category because of their willingness to engage with human rights or social justice issues. Some institutions may also feature the key characteristics of two categories: for example, the Peace and Sport organization is a Monaco-based NGO that supports SDP initiatives, but also exhibits many features of government because it receives strong supported from Prince Albert of Monaco, a long-standing member of the International Olympic Committee, and its organization of conferences and promotion of networking opportunities.

Currently, there is substantial cooperative work across the first three categories: that is, among NGOs, (inter)governmental agencies, sport governing bodies and institutions, and transnational corporations (TNCs). Much of this work features the planning, financing, and implementing of SDP projects. For example, one scenario might involve a UN agency highlighting a particular major problem, such as a large number of refugees or a major health issue; then an international NGO and a local NGO may collaborate to develop a sports project, with logistical and advocacy support from the UN agency; and finally, a TNC and a sport federation may provide funding and other resources (such as sports equipment) to support the project. A further illustration is provided by the SDP initiative with which I am working. This project is located in Europe and funded by the European Commission with the objective of empowering European football supporters to promote anti-discrimination messages and practices. The project partners include several international NGOs in sport, several national football associations, the international football players' union, and a group of academics.[19]

We also find that extensive forms of social capital are established across the first three categories, notably as officials within NGOs, (inter)governmental agencies, TNCs, and sport federations attend a regular series of international conferences on SDP. These events also serve to publicize SDP work and provide platforms for the shaping of future SDP agendas. Such events and networks have been particularly prominent since 2005, which was named the "International Year of Sport and Physical Education" by the UN, with a very strong focus on SDP activity. Conversely, more radical NGOs and social movements have tended to have relatively restricted roles or to have been absent from these networks and events, with the result that these forces have been marginalized within the SDP sector.

19 "Pro Supporters—Prevention Through Empowerment," Fonds Wiener Institut für Internationalen Dialog und Zusammenarbeit, http://ec.europa.eu/sport/preparatory_actions/documents/annexe-i-066.pdf.

Development and Peace Initiatives: The Attractions of Sport

Having provided some detail on the different kinds of agencies and goals across the SDP sector, it is useful to set out what the strengths of sport might be for those institutions that seek to undertake development and peace work. These perceived benefits or attractions can be summarized as follows:

- As global cultural forms, sports are played worldwide and are familiar or easily taught to people in most settings. Sports are thus an immediate way of building contact with projected client groups.
- SDP work typically targets young people, as they are critical to building long-term social change and development. Sports participation appeals particularly to young people, thereby offering project workers an effective way of reaching this social cohort.
- Sports are already employed in schools and wider social settings as educational tools.
- Where organized in such a way as to promote full social inclusion and personal enjoyment, sports have the potential to secure social and psychological benefits for participants, such as facilitating positive and enjoyable self-expression, developing personal and interpersonal creativity, and fostering team building and group solidarity.
- Sports may enable new social contacts and relationships to be established between different groups within play-focused contexts.
- Sports may promote the wider socialization and education of young people into competitive, rule-governed behavior.
- Sports may feature individuals at local, national, and global levels who have high volumes of symbolic capital and are thus effective in communicating messages.
- The official ideologies and discourses that envelop sports tend to have strong universalist messages.

SDP projects that are centered on peace building tend to view sport as offering a particular set of positive sociocultural and political characteristics that may be helpful in contexts where the targeted user groups have been caught up in violent conflicts. These perceived benefits can be summarized as follows:

- Sports are understood as offering particularly effective meeting spaces for "breaking the ice" between those who have been in conflict. Sports may provide one of the first post-war contact points for such conflicts, while also enabling third parties to be involved, for example in the role of mediator (perhaps as a referee or umpire). For example, sports projects in Bosnia provide one of the few ways in which young people from different Serb and Bosniak (Muslim) communities may interact, despite the fact that these participants may live in villages or towns that are only 15–20 kilometers apart.
- Sports may provide a playful, competitive, rule-governed context for relations to be built with "the other." The presence of a confirmed set of rules in sport, which are agreed upon by the participants and which underpin their interaction, is particularly important for facilitating play and, more seriously, for offering a basis for future, rule-governed interaction off the field of play. Participants may benefit in particular by being responsible for making and enforcing the rules of play, by entering into dialogue, and by negotiating. For example, in war-torn regions of West Africa, sports projects may provide former

child soldiers with a nonviolent social field in which they may enter into these forms of rule-governed interaction.

- Sport-based interventions may help to routinize forms of contact and interaction with former enemies, and to challenge the demonization of the absent or imagined "other." Sports are particularly effective in reaching and engaging with the next generation of potential combatants, while encouraging older generations to allow young people to take ownership of future relationships with peers on "the other side." For example, in Sri Lanka, some sports projects engage directly with different generations in towns and villages, in order to promote wider understanding between different communities, particularly with respect to the treatment of Tamils.
- The universalist messages within sports typically convey support for internationalism and peaceful relations between competitors. While often closely linked to the branding and ideologies of major sports federations, messages (such as those regarding "fair play") may also be evident in the everyday playing ethics of different sports communities.
- Sports may be used to resocialize and to rehabilitate people who have been traumatized, or physically or emotionally damaged by war. Examples of this would include the use of sport to help in the social inclusion and personal rehabilitation of land mine victims in West Africa or Cambodia.
- Sports may contribute more broadly to the reconstruction of societies within the post-war context, for example, by providing a focus for the re-establishment of civil society associations, and for leisure and recreational facilities.
- Sports may also demonstrate to nonparticipants, such as parent groups, how "normal" social relations with other groups and communities may be achieved.

This final point may serve to illustrate the "ripple effect," whereby the impacts of peace-building education projects spread to wider social groups, beyond the immediate participants in such programs. Gavriel Salomon developed and applied the idea of the ripple effect in his study of Israeli–Arab peace education programs, and their potential impacts on wider communities; his colleague Baha Zoubi has employed the concept in his study of binational (Israeli and Arab) participation in football clubs in Israel.[20]

This summarizes the perceived benefits of sport for different development and peace initiatives and agencies. However, to develop an adequate understanding of sport's social impacts and possibilities, we need to recognize the complex and highly uneven historical and sociopolitical relationships of sport to development and peace. This is perhaps best demonstrated through a brief examination of sport's nexus to processes of peace, conflict, and subjugation.

Sport, Peace, and Violence: A Complex History

If we turn to examine the positive side of sport's historical association with peace and development, one focus may fall on the Olympic Games. In Ancient Greece, the Olympic Truce was established as early as the ninth century BC, with the aim of suspending military conflicts and enabling athletes

---

20 Gavriel Salomon, "Four Major Challenges Facing Peace Education in Regions of Intractable Conflict," Peace and Conflict 17 (2011): 46–59; Baha Zoubi, The Direct and Indirect Influence of Jewish and Arab Participation in Bi-National Soccer Clubs on the Attitudes and Perceptions of Their Family Members and Friends toward the Other Side (unpublished PhD diss., University of Haifa, 2011).

and spectators to enjoy safe passage to the games. The Olympic Truce was subsequently revived by the IOC and, since 1993, via UN Resolutions 48 and 11, the Truce has been supported by the United Nations prior to each Olympic Games.[21] Baron Pierre de Coubertin, the inspiration for the modern Olympics, believed that the competition would promote internationalism by bringing different nations and peoples into contact.[22] Further historical illustrations of peace building through sport include the story of the 1914 Christmas Truce between British and German soldiers during which hostilities between the two sides were suspended. Some reports indicate that the soldiers met in no-man's-land to exchange greetings, sing songs, and play football.

On the other hand, we need also to recognize the long-running associations between sport, warfare, and violent conflicts. We might consider here the 100-hour so-called Football War, which erupted between Honduras and El Salvador in 1969. Relations between the two nations had long been tense due to disputes over land, the treatment of cross-border migrants (particularly of Salvadorans in Honduras), and the strong nationalism of politicians and national media. El Salvador and Honduras contested three key football matches which were qualifying fixtures for the 1970 World Cup finals in Mexico; all three fixtures generated significant violence between rival supporters and communities, with the third and final game providing the spark for the declaration of military conflict, which lasted around four days and was understood to have claimed up to 3,000 lives.[23] The Yugoslav civil war was preceded by widespread rioting among football fans, players, and police at a fixture between Dinamo Zagreb and Red Star Belgrade in 1990. Many of the supporter movements were subsequently transformed into paramilitary units during the civil war.[24] These provide relatively recent illustrations of modern sport's long association with aggressive militarism, as reflected in the long-running and widespread use of sporting disciplines to prepare members of the armed forces physically and psychologically for future conflicts.

More broadly, we might consider the long-standing presence of hooligan subcultures, or outbreaks of hooliganism and violence at football fixtures at both national and club levels, which have occurred throughout almost the entire history of the modern game. As I write, Egypt has been gripped by a major social crisis following the death of 74 spectators and the injury of hundreds more at a club fixture between Al-Masry and Al-Ahly; there has been substantial subsequent comment on the possible complicity, or worse, of the security forces in facilitating the violence.[25]

Sport has also been a device of social intervention for serving the political interests of dominant social groups.

Finally, we might also note modern sport's role in enabling forms of social subjugation, pacification, and integration to be imposed upon diverse populations. Otherwise stated, sport has also been a device of social intervention for serving the political interests of dominant social groups. For example, in Britain, modern sports were established and promoted through the late nineteenth and early twentieth centuries in part to pacify unruly upper- and middle-class schoolboys within private (fee-paying) schools, and also to help the social integration and political pacification of the lower

21 "Observance of the Olympic Truce," Res. 48/11, Forty-eighth session, United Nations General Assembly, November 2, 1993, http://www.un.org/ga/search/view_doc.asp?symbol=A/RES/48/11.

22 William J. Morgan, "Cosmopolitanism, Olympism, and Nationalism: A Critical Interpretation of Coubertin's Ideal of International Sporting Life," Olympika: The International Journal of Olympic Studies 4 (1995): 79–92.

23 Ryszard Kapuscinski, The Soccer War (London: Vintage, 1992).

24 Srdjan Vrcan and Drazen Lalic, "From Ends to the Trenches and Back," *in* Football Cultures and Identities, ed. *Gary Armstrong and* Richard Giulianotti (Basingstoke: Palgrave, *1999*).

25 "Egyptian Police Incited Massacre At Stadium, Say Angry Footballers," Observer, February 5, 2012.

classes within the bourgeois social order.[26] In the colonies, the British games revolution helped to build social relations and social capital among the colonial classes and indigenous elites, and also to promote ideologies of "muscular Christianity" and Anglocentric "fair play" that served to normalize colonial rule.[27] Elsewhere, we might consider the connections between football and political populism, notably in mobilizing support for rightist or military regimes, such as in Latin America during various periods of the twentieth century.[28] Finally, in recent times, the sport of football has provided the crucial social laboratory for the testing of new techniques and technologies of social control; in the United Kingdom, for example, closed-circuit television systems were effectively pilot tested in football stadiums in the late 1980s and early 1990s before being rolled out across most urban centers.[29]

The historical record reveals that sport's relationship to peace building and conflict resolution is, at best, highly uneven. Consideration of this record also provides us with a more general reminder that any adequate analysis of the SDP sector should avoid slipping into what I have termed "sport evangelism," wherein sport is assumed to be inherently good and an innate source of positive and peaceful social relations.[30] We need to recognize instead the crucial role of social context in determining sport's relationship to development and peace. The social context shapes the diverse meanings and uses to which sport is put; it underpins the ways in which sport, as a cultural form and as a force for diverse kinds of social solidarity, is embedded within the wider social order; and, it is itself shaped by matrices of power relations between elites and wider publics.

With those points in mind regarding the historical and social context, we may turn to consider some of the distinctive features that are evidenced in the more progressive SDP projects.

Progressive SDP Projects: Key Features

Projects that appear to have the most progressive social qualities and impacts in the SDP field tend to have several key features. The discussion here is perhaps most applicable to SDP projects that are run by NGOs in the Global South, but what follows is also relevant to multi-agency projects and those initiatives that are enacted in the Global North.

First, *sustainability* is critical to the project's potential success. Sustainability may be secured through harnessing or developing sufficient financial support or human resources to enable the project to operate beyond its initial life, ideally over several years. Thus, solid financing may enable the project to be implemented over a significant period of time, while the training of local people may also promote the project's longer and more diffuse impacts, as local people learn the skills and techniques for implementing their own projects, some of which may require little or no resources. In the context of peace-building SDP projects, social contacts involving members of divided communities need to be sustained over a significant period of time in order to increase opportunities for the formation of deeper relationships and to facilitate extended challenges to the demonization of "the other."

26 John Hargreaves, Sport, Culture and Power (Cambridge: Polity, 1986); J.A. Mangan, The Games Ethic and Imperialism (London: Vintage, 1986).
27 John MacAloon, ed., Muscular Christianity in Colonial and Post-Colonial Worlds (London: Routledge, 2007).
28 Tony Mason, Passion of the People? Football in South America (London: Verso, 1994).
29 Richard Giulianotti, "Social Identity and Public Order: Political and Academic Discourses on Football Violence," in Football Violence and Social Identity, ed. Richard Giulianotti, Norman Bonney, and Mike Hepworth (London: Routledge, 1994); Richard Giulianotti and Gary Armstrong, "From Another Angle: Police Surveillance and Football Supporters," in Surveillance, CCTV & Social Control, ed. Clive Norris, Gary Armstrong, and Jay Moran (Aldershot: Gower/Ashgate, 1998).
30 Giulianotti, "Human Rights," 356.

Second, it is particularly beneficial if SDP agencies are committed to the *empowerment* of their user communities in a way that enables the latter to take ownership of SDP initiatives. To achieve this goal, it certainly helps if SDP projects are strongly embedded within the host community, and thus able to engage in dialogue with local communities in the planning, implementation, and evaluation of projects. Grassroots NGOs are best placed to conduct this work, notably in enabling local communities to take ownership of the projects. As the project unfolds, this form of social empowerment should enable targeted user groups to take responsibility for, and to make informed choices regarding, the future forms of development and peace-building work that they wish to implement.

Third, the SDP project needs to be carefully located within the *wider social, political, and cultural context*. For example, with regard to peace-building initiatives, the project is most likely to succeed where there exists a positive environment for its work to be conducted, particularly in post-conflict situations where significant cultural, social, and symbolic capital can be secured by engaging with influential individuals and groups. Moreover, the project should also be carefully located with regard to other relevant stakeholders. For example, peace-making projects and initiatives must be considered in relation to work being undertaken by other agencies in the same region.

Fourth, when examining and assessing their long-term impacts, the most progressive projects draw on a *diversity of monitoring and evaluation* techniques, which might include the use of both quantitative and qualitative methods. At the same time, these projects recognize that isolating and demonstrating the direct social effects of their work can be problematic. Moreover, the SDP agency must not slip into "sport evangelism," recognizing instead the complex historical and contextual relationships of sport to development and peace.

Finally, SDP agencies or institutions offer perhaps the most progressive responses to development and peace-building problems within different regions when they are able to *engage fully with different stakeholders* across the sector. In particular, working with new social movements and comparatively radical NGOs, which are particularly interested in social justice issues or civil rights, may help both to draw the SDP project into a deeper relationship with the local community and to explore how development and peace are more effectively secured in the long term through engaging fully with difficult questions of social justice and human and civil rights.

Concluding Comments

The SDP sector is one of the fastest-growing and most vibrant fields of activity involved in development and peace building, and is highly salient to academic research into the transnational aspects of sport. Four main types of stakeholder agencies may be identified, each with different objectives and modus operandi within the SDP sector. Sport is understood to have a variety of benefits for the implementation of development and peace projects, but at the same time we need to avoid assuming an essentialist or evangelist perspective. The most constructive and progressive SDP initiatives are sustainable over time and more oriented toward the empowerment of local user groups, the use of imaginative evaluation methods, engagement with other SDP agencies, and acknowledgement of the complexities of their operational contexts.

Overall, SDP agencies are at their best when the officials employ what I termed in 2008 a "critical reflexivity" in their work: by this, I am referring to how agency officials may reflect critically on how they engage with different user groups, in order to improve their own practices and service delivery.[31] More broadly, since 2009, I have argued that SDP projects tend to draw on three main models or approaches in their philosophies and their work, namely the *technical*, the *practical*, and the *critical*.[32] The *technical* model tends to take a strongly interventionist approach toward SDP work, and has relatively little open dialogue with local user groups. The *practical* and *critical* approaches, in which the best SDP work tends to occur, are more appreciative of different cultural contexts and are more committed to empowering local user groups.

In recent years, attendance at conferences and events on SDP indicates that the sector has become somewhat standardized and routinized, and would benefit from exploring new themes, principles, and strategies. One way ahead would be to draw critical NGOs and social movements more fully into the main networks within the sector. These kinds of institutions or agencies have been particularly active in the past in highlighting major social problems that have been subsequently and positively addressed, such as the use of child labor in the manufacturing of sports equipment. Drawing critical NGOs and social movements into transnational SDP networks would also encourage other SDP institutions to adopt a stronger form of critical reflexivity and to explore practical or critical approaches in the implementation of future projects.

31 Richard Giulianotti, "Sport, Globalization and Development: Making the Global Civil Society," International Sociology of Sport Association annual conference (paper, Kyoto, Japan, July 26–29, 2008).

32 Richard Giulianotti, "Sport, Peace and Development: Exploring the Role of Sport within the Emerging Transnational Civil Society," 6th conference of the European Association for the Sociology of Sport (keynote speech, Rome, May 27–31, 2009); Giulianotti, "Sport, Peacemaking and Conflict Resolution."

30

THE FIRE THIS TIME

A CONTEXT FOR UNDERSTANDING THE BLACK MALE ATHLETE PROTESTS AT MISSOURI

Scott Brooks

On Nov. 9, the University of Missouri's system president resigned and the Columbia campus chancellor was demoted after a number of the school's Black football players joined #ConcernedStudent1950's protest and refused to play. This should not come as a surprise considering today's sports industrial complex and Black athlete activism. The Black players who decided to protest were joining a movement on campus and in wider society that they not only could understand, but felt.

A component of the sports industrial complex is the separation of athlete from campus and wider society; big-time collegiate athletes are set apart and earn special treatment, Mizzou is no exception. The athletic world is largely across the street, at a complex just for athletes with a dining hall, training equipment and fields, lockers, parking, doctors, trainers, coaches, and administrators. Activism is not new, and Black athletes have brought it back in vogue.

This is not simply for self-aggrandizement; the broad media coverage of police brutality against Black males and other incidents setting the #BlackLivesMatter movement aflame disrupted the athletic identity that usually insulates elite Black male athletes and limits their connection with other Black people. They are different from the rest of us and, yet, still the same.

Here's an example of what I mean.

It was a Monday in fall of 2012, my very first semester here at Mizzou. I was teaching Introduction to Black Studies and we were entering the final stretch of the semester. The group project was all that was left—a campus study on aspects of Black student life. One component of the study was observation. I asked the class about their progress and grew concerned they weren't getting out and doing the necessary fieldwork. I decided on the fly that we'd get out of the classroom, observe some students, and discuss what we'd seen. There were moans and groans, but I walked out and told them to meet me at the Memorial Student Union. I got there and found a seat.

Scott Brooks, "The Fire This Time: A Context for Understanding the Black Male Athlete Protests at Missouri," *Phi Kappa Phi Forum*, vol. 96, no. 2, pp. 18-21.

The Union's main floor has a large atrium with two- and four-seat tables, loveseats, and couches. There's a Starbucks and a to-go eatery. I watched the class enter and try to find seats; it was about three-quarters full. Some of the students, reluctant to take observations, walked around in groups of three or four until they found seats. For 15 minutes, I watched the students blending in to varying degrees, some sitting in silence while others spoke with each other and non-classmates. Then, I got up, moved towards an exit and signaled with a head nod for them to meet me outside, and walked to the patio. When we sat down, one student—one of two football players in the class—was noticeably upset. I asked what was bothering him and he said, "I didn't like it."

"What?" I asked.

"That wasn't cool. You had us going in there looking like inner city kids from the Y(MCA) on a field trip."

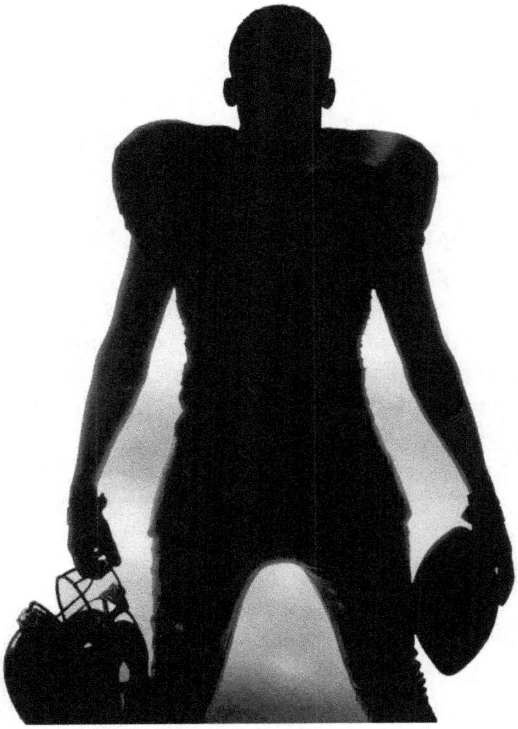

"How so?"

"I mean, people were looking at us like we were aliens."

"Whaddyamean?"

Another student chimed in, "Some got up and left. Two girls pulled their tables together so that we couldn't sit next to them."

"Yeah, they told us that the seats was taken and they wasn't. I know they wasn't 'cause I watched and nobody showed up," the footballer said.

"So why you mad with me?" I asked. "Two days ago (on Saturday) 50,000-plus (fans) was cheering for you and now they treat you like you don't belong? And you look like a football player—look at what you wearing. Maybe you're getting a slice of what it feels like to be a regular Black student."

Other students nodded and shrugged in agreement. It was one thing for the football player to enjoy higher status, but quite another to get lost in it and forget something as basic as the marginalization that many Blacks experience on a predominantly White campus.

His discomfort should not be surprising: He lives a different Black student experience.

> Some Black athletes are worshipped as heroes in certain settings; ridiculed and resented regarding their educational engagement in other spaces; and alienated by a system that puts them under surveillance as a means to keep them compliant. …

This is on purpose, a means of keeping him away from the *real* students and to keep him from challenging himself academically—and to keep him focused on his job of playing football. In this way, my student was acknowledging a racism particular to the Black student athlete. Some Black athletes are worshipped as heroes in certain settings; ridiculed and resented regarding their educational engagement in other spaces; and alienated by a system that puts them under surveillance as a means to keep them compliant and that largely controls their time, relationships, and outputs. Graduate assistants patrol halls to conduct classroom checks, tracking and reporting athlete attendance (largely only football players). Journalists peruse the police dockets daily to see if any athletes have made the list of arrestees. And football players are strongly discouraged from joining organizations away from athletics, like #CS1950 and fraternities. They don't have time for the extracurricular activities that are the benefits of attending a prestigious college and university. Their time is accounted for—their home, family, and job are their sport.

In addition to joining a student movement that highlighted the shared phenomenon of *living while Black*, our Black male college athletes have contemporary sports heroes and models to emulate. Black male athlete activism is not new. One could begin with Tom Molineaux and his aspiration to be a prizefighter to purchase his freedom from slavery. Many have written about or studied Jack Johnson, another prizefighter who bucked the status quo and battled desegregating the heavyweight world championship. Of course, there's Muhammad Ali and his refusal to fight in the Vietnam War. And Ali's activism leads right into the Olympic Project for Human Rights and the broader statement by Black athletes including Jim Brown, Bill Russell, Kareem Abdul-Jabbar and others.

A few more recent and relevant moments:

- March 2012: LeBron James, Dwyane Wade and members of the 2012 Miami Heat post a photo on Twitter with hoodies and heads lowered in mourning for Trayvon Martin.
- 2013: College football players around the country wrote "APU"—All Players United—on their gear in protest of collegiate amateurism.
- April 2014: Los Angeles Clippers' players wear their warm-up shirts inside out and put their shirts on the middle of the floor to cover the team logo after owner Donald Sterling's hate-filled rant.
- November 2014: Some players of the St. Louis Rams run out for introductions with their hands raised, in the "hands up, don't shoot" pose in solidarity with #BlackLivesMatter after Michael Brown's shooting death in nearby Ferguson, Missouri.

Thus, the action of Black members of Mizzou's football team is in step with the current climate of Black athlete protests. "Let this be a testament to all of the athletes across the country that you do have power," pronounced Tigers defensive end Charles Harris (Nov. 11, 2015, espn.com). Harris and others considered their action a rallying cry. The impact goes beyond sports: Students in support and against were motivated to speak more openly; universities have renewed support for diversity in hiring, admissions, and treatment of students; several university presidents have restated their positions on freedom of speech and civility; and sports scholars have pronounced the Black football protest a part of history to be taught in courses.

This is the blessing and the curse of the collegiate arms race. The fight to find and secure the best talent in order to win football games makes each big-time sports school vulnerable to the actions of their star athletes, who together can shut down an institution of higher learning because of the millions of dollars at stake for sports. Missouri is only a canary in the mine; there is a huge problem in our collegiate system where millions of dollars are at stake each and every kickoff. The business of the university is football. Because of this, Black football players as the "preferred workers" and cornerstones of the workforce can bring that business to a halt by saying that they won't play.

The Black players at Mizzou may have won a battle, but the war is far from over. Institutions don't generally lose to individuals, especially in small groups. Instead they reload, retrench, and get back to the status quo, wiser and better able to thwart revolts. There are no final victories; to cause real change, athletes will have to do more, connect with other global movements for change.

We will have to watch the next couple of seasons to see any long-term effects. How will the athletics department and Mizzou's new head football coach embrace what has happened? What will the locker room be like and who will be present? Some players will graduate or try out for the NFL. Others will transfer, be dropped, or quit. The power is in the hands of departments and coaches who sign athletes to one-year renewable scholarships. Some players, seen as "troublemakers" for their part in the protest, will not be asked to return, labeled as uncoachable or a poor fit. The administration will work to prevent future protests. It is likely they will cover "appropriate forms of protest" in new student-athlete orientations. Coaches have learned to speak about the protest as necessary, inspiring, and a growth opportunity that need not be repeated; and committees have been created to pay closer attention to the needs of Black athletes and serve as a space for their concerns. In short, the institution isolates the problem, creates a means for managing it, and then, trains people and recruits people who can manage themselves accordingly. Ultimately, this stamps down protest, at least for a while.

How long do we continue to sit idle and watch the casualties of this arms race?

> The Black players at Mizzou may have won a battle, but the war is far from over. Institutions don't generally lose to individuals, especially in small groups. Instead, they reload, retrench, and get back to the status quo. ...

TRIUMPH OVER TRAUMA

INJURED WAR VETERANS OVERCOME INSURMOUNTABLE ODDS BY USING RECREATION TO STAY FIT AND ON TOP OF THEIR GAME

Andrew Carnahan

Born in Pittsburgh, James Stuck was a natural athlete and a soccer player. He enlisted in the military after a brief stint at LaRoche College, training at Fort Benning, Ga., and Fort Kennedy, Ken., before being deployed to Iraq in September 2005.

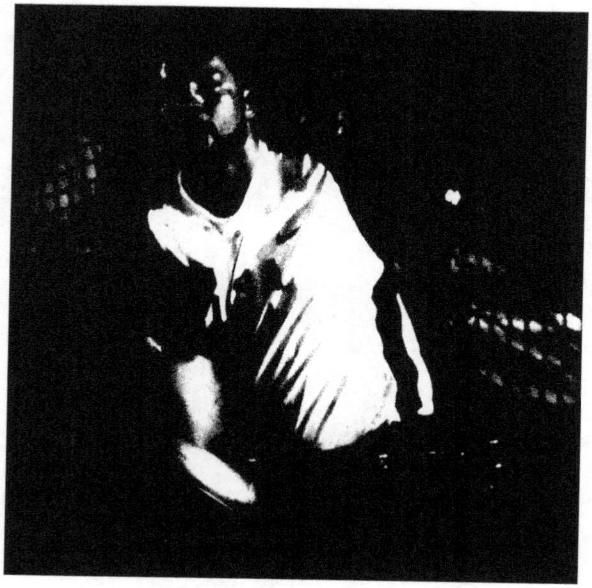

Stuck returned to the United States facing some life-changing challenges. Three months into his deployment, his convoy had been hit by a roadside bomb in Kirkuk, Iraq. His lower leg was crushed in the blast and had to be amputated. He spent most of the next year in rehabilitation at Walter Reed Army Medical Center.

Stuck says he was introduced to adaptive sports through a Paralympic Military Summit, an opportunity for injured war veterans to learn about and try a variety of activities in the hopes to encourage daily physical activity. "The whole idea of a military summit is to get wounded soldiers and disabled vets confident in different sports," Stuck says.

He began playing sitting volleyball at the U.S. Olympic Committee's Paralympic Military Sports Camp in 2006. Stuck took quickly to the sport, aided by his long reach, and made the U.S. Paralympics Men's Sitting Volleyball National Team that same year. Although he is back in college—now at the University of Central Oklahoma—he is still training with team members, recently returning with a silver medal from the Parapan Olympic Games in Rio de Janeiro, Brazil.

Andrew Carnahan, "Triumph Over Trauma," *Parks & Recreation*, vol. 43, no. 8, pp. 51-53.

He lights up when he talks about participating in sports after his injury. "It's a huge, huge influence. It makes you more confident being out in public and seeing other amputees out and about doing the same thing." Stuck credits the sport with boosting his confidence, but he also says it's about more than just participating in the games. "The sports are huge, but what goes along with it are the bonds that you make with people."

The mental and physical benefits of organized sports and recreation play a vital role in getting veterans readjusted and thriving back at home. Carlos Leon is a former Marine and Paralympic athlete, and recently set a new, unofficial world record in the discus at the 2008 U.S. Paralympic Track and Field Team Trials. He says the importance of simply having something to do after an injury cannot be underestimated. "It gives you something to strive for. You can only be good if you try."

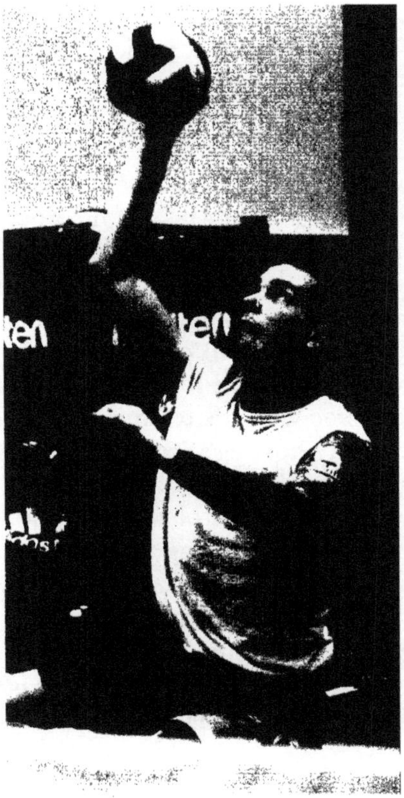

JAMES STUCK, serving in a game of sitting volleyball, won a silver medal at the Parapan Olympic Games in Brazil.

The sense of purpose that comes from participating in sports can be vital to veterans dealing with serious injuries. Partaking in sports and recreation is a simple yet indispensable outlet to give injured veterans a way to return to activities they participated in before they were injured. In addition, recreation can give them a sense of belonging they might have lost post-injury. Leon credits his participation in sports with giving him a positive attitude and allowing him to avoid the depression that people often face after suffering a life-changing injury.

Leon says an additional advantage is the fitness that his sport provides. "I can't remember the last time I was sick," says Leon. "I've never been healthier in my life." The benefits of exercise can be garnered at any level of participation and is not just seen in veterans who become elite athletes.

Recreation is also important for veterans returning from combat duty—injured or not—because they often need to adjust to returning home after a stressful situation. Returning war veterans are particularly susceptible to complications from war experiences and the potential for unhealthy inactivity. According to the U.S. Department of Veterans Affairs, as many as 20 percent of veterans returning from Iraq may suffer from Post-Traumatic Stress Disorder (PTSD), which can result in depression and can lead to a dangerously sedentary lifestyle.

Recreation provides an outlet for stress, helping to balance mental and physical health. Physically injured soldiers are dealing with many serious issues, and sports can be a channel to refocus their energy on a positive activity in which they receive positive reinforcement for their participation. For veterans suffering from PTSD or other mental illnesses, participating in sports can be important. The sense of purpose, healthy exercise, and camaraderie complement other programs designed to improve their lives. Organized community-based programs can play a vital role in getting veterans engaged in physical activities when they return home and as they recover from injury.

Stuck says that his athletic participation proved to him that he could bounce back. "It's important to me because it shows that I was able to recover from my injury and I've been able to do all the sports I used to do, and I've discovered new sports," he says.

Therapeutic recreation, which combines recreation with treatment and education, can play an important role in improving the health and well-being of veterans. Service members tend to be athletic and are used to being active, so they often take naturally to sports as a form of therapy. Adaptive sports allow physically disabled veterans to remain active, and organized events can allow them an opportunity to compete at an advanced level. More important than one-time events is for park and recreation agencies to provide regular programming for veterans with physical disabilities that in turn will benefit additional individuals in the community with physical disabilities.

Many military, sports, and recreation groups realize the potential for sports and recreation to benefit our veterans. Several organizations, including the U.S. Olympic Committee Paralympics Division, the National Recreation and Park Association, and BlazeSports, have teamed up to form a Warrior Transition Unit task force to provide a framework for adaptive athletics for injured service members. Currently the task force is working with Fort Lewis in Washington to develop sport and recreation activities for the more than 780 wounded warriors at the base. From the work at Fort Lewis and other pilot sites, the task force will develop a framework for all installations to develop sport and recreation programs that will assist in the recovery of injured service members.

Athletes who want to take their sport to the next level can apply to participate in the Veterans Paralympic Performance Program. The U.S. Olympic Committee, Department of Veterans Affairs, and other partners formed VP3 to provide athletes with the chance to train fulltime for the Paralympics. This program allows Stuck to fulfill his dreams by training full time with his teammates and Paralympic coaches at the University of Central Oklahoma, one of six sites hosting VP3 programs.

VP3 not only allows individuals such as Stuck to pursue their sport, but also brings attention to the power of injured veterans to achieve great things despite their disabilities. The athletes who train for the Paralympics serve as role models for other injured veterans who are learning to deal with their injuries.

U.S. Paralympics reaches out to veterans through its U.S. Military Paralympic program. Paralympic Military Sports Camps provide veterans with a chance to meet Paralympic athletes and participate in sports clinics. By working with NRPA and local park and recreation agencies, U.S. Paralympics is also working to expand Paralympic Sport Clubs in communities, with the goal of having programs in 250 cities by 2012.

While all of these national organizations and programs are helping to catalyze an increased focus on recreation for veterans, local and regional groups need to be involved. Many veterans do not live on or near a military base, so their local park and recreation centers are their source for sport and recreation, and an avenue to assist them in returning to normal life.

As for physically disabled veterans who are thinking of participating in sports, Leon says, "Don't be afraid to try. Don't be scared to fail." He says that he struggled when he first started trying sports after his injury, but eventually he found track and field and went on to set a world record in the discus. James Stuck advises veterans, "Just go out and do it. Don't hold back."

FURTHER READING

Read LeBron James and Carmelo Anthony's Power Speech on Race at the ESPY Awards

Melissa Chan

If you have a digital edition of this book, please click on the link below to access the article:

http://time.com/4406289/lebron-james-carmelo-anthony-espy-awards-transcript/

If you have a print edition of this book, please use your cell phone to scan the QR code below to access the article:

Social Activism Is Part of the Washington Mystics' DNA

Julian Karron

If you have a digital edition of this book, please click on the link below to access the article:

https://sports.yahoo.com/social-activism-part-washington-mystics-195914213.html

If you have a print edition of this book, please use your cell phone to scan the QR code below to access the article:

CPSIA information can be obtained
at www.ICGtesting.com
Printed in the USA
LVHW010418080420
652527LV00005B/11

9 781793 507471